中文翻译版

糖尿病社会心理评估及干预

Psychosocial Care for People with Diabetes

主　编　Deborah Young-Hyman，PhD

　　　　Mark Peyrot，PhD

主　译　刘彦君

科 学 出 版 社

北 京

图字：01-2016-2054 号

内 容 简 介

　　本书就糖尿病患者的社会心理问题及其调整的方法进行了较为翔实的介绍。作为美国糖尿病学会出版的书籍，它具有一定的权威性和指导价值。本书主要内容包括：糖尿病患者主要的异常行为及其形成的原因，特别介绍了一些糖尿病患者相关的主要社会心理问题及其对糖尿病病情控制的影响，讲解了如何识别糖尿病患者的社会心理问题，改变异常行为习惯的方法有哪些，改变行为异常的阶梯治疗方法，如何在不同的阶段对患者实施相应的指导和帮助，同时，介绍了社会心理问题评估的相关指南和共识，帮助医护人员规范对糖尿病患者社会心理问题的识别和干预。

　　本书对糖尿病临床实践有较强的指导意义，适合糖尿病临床工作者参考使用。

图书在版编目(CIP)数据

糖尿病社会心理评估及干预 /（美）扬-海曼（Deborah Young–Hyman）等主编；刘彦君等译. —北京：科学出版社，2016.11

书名原文：Psychosocial Care of People with Diabetes

ISBN 978-7-03-050300-8

Ⅰ. 糖… Ⅱ. ①扬… ②刘… Ⅲ. ①糖尿病–病人–社会心理–心理测验 ②糖尿病–病人–社会心理–心理干预 Ⅳ. ①R587.1 ②R395

中国版本图书馆 CIP 数据核字(2016)第 256061 号

责任编辑：康丽涛 / 责任校对：李　影
责任印制：徐晓晨 / 封面设计：陈　敬

Deborah Young-Hyman,PhD Mark Peyrot,PhD：Psychosocial Care for People with Diabetes
ISBN 978-1-58040-439-6 (alk. paper)
Copyright©2012 by the American Diabetes Association®

科 学 出 版 社 出版
北京东黄城根北街 16 号
邮政编码：100717
http://www.sciencep.com

北京建宏印刷有限公司 印刷
科学出版社发行　各地新华书店经销
*

2016 年 11 月第 一 版　开本：890×1240　1/32
2018 年 5 月第二次印刷　印张：6 3/4
字数：296 000
定价：68.00 元
（如有印装质量问题，我社负责调换）

《糖尿病社会心理评估及干预》
翻译人员

主　　译　刘彦君

副 主 译　李　翔　史琳涛

译　　者　(按姓氏笔画排序)

王丹丹　牛文芳　石静琳　史琳涛

冯　莉　朱　平　刘彦君　李　翔

李晓瑾　赵德明　黄　雪　翟筱涵

List of Contributors

Barbara J. Anderson, PhD, is Professor of Pediatrics and Associate Head of the Psychology Section at Baylor College of Medicine in Houston, TX.

Brooke A. Bailer, PhD, is a Postdoctoral Fellow at the Center for Weight and Eating Disorders in the Department of Psychiatry at the Perelman School of Medicine of the University of Pennsylvania in Philadelphia, PA.

Daniel J. Cox, PhD, ABPP, is a clinical psychologist and professor in the Department of Psychiatry and Neurobehavioral Sciences and the Department of Internal Medicine at the University of Virginia in Charlottesville, VA.

Mary de Groot, PhD, is an Associate Professor of Medicine at the Indiana University School of Medicine in Indianapolis, IN.

Linda M. Delahanty, MSRD, is Chief Dietitian and Director of Nutrition and Behavioral Research at Massachusetts General Hospital Diabetes Center in Boston, MA.

Lucy F. Faulconbridge, PhD, is the Director of Research at the Center for Weight and Eating Disorders in the Department of Psychiatry at the Perelman School of Medicine of the University of Pennsylvania in Philadelphia, PA.

Linda Gonder-Frederick, PhD, is an Associate Professor in the Department of Psychiatry and Neurobehavioral Sciences at the University of Virginia School of Medicine in Charlottesville, VA.

Felicia Hill-Briggs, PhD, is Associate Professor in the Department of Medicine and Department of Physical Medicine and Rehabilitation, Johns Hopkins School of Medicine; Associate Professor in the Department of Health, Behavior, and Society, Johns Hopkins Bloomberg School of Public Health; and a member of the Core Faculty at the Welch Center for Prevention, Epidemiology & Clinical Research, Johns Hopkins Medical Institutions, in Baltimore, MD.

Clarissa S. Holmes, PhD, is a Professor of Psychology, Pediatrics and Psychiatry at Virginia Commonwealth University in Richmond, VA. She also has an appointment as an Adjunct Professor of Psychiatry at Georgetown University in Washington, DC.

Suzanne Bennett Johnson, PhD, is Distinguished Research Professor at Florida State University College of Medicine in Tallahassee, FL, and President of the American Psychological Association.

Lori Laffel, MD, MPH, is Chief of the Pediatric, Adolescent and Young Adult Section and an Investigator in the Section on Genetics and Epidemiology at the Joslin Diabetes Center, and an Associate Professor of Pediatrics at Harvard Medical School in Boston, MA.

David G. Marrero, PhD, is the J.O. Ritchey Professor of Medicine and Director, Diabetes Translational Research Center at the Indiana University School of Medicine in Indianapolis, IN.

Mark Peyrot, PhD, is Professor in the Department of Sociology, Loyola University Maryland in Baltimore, MD.

Richard R. Rubin, PhD, is Professor in the Departments of Medicine and Pediatrics at The Johns Hopkins University School of Medicine in Baltimore, MD.

Christopher M. Ryan, PhD, is Professor of Psychiatry at the University of Pittsburgh School of Medicine in Pittsburgh, PA.

David B. Sarwer, PhD, is the Director of Clinical Services at the Center for Weight and Eating Disorders in the Department of Psychiatry at the Perelman School of Medicine of the University of Pennsylvania in Philadelphia, PA.

Jaclyn A. Shepard, PsyD, is an Assistant Professor in the Department of Psychiatry and Neurobehavioral Sciences at the University of Virginia School of Medicine in Charlottesville, VA.

Harsimran Singh, PhD, is a Research Scientist in the Department of Psychiatry and Neurobehavioral Sciences at the University of Virginia School of Medicine in Charlottesville, VA.

Paula M. Trief, PhD, is a Professor in the departments of Psychiatry and Medicine at SUNY Upstate Medical University in Syracuse, NY, where she also serves as Senior Associate Dean for Faculty Affairs and Faculty Development.

Thomas A. Wadden, PhD, is the Director of the Center for Weight and Eating Disorders in the Department of Psychiatry at the Perelman School of Medicine of the University of Pennsylvania in Philadelphia, PA.

Jill Weissberg-Benchell, PhD, CDE, is an Associate Professor of Psychiatry at Northwestern University's Feinberg School of Medicine at the Ann and Robert H. Lurie Children's Hospital of Chicago in Chicago, IL.

Garry Welch, PhD, is Director of Behavioral Medicine Research at Baystate Medical Center in Springfield, MA, and Research Associate Professor at Tufts University School of Medicine in Boston, MA.

Judith Wylie-Rosett, EdD, RD, is Professor and Head of the Division of Health Promotion and Nutrition Research in the Department of Epidemiology and Population Health at Albert Einstein College of Medicine of Yeshiva University in Bronx, NY.

Tim Wysocki, PhD, is Principal Research Scientist and Director of the Center for Pediatric Psychology Research in the Department of Biomedical Research at Nemours Children's Clinic in Jacksonville, FL.

Deborah Young-Hyman, PhD, CDE, is a diabetes/obesity expert at the Georgia Prevention Center, Institute for Public and Preventive Health, Medical College of Georgia, in Augusta, GA.

Sofija E. Zagarins, PhD, is a Postdoctoral Research Fellow in the Department of Behavioral Medicine Research at Baystate Medical Center in Springfield, MA, and a Visiting Assistant Professor in the Department of Public Health at the University of Massachusetts in Amherst, MA.

致 谢

感谢所有为该书的编写做出贡献的工作人员，包括曾经及现在，在美国糖尿病学会工作的人员，尤其感谢 Nathaniel Clark。感谢参与校正美国糖尿病学会关于社会心理学关怀标准的工作人员，以及为该书的审批及印刷提供经费赞助的人。我们还想感谢 Robert Anderson，William Polonsky 和 Paul Ciechanowski 这些糖尿病专家为该书做出的贡献。

再次感谢不知疲倦长期工作在行为糖尿病研究和治疗领域的专家 Barbara Anderson 和 Pichard Rubin，他们编写了本书的重要部分。最后，感谢美国糖尿病学会的编辑维克多·范·德伊伦，在他的协助、鼓励、支持下，这本书才得以编写出版。

马克·佩罗
德博拉·扬·海曼
2012 年 9 月 1 日

前　言

　　众所周知，糖尿病是一种慢性病，需要医护人员、患者及患者家属共同参与管理，糖尿病及糖尿病的日常管理严重影响着患者的日常生活，包括患者的情绪，反过来，生活事件也影响着患者对糖尿病病情的控制。糖尿病本不是社会心理问题，但糖尿病的医学管理却与患者的社会心理错综复杂地交织在一起。社会心理问题内容广泛，包括诸多相互独立的因素，如抑郁的控制；如何有效地与患者交流；如何从患者的角度和患者的目标、生活背景、生活态度及其对糖尿病相关知识的了解，帮助患者进行有效、长期的自我血糖管理；以及如何将糖尿病的管理融入患者的生活。

　　至今，仅有很少的指南能帮助临床医师解决棘手的、关于糖尿病患者社会心理的问题。虽然此类问题已经包括在美国糖尿病学会每年发表的《临床实践建议》，但在该建议中仅简要地提及该部分内容。《临床实践建议》中指出，建议评估患者的社会心理状况。糖尿病管理的结局不仅包括医疗结局，还包括健康的社会心理。

　　糖尿病患者相关的社会心理问题已经引起社会的关注，诸多文献论述了糖尿病结局与社会心理因素的关系。《糖尿病社会心理评估及干预》提出对心理因素的干预应作为日常干预的一部分，专业医师应评估糖尿病患者相关的社会心理问题。该书论述了在日常工作中，临床医师遇到的糖尿病患者的心理问题，以及患者在生活中遇到的影响糖尿病管理的各种心理因素，如患者的生活状态、医患关系、患者承担自我血糖管理及生活方式改变的责任。该书着重论述了糖尿病治疗的方法（如胰岛素泵、自我血糖监测、医学营养治疗和体育锻炼），患者的依从性，年龄相关性问题，患者对患病的心理调整，以及特定问题的评估和建议。临床建议是基于已发表的文献及专家的意见而提出的。

　　该书分为四篇：行为健康、患者自我管理、治疗技术的应用、生命相关问题。虽然这四篇相互关联，相互重叠，但把它们分成独立的章节也是非常有必要的。第一篇为行为健康，从专业行为医师的角度，给临床医师提供指南及参考。行为医师对协助临床医师帮助患者改变行为习惯、维持良好的行为习惯起着重要作用。同样的，患者自我血糖管理是糖尿病管理的重要组成部分，故而，该书第二篇为患者自我管理。第三篇为治疗技术的应用，该篇主要论述行为和社会心理因素在应用技术设备帮助糖尿病管理中的作用。最后，生命相关问题论述了在糖尿病患者基本生命过程中，对患者的糖尿病及糖尿病管理应考虑的因素。

　　第一篇为行为健康，论述了抑郁及饮食失调，这些都可以归为社会心理失调。与健康人群对比，抑郁和饮食失调在糖尿病患者中呈高发病率，并且均可达到亚临床和临床诊断水平。近期已经开始研究糖尿病与抑郁、饮食失调的关系。因而，给予出现抑郁和饮食失调的患者关注是成功控制疾病的必要因素。低血糖不仅仅是一种单纯的行为健康问题，第三章论述了低血糖的发生、发生频次及所导致的后果与患者行为有密切关系。低血糖症和糖毒性（高血糖症），与糖尿病患者在整个生命过程中的意识功能相关。第四章和第五章论述了高血糖与神经认知功能的关系，包括神经认知功能中关于完成适当任务的能力、脑功能，以及适当任务完成能力、脑功能可能被高血糖损害，而这一病变是脑结构改变所致。该章的内容主要集中在患者完成自我血糖管理的能力及当怀疑认知功能损害时应该采取的措施。

　　第二篇为患者自我管理，内容主要是糖尿病知识、技巧、行为，以及生活方式的调整以帮助患者实现疾病的管理。作者着重强调了医护人员、患者及患者的身体状态、人际关系和社会环境之间的相互作用。第六章论述了自我血糖监测的各种方法，为调整各种治疗方案提供了依据。第九章论述了基于研究证据和已经被广泛接受的理论,如何利用资源(第九章，关于运动)，责任程度（第七章，关于依从性），计划性干预（第八章，关于营养），这些因素影响患者接受并坚持自我血糖管理。

　　第三篇为治疗技术的应用，论述了各种治疗方案及其优势，如胰岛素泵（第十章），动态血糖监测的技术优势；肥胖外科手术能改善肥胖患者的2型糖尿病病情（第十二章）。这些技术较新，长期的影响还有待观察研究。然后，该篇建议对应用该技术相关的患者进行社会心理问题的筛查和监测。虽然，这些先进的治疗技术理论上可以应用在所有糖尿病患者身上，然而，应用这些治疗技术的适当性和心理问题的监测仍未引起关注或实现标准化。该篇重点为帮助临床医师参考患者的社会心理状态，选择合适的时机给予患者强化的治疗方案；并建议应该监测患者的社会心理健康及改变。

最后一篇是关于生命相关问题，论述了在患病的整个生命过程中患者身体和心理的改变。虽然可通过外科手术或移植（该技术目前仍处于实验阶段）来延缓糖尿病进程，但糖尿病是慢性、进展性疾病。因此，疾病的控制会变得越来越困难，针对患者的治疗越来越有限(第十三章)。该部分内容分为三章讨论了如何在整个生命过程包括儿童期、青春期(第十四章)、成人期（第十五章）、残疾期（多发生在老年）(第十六章)给予此类特殊患者更多的关怀。越来越多的儿童被诊断为 2 型糖尿病，糖尿病治疗方法的不断进步，患者可以带病生存更久的时间，故而，患者个人的生活与疾病的进展相互交织，这种情况下需要给予患者更多的关注。

该书的作者们希望该书能够给予医护人员帮助，并影响到关于糖尿病的治疗及研究，以及保险公司的赔偿政策。另外，作为临床机构，系统、全面地记录患者的信息，有利于获得足够的资源而有效地应对糖尿病患者的社会心理需求。近年来，药物和技术的进步，已经开发出越来越多的治疗方案，这将改善患者的医疗结局。然而，这些治疗的完成都必须基于患者对糖尿病知识的了解，患者战胜疾病的信心、态度及患者的健康生活方式行为，而且还包括医护人员对于如何克服患者的社会心理障碍，从而帮助糖尿病患者及其家属改善生活质量，促进患者对健康的了解。

目　　录

第一篇　行　为　健　康

第二篇　患者自我管理

第三篇　治疗技术的应用

第四篇　生命相关问题

第一篇
行为健康

第一章
抑郁和糖尿病

Mary de Groot，PhD

抑郁的评估和诊断

抑郁是指包括悲伤、情绪低落、兴趣缺失和自主神经症状（如食欲、睡眠改变）在内的一系列障碍和症候群，以及间隔时间内出现的认知障碍。严重抑郁障碍（major depressive disorder，MDD）是指出现以下症状中的 5 个或以上并持续至少 2 周以上：压抑或悲伤、丧失日常生活的愉悦感或兴趣、体重或食欲改变、嗜睡或失眠、疲劳、精神运动性激越或者迟滞、无用或负罪感、注意力下降，和（或）自杀的意念或未遂。发作可以是反复发作或单次发作。

亚综合征型抑郁或轻度抑郁障碍包括心境恶劣（2 年间轻度抑郁持续时间超过一半）、情绪压抑伴调节障碍（对于由确定的社会心理刺激如重大生活事件或医疗事件所产生的抑郁，其持续时间少于 6 个月），以及未做特殊说明的抑郁障碍（抑郁症状可导致社交或职业受影响但不符合其他诊断标准）。

糖尿病相关的心理痛苦与抑郁谱系障碍明显不同，因为其直接与糖尿病的管理和（或）社会支持直接相关（如针对自我管理行为，与家人进行互动）。心理痛苦与糖尿病共生和管理的经验明确相关。糖尿病相关的心理痛苦可以与抑郁症状或发作同时存在，亦可单独存在。尽管糖尿病相关的心理痛苦是社会心理干预的一个合适目标，但其还不被认为是一种精神疾病。

对一些全国性的调查进行分析表明糖尿病患者 MDD 或轻度抑郁障碍的人口学和心理社会学相关因素包括：女性、低龄、BMI > 30 kg/m^2、高学历、贫困、吸烟、胰岛素治疗、高糖化血红蛋白（HbA1C）、单身、健康状况感知较差和并发症数量较多。症状的出现可以是渐进的，也可与某种易被患者识别的外部事件密切相关。

鉴别诊断

MDD 的诊断需要排除原发性精神疾病（如精神分裂症、情感分裂性精神障碍、妄想症）或存在重度躁狂或轻度躁狂分别导致的 I 型或 II 型双向障碍。焦虑谱系障碍（包括惊恐障碍、场所恐惧症、特殊恐惧症、社交恐惧症、强迫症、广泛性焦虑症）可以与抑郁谱系障碍同时发生（表 1-1）。

表 1-1　重度抑郁的 DSM-IV 标准

A. 在连续两周内有下述 5 项（或更多）症状，并且是原有功能的改变；其中至少 1 项症状为心境抑郁或兴趣或愉悦感丧失

　1. 几乎每日大部分时间心境抑郁（主观体验或由其他人观察到）

　2. 几乎每日大部分时间对所有的或几乎所有活动的兴趣或愉悦感显著降低（主观体验或他人观察到）

　3. 没有节食时体重明显下降或体重增加，或几乎每日都有食欲减退或增加

　4. 几乎每日都有失眠或嗜睡

　5. 几乎每日都有精神运动性激越或者迟滞（不仅主观感到坐立不安或者迟滞，其他人也能观察到）

　6. 几乎每日都感到疲倦或缺乏精力

　7. 几乎每日都感到自己无用，或者有不恰当的过分内疚（可以达到罪恶妄想程度；不仅是为患病而自责或者内疚）

　8. 几乎每日都有思维能力或注意力集中能力下降，或者犹豫不决（主观体验或其他人观察到）

　9. 反复出现死亡的想法（不只是害怕死亡），反复出现自杀的意念但没有特定计划，或有自杀未遂，或有特定的自杀计划

B. 症状不符合混合发作标准

C. 症状引起具有临床意义的苦恼或者社交、职业或其他重要功能的损害

D. 症状不是由于物质（如成瘾药物、处方药物）或者躯体情况（如甲状腺功能减退）的直接生理效应所致

E. 症状不能用丧亲反应（即失去亲人的反应）来解释，症状持续 2 个月以上，或者症状的特征为显著的功能损害、病态地沉浸于自己的无用感、自杀意念、精神病性症状或精神运动性迟滞

抑郁的判定

抑郁可以通过自我报告症状量表如 Beck 抑郁量表（BDI）-Ⅱ、9 条目患者健康问卷抑郁量表（PHQ-9）或抑郁量表流行病学研究中心（CESD）来充分评估。这些方法在项目的数量和内容上不尽相同，可以选择性地用于不同目的的研究（如临床筛查或临床研究）。这些都是为一般人群设计的（他们不是糖尿病患者），其有效性和可信度已得到证实。对于每一种量表，与有临床意义和抑郁诊断相一致的临床切点分值已在精神病患者身上运用并得到证实。BDI 已经证实可以应用于 1 型和 2 型糖尿病患者。应该注意的是，BDI-Ⅱ和 PHQ-9 收集了有关自杀意念和（或）自杀倾向及自杀计划的特有信息。这些测量量表可应用于如下环境：医生在患者完成量表后即刻评估患者反应；患者自我伤害风险的随访评估；用于转诊患者。

有效评估抑郁的精神科访谈协议的范围涉及半结构式访谈，如情感障碍和精神分裂症量表（SADS-L）和 DSM-Ⅳ-TR 结构式的临床访谈（SCID）；以及可以通过计算机来进行诊断评分的结构式访谈，如复合性国际诊断交谈表（CIDI）和诊断性会谈量表（DIS）。DIS 已经证实可以应用于 1 型和 2 型糖尿病患者。这些访谈需要医师在精神病理学及访谈评估方面进行专业培训。SCID 的临床版本已证实可行，但是这些访谈更常用于临床研究的背景中。

检测糖尿病相关痛苦有两个量表：糖尿病问题量表（PAID）及糖尿病痛苦量表（DDS）。与自我报告的抑郁调查问卷相比，这些量表有共同的差异，也有独特的差异。

抑郁与糖尿病共病的患病率

研究 1 型和 2 型糖尿病患者当中重症抑郁和（或）抑郁症状的横断面患病率已屡见不鲜。Meta 分析显示 1 型糖尿病患者中抑郁或者抑郁症状的患病率比非糖尿病对照患者高（21.6%vs.11.4%）。同样，Meta 分析显示 2 型糖尿病患者中抑郁或者抑郁症状的患病率也比非糖尿病对照患者高（27%vs.17.6%）。抑郁评估方法和阈值在这些文献当中变化范围很大，MDD 和抑郁症状的患病率也一样（例如，精神方面访谈的抑郁患病率是 11%，而自我报告调查问卷的患病率是 31%）。通过允许访谈者决定时间、来源、对患者认可的个人抑郁症状（如可预料的丧亲反应 vs 重症抑郁障碍）可供选择的诊断解释，精神访谈提供更大的诊断精确度，因此有更低的患病率。这些特性不能通过自我报告量表产生，所以任何原因引起的抑郁症状均可能通过受访者得到。

总的来说，T1D 与 T2D 患者的抑郁症患病率比一般人群高出两倍（有一个例外：Pouwer 2003）。女性糖尿病患者被报道存在抑郁症状的数量是男性糖尿病患者的 1.6 倍，一项研究发现在较年轻女性（＜40 岁）中这种关联性更强。现已发现男性 T1D 患者的抑郁症患病率超过非糖尿病对照群。虽然大多数研究是针对中产阶级白人进行分析；但抑郁症状患病率在不同种族、民族或国际样本人群中似乎没有显著变化。但使用合理控制的前瞻性研究设计很少。

对伴有 T1D 的儿童和青少年的心理特征进行合理控制的前瞻性纵向研究，其混合的研究结果显示共病抑郁症的患病率上升。一些研究观察到患病率上升，而其他研究则显示抑郁症患病率与健康对照组相比没有差别。一项研究显示，女性糖尿病患者比男性糖尿病患者或精神病患者表现出更大的抑郁症复发风险。在一个青年（10～21 岁）样本人群中，男性 T2D 患者自我报告抑郁症状的风险要高于男性 T1D 患者。抑郁症状似乎增加了血糖控制恶化、早期糖尿病性视网膜病变的发生，以及增高的青少年住院治疗和急诊就诊的风险。

很少有研究调查成人 T1D 和 T2D 抑郁症自然发展的过程。在超过 1～5 年的前瞻性纵向研究随访结果显示，无论治疗与否，抑郁症状和情感障碍会高水平的持续存在（如 73%～79%患者仍存在抑郁）。例如，一项试验表明，对曾进行 8 周抗抑郁药物治疗的患者进行 5 年的随访，结果发现有 92%的患者经历了持续或复发的重症抑郁，58%的患者在治疗的 12 个月内复发。

抑郁症对糖尿病和社会心理结局的影响

在被诊断为 T1D 和 T2D 的样本人群中发现抑郁症与较差的血糖控制情况和糖尿病并发症相关。在 25 个横断面研究的 Meta 分析中观察到高血糖与抑郁症状存在中小程度的效应值。最近的横断面研究在西班牙成年人、T1D 儿童和有 MMD 病史的绝经妇女群体中也反映了这一发现。抑郁症状改变的前瞻性研究并未表明抑郁可预测不同种群的中老年患者血糖控制的改变。在 1 型和 2 型糖尿病患者中，自我管理行为的依从性似乎没能成为抑郁症状和血糖控制的调停者。27 项研究的 Meta 分析发现在 1 型和 2 型糖尿病样本中，抑郁症与日益恶化的长期糖尿病慢性并发症（如大血管病变、神经病变、肾脏病变、视网膜病变、微血管病变）的关联中存在中等效应值。最近的研究显示抑郁症与糖尿病神经病变的关系与这些发现一致。

与抑郁症共病相关的阴性结果的累积证据包括：糖尿病自我管理依从性降低，如饮食推荐、运动行为和口服降糖药；生活质量降低；社会支持减少；与重症抑郁的非糖尿病患者相比，功能丧失及显著的失业和工作能力丧失增加；1 型糖尿病儿童住院治疗增加；相关变量（如年龄、糖尿病并发症）调整后过早的死亡率。轻度抑郁症可能与自我报告健康状况的降低、认知受限（如困惑、记忆丧失、决策困难）和糖尿病症状相关，当然还需要其他证据进一步来阐明这种关系。

分析糖尿病和抑郁症共病的经济影响表明与单纯患糖尿病的患者相比，共患这两种病的个体有更高的门诊医疗需求、更多的处方花费和全面的医疗保健花费。

抑郁症是糖尿病的预警

已经发现，抑郁症和糖尿病有双向性的关联。其中，在前瞻性的纵向队列研究中发现抑郁症能够增加 2 型糖尿病发展的风险。同时，糖尿病的存在会增加诊断后抑郁症发展的风险。一些研究发现，存在重度抑郁或者中度抑郁症状会使随后的 2 型糖尿病的风险增加 2 倍。然而，在校正一些相关变量如体质指数和教育程度后，其他研究报道了在相似的时间内较小的或非显著的危险评估。一项 9 个研究的 Meta 分析发现，对于有终生抑郁症状病史的患者，其 2 型糖尿病发生的风险会增加 37%。第三次全国健康和营养调查（NHANES III）的证据表明，有终生重症抑郁症状病史的 40 岁以下的女性增加了代谢综合征的风险，但是这个发现仍需其他研究来证实。

治疗方法和提供者

糖尿病患者抑郁症可以应用传统的治疗方式有效治疗，如抗抑郁药物治疗、个体认知行为治疗（CBT）和问题-解决导向治疗（PST）。随机安慰剂对照试验显示三环类（如去甲替林）和选择性 5-羟色胺再摄取抑制剂（SSRI）抗抑郁药物（如氟西汀、舍曲林、帕罗西汀）可有效治疗抑郁症。一项以糖尿病和重症抑郁共病为样本人群的非对照随机比较研究显示氟西汀和帕罗西汀均能改善抑郁。已经发现，去甲替林（25～50mg/d）在治疗后血糖控制中有增高血糖效应。当检测安非拉酮时，发现氟西汀（40mg/d——最大剂量）、舍曲林（50mg/d——最大剂量）、帕罗西汀（20mg/d）和安非拉酮缓释剂（150～450mg /d）与升高血糖及 BMI 有关。应用舍曲林维持治疗与安慰剂相比，能够有效延长抑郁缓解期，同时在抑郁症状缓解的 1 年中，舍曲林和安慰剂组均维持降低血糖作用。在这项研究中，与对照组和老年组比较，使用舍曲林的年轻者（＜55 岁）能更长时间地维持症状缓解期。

在随机对照研究中，与糖尿病教育干预组比较，CBT 组能有效治疗 2 型糖尿病患者的抑郁。在 6 个月的随访评估中发现，CBT 组可改善 HbA1C 且效果超过对照组。

最近的研究显示了应用 PST 合作护理方法的有效性。在路径研究中，1 型和 2 型糖尿病参试者入选标准为重症抑郁或心境恶劣（持续 2 年或以上的低程度郁闷心情），他们来自 9 个初级护理健康中心并被随机分为初级护理中心联合个体管理干预治疗或常规护理（UC）。进行个体管理干预治疗的患者，接受了应用教育、抗抑郁药物和（或）PST（由受过临床专业训练的护理人员执行）的逐步护理方法。在超过 12 个月的随访中，接受干预治疗的患者严重抑郁症减少，患者全面改善率提高，对护理的满意度提高。在随访中，对于有两种或以上糖尿病并发症的患者，干预组比 UC 组的抑郁结局有更显著改善。并发症少于两种的糖尿病患者，干预组与 UC 组的抑郁结局相当。与 UC 比较，患者依附 PST 这种模式治疗与抑郁症治疗成功相关。总的来说，从基线到 6 个月或 12 个月的随访评估中，血糖控制或糖尿病自我管理行为均无改善。在干预组，发现 BMI 小幅度降低和口服降糖药非依从性的增加。没有接受糖尿病特殊教育或糖尿病自我管理依从性支持的参试者可能对改善血糖结局有贡献。这种治疗方法为糖尿病抑郁症共病的治疗提供了高成本效益的方法，即将有限的额外费用用于干预治疗，可显著减少非精神疾病相关的费用。

寻找糖尿病患者合并抑郁症的有效治疗方法总是不尽如人意，存在各种障碍，包括精神疾病耻辱感和患者已知无力或不可避免的慢性疾病结果所表现的抑郁症状；发觉在医疗或精神健康护理中的歧视，从而导致不同种族和民族应用抗抑郁治疗方法的不同；初级护理工作者缺乏筛查和合适的诊断；初级护理提供者缺乏对抗抑郁药物剂量调整的知识；缺乏除抗抑郁药物治疗之外的心理疗法服务。在接受抑郁治疗的患者中，患者对抗抑郁药物的使用和精神健康提供者的满意度也是有利因素。

深入研究的建议

基于可用的文献，许多方面值得额外的研究来进一步明确病因学、病程、结果、抑郁与糖尿病共病的治疗。

1. 对导致 1 型和 2 型糖尿病患者抑郁显著增加的生理因素所知甚少。进一步的研究需要来评估糖尿病抑郁患者的神经化学物质、激素、免疫/炎症和神经病学因素。

2. 虽然有大量的证据表明 1 型和 2 型糖尿病患者抑郁患病率的增加，但大多数的研究为横断面和非对照设计。前瞻性、对照的研究需要更好地描述临床糖尿病抑郁的病程和影响，以及抑郁在代谢综合征和 2 型糖尿病发展中的独特贡献。临床定义和阈值应该被用来区分短期的情绪状态（如对糖尿病的诊断或一种并发症发展的适应）和糖尿病相关的心理痛苦的抑郁症状。

3. 目前，缺乏文献陈述 2 型糖尿病儿童和妊娠期糖尿病女性患者中抑郁症的比率和相关性。

4. 虽然有强有力的证据证明一种三环类抗抑郁药物和四种 SSRI 药物的疗效，但在成人和儿童糖尿病患者中，还需更多的研究来评价它们短期和长期的疗效，以及 5-羟色胺和去甲肾上腺素再摄取抑制剂抗抑郁药物与血糖控制之间的相关性。

5. 额外的研究需要来评估运动作为 1 型和 2 型糖尿病患者抑郁症治疗方式的有效性。

6. 额外的研究需要来调查糖尿病患者预防抑郁症发生的有效方法。

7. 额外的研究需要来确立所有 1 型和 2 型糖尿病患者抑郁症治疗模式的成本效益。

筛查和护理的建议

抑郁症是 1 型和 2 型糖尿病患者的常见共存症。下列是基于文献和专家意见关于临床护理的建议。

1. 建议对糖尿病患者的每一次访视都进行抑郁筛查,辅以回顾患者反应的流程并描述显著的临床症状。对于表现为血糖升高、糖尿病并发症恶化,报告有终身抑郁症病史及可能因此处于未来抑郁发作高风险的患者,需给予更多的关注。研究者可使用多种简明的筛查工具来发现糖尿病患者的抑郁症状。

2. 医疗工作者推荐保持一个较低的抑郁症治疗门槛,一旦确诊,需推进严格序贯的抑郁症治疗。合理调整抗抑郁药物剂量,维持治疗的良好监测,健康护理人员给予常规的精神健康护理。根据糖尿病患者抑郁症的持续和反复及相关的不良医疗管理,建议抑郁症和糖尿病护理工作者相互协调来确保合适的抑郁症治疗和后续护理。

3. 证据支持逐步护理方法(药物治疗和心理治疗)的使用,以及监测维持治疗以达到症状缓解和血糖控制的提高。

4. 建议在健康护理中心使用联合心理治疗和抗抑郁药物为一体的合作护理方式。这一干预范例已经证实可减少社会歧视这类障碍,对糖尿病患者抑郁症治疗有效,并且在健康医疗机构呈现出良好的成本效用。

5. 推荐将抑郁症课程加入糖尿病教育,并且常规地与患者沟通糖尿病结局中抑郁症的作用,以减少患者对精神疾病相关的耻辱感的感知并提高患者治疗选择权的意识。

6. 在医疗护理机构中推荐抑郁症筛查措施与临床治疗结局相结合。

参 考 文 献

Ali S, Stone MA, Peters JL, Davies MJ, Khunti K: The prevalence of co-morbid depression in adults with type 2 diabetes: a systematic review and meta-analysis. *Diabet Med* 23:1165–1173, 2006

American Psychiatric Association: *Diagnostic and Statistical Manual of Mental Disorders - DSM-IV-TR.* 4th ed. Washington, D.C., American Psychiatric Association, 2000

Anderson RJ, Freedland KE, Clouse RE, Lustman PJ: The prevalence of comorbid depression in adults with diabetes: a meta-analysis. *Diabetes Care* 24:1069–1078, 2001

Arroyo CG, Hu FB, Ryan L, Kawachi I, Colditz G, Speizer F, Manson J: Depressive symptoms and risk of type 2 diabetes in women. *Diabetes Care* 27:129–133, 2004

Asghar S, Hussain A, Alit SMK, Khan AKA, Magnusson A: Prevalence of depression and diabetes: a population-based study from rural Bangladesh. *Diabet Med* 24:872–877, 2007

Barnard KD, Skinner TC, Peveler R: The prevalence of co-morbid depression in adults with type 1 diabetes: systematic literature review. *Diabet Med* 23:445–448, 2006

Beck AT, Steer RA, Brown GK: *BDI-II Beck Depression Inventory Manual.* 2nd ed. San Antonio, TX, The Psychological Corporation, Harcourt, Brace & Company, 1996

Bruce DG, Davis WA, Davis TME: Longitudinal predictors of reduced mobility and physical disability in patients with type 2 diabetes. *Diabetes Care* 28:2441–2447, 2005

Carnethon MR, Biggs M, Barzilay JJ, Smith N, Vaccarino V, Bertoni AG, Arnold A, Siscovick D: Longitudinal association between depressive symptoms and incident type 2 diabetes mellitus in older adults: the Cardiovascular Health Study. *Arch Intern Med* 167:802–807, 2007

Carnethon M, Kinder L, Fair J, Stafford R, Fortmann S: Symptoms of depression as a risk factor for incident diabetes: findings from the National Health and Nutrition Examination Epidemiologic Follow-Up Study, 1971–1992. *Am J Epidemiol* 158:416–423, 2003

Ciechanowski PS, Russo JE, Katon WJ, Von Korff M, Simon GE, Lin EHB, Ludman EJ, Young BA: The association of patient relationship style and outcomes in collaborative care treatment for depression in patients with diabetes. *Med Care* 44:283–291, 2006

Ciechanowski PS, Katon WJ, Russo JE: Depression and diabetes: impact of depressive symptoms on adherence, function, and costs. *Arch Intern Med* 160:3278–3285, 2000

Clouse RE, Lustman PJ, Freedland KE, Griffith LS, McGill JB, Carney RM: Depression and coronary heart disease in women with diabetes. *Psychosom Med* 65:376–383, 2003

de Groot M, Doyle T, Hockman E, Wheeler C, Pinkerman B, Shubrook J, Gotfried R, Schwartz F: Depression among type 2 diabetes rural Appalachian clinic attenders. *Diabetes Care* 30: 1602–1604, 2007

de Groot M, Pinkerman B, Wagner J, Hockman E: Depression treatment and satisfaction in a multicultural sample of type 1 and type 2 diabetic patients. *Diabetes Care* 29:549–553, 2006

de Groot M, Anderson RJ, Freedland KE, Clouse RE, Lustman PJ: Association of depression and diabetes complications: a meta-analysis. *Psychosom Med* 63:619–630, 2001

Eaton WW, Armenian H, Gallo J, Pratt L, Ford DE: Depression and risk for onset of type 2 diabetes. *Diabetes Care* 19:1097–1102, 1996

Egede LE: Diabetes, major depression and functional disability among U.S. adults. *Diabetes Care* 27:421–428, 2004

Egede LE, Zheng D: Independent factors associated with major depressive disorder in a national sample of individuals with diabetes. *Diabetes Care* 26:104–111, 2003

Egede LE: Beliefs and attitudes of African Americans with type 2 diabetes toward depression. *Diabetes Educ* 28:258–268, 2002a

Egede LE, Zheng D, Simpson K: Comorbid depression is associated with increased health care use and expenditures in individuals with diabetes. *Diabetes Care* 25:464–470, 2002b

Engum A: The role of depression and anxiety in onset of diabetes in a large population-based study. *J Psychosom Res* 62:31–38, 2007

Erdman HP, Klein MH, Greist JH, Skare SS, Husted JJ, Robins LN, Helzer JE, Goldring E, Hamburger M, Miller JP: A comparison of two computer-administered versions of the NIMH Diagnostic Interview Schedule. *J Psychiatr Res* 26:85–95, 1992

Evans D, Charney DS, Lewis L, Golden RN, Gorman JM, Krishnan KRR, Nemeroff CB, Bremner JD, Carney RM, Coyne JC, Delong MR, et al.: Mood disorders in the medically ill: scientific review and recommendations. *Biol Psychiatry* 58:175–189, 2005

Finkelstein, EA, Bray JW, Chen H, Larson MJ, Miller K, Tompkins C, Keme A, Manderscheid R: Prevalence and costs of major depression among elderly claimants with diabetes. *Diabetes Care* 26:415–420, 2003

Fisher L, Skaff MM, Mullan JT, Arean P, Mohr D, Masharani U, Glasgow R, Laurencin G: Clinical depression versus distress among patients with type 2 diabetes: not just a question of semantics. *Diabetes Care* 30:542–548, 2007

Fisher L, Chesla CA, Mullan JT, Skaff MM, Kanter RA: Contributors to depression in Latino and European-American patients with type 2 diabetes. *Diabetes Care* 24:1751–1757, 2001

Gary TL, Baptiste-Roberts K, Crum RM, Cooper LA, Ford DE, Brancati FL: Changes in depressive symptoms and metabolic control over 3 years among African Americans with type 2 diabetes. *Int J Psychiatry Med* 35:377–382, 2005

Gary TL, Crum RM, Cooper-Patrick L, Ford D, Brancati FL: Depressive symptoms and metabolic control in African-Americans with type 2 diabetes. *Diabetes Care* 23:23–29, 2000

Gaynes BN, Burns B, Tweed D, Erickson P: Depression and health-related quality of life. *J Nerv Ment Dis* 190:799–806, 2002

Golden SH, Williams JE, Ford DE, Yeh H, Sanford CP, Nieto FJ, Brancati FL: Depressive symptoms and the risk of type 2 diabetes. *Diabetes Care* 27:429–435, 2004

Goodnick PJ, Kumar A, Henry JH, Buki VM, Goldberg RB: Sertraline in coexisting major depression and diabetes mellitus. *Psychopharmacol Bull* 33:261–264, 1997

Grandinetti A, Kaholokula J, Crabbe K, Kenui C, Chen R, Chang H: Relationship between depressive symptoms and diabetes among native Hawaiians. *Psychoneuroendocrinology* 25:239–246, 2000

Grey M, Whittemore R, Tamborlane W: Depression in type 1 diabetes children: natural history and correlates. *J Psychosom Res* 53:907–911, 2002

Gross R, Olfson M, Gameroff M, Carasquillo O, Shea S, Feder A, Lantigua R, Fuentes M, Weissman M: Depression and glycemic control in Hispanic primary care patients with diabetes. *J Gen Intern Med* 20:460–466, 2004

Gulseren L, Gulseren S, Hekimsoy Z, Mete L: Comparison of fluoxetine and paroxetine in type II diabetes mellitus patients. *Arch Med Res* 36:159–165, 2005

Helzer JE, Robins LN: The Diagnostic Interview Schedule: its development, evolution and use. *Soc Psychiatry Psychiatr Epidemiol* 23:6–16, 1988

Hermanns N, Kulzer B, Krichbaum M, Kubiak T, Haak T: How to screen for depression and emotional problems in patients with diabetes: comparison of screening characteristics of depression questionnaires, measurement of diabetes-specific emotional problems and standard clinical assessment. *Diabetologia* 49:469–477, 2006

Ismail K, Winkley K, Stahl D, Chalder T, Edmonds M: A cohort study of people with diabetes and their first foot ulcer: the role of depression on mortality. *Diabetes Care* 30:1473–1479, 2007

Jacobson AM, de Groot M, Samson JA: The effects of psychiatric disorders and symptoms on quality of life in patients with type I and type II diabetes mellitus. *Qual Life Res* 6:11–20, 1997a

Jacobson AM, Hauser ST, Willet JB, Wolfsdorf JI, Dvorak R, Herman L, de Groot M: Psychological adjustment to IDDM: 10-year follow-up of an onset cohort of child and adolescent patients. *Diabetes Care* 20:811–818, 1997b

Jones LE, Clarke W, Carney CP: Receipt of diabetes services by insured adults with and without claims for mental disorders. *Medical Care* 42:1167–1175, 2004

Katon W, Lin EHB, Kroenke K: The association of depression and anxiety with medical symptom burden in patients with chronic medical illness. *General Hospital Psychiatry* 29:147–155, 2007

Katon W, Unutzer J, Fan M, Williams JW, Schoenbaum M, Lin EHB, Hunkeller EM: Cost-effectiveness and net benefit of enhanced treatment of depression for older adults with diabetes and depression. *Diabetes Care* 29:265–270, 2006

Katon W, Rutter C, Simon G, Lin EB, Ludman E, Ciechanowski P, Kinder L, Young G, von Korff M: The association of comorbid depression with mortality in patients with type 2 diabetes. *Diabetes Care* 28:2668–2672, 2005

Katon W, Simon G, Russo J, von Korff M, Lin E, Ludman E, Ciechanowski P, Bush T: Quality of depression care in a population-based sample of patients with diabetes and major depression. *Med Care* 42:1222–1229, 2004a

Katon W, Von Korff M, Ciechanowski P, Russo J, Lin E, Simon G, Ludman E, Walker E, Bush T, Young B: Behavioral and clinical factors associated with depression among individuals with diabetes. *Diabetes Care* 27:914–920, 2004b

Katon W, Von Korff M, Lin E, Simon G, Ludman E, Russo J, Ciechanowski P, Walker E, Bush T: The Pathways Study, a randomized trial of collaborative care in patients with depression and diabetes. *Arch Gen Psychiatry* 61:1042–1049, 2004c

Kinder LS, Carnethon MR, Palaniappan LP, King AC, Fortmann SP: Depression and the metabolic syndrome in young adults: findings from the Third National Health and Nutrition Examination Survey. *Psychosom Med* 66:316–322, 2004

Kinder LS, Katon WJ, Ludman E, Russo J, Simon G, Lin EHB, Ciechanowski P, Von Korff M, Young B: Improving depression care in patients with diabetes and multiple complications. *J Gen Intern Med* 21:1036–1041, 2006

Knol MJ, Twisk JW, Beekman AT, Heine RJ, Snoek FJ, Pouwer F: Depression as a risk factor for the onset of type 2 diabetes mellitus: a meta-analysis. *Diabetologia* 49:837–845, 2006

Kokkonen J, Kokkonen ER: Mental health and social adaptation in young adults with juvenile-onset diabetes. *Nord J Psychiatry* 49:175–181, 1995

Kovacs M, Obrosky DS, Goldston D, Drash A: Major depressive disorder in youths with IDDM: a controlled prospective study of course and outcome. *Diabetes Care* 20:45–51, 1997

Kovacs M, Mukerji P, Drash A, Iyengar S: Biomedical and psychiatric risk factors for retinopathy among children with IDDM. *Diabetes Care* 18:1592–1599, 1995

Kroenke K, Spitzer RL, Williams JBW: The PHQ-9: validity of a brief depression severity measure. *J Gen Intern Med* 16:606–613, 2001

Lawrence JM, Standiford DA, Loots B, Klingensmith GJ, Williams DE, Ruggiero A, Liese AD, Bell RA, Waitzfelder BE, McKeown RE: Prevalence and correlates of depressed mood among youth with diabetes: the SEARCH for Diabetes in Youth study. *Pediatrics* 117:1348–1358, 2006

Lin EHB, Katon W, Rutter C, Simon GE, Ludman EJ, Von Korff M, Young B, Oliver M, Ciechanowski PC, Kinder L, Walker E: Effects of enhanced depression treatment on diabetes self-care. *Ann Fam Med* 4:46–53, 2006

Lustman PJ, Williams MM, Sayuk GS, Nix BD, Clouse RE: Factors influencing glycemic control in type 2 diabetes during acute- and maintenance-phase treatment of major depressive disorder with bupropion. *Diabetes Care* 30:459–466, 2007

Lustman PJ, Clouse RE, Nix BD, Freedland KE, Rubin EH, McGill JB, Williams MM, Gelenberg AJ, Ciechanowski PS, Hirsch IB: Sertraline for prevention of depression recurrence in diabetes mellitus: a randomized, double-blind, placebo-controlled trial. *Arch Gen Psychiatry* 63:521–529, 2006

Lustman PJ, Clouse RE, Ciechanowski PS, Hirsch IB, Freedland KE: Depression-related hyperglycemia in type 1 diabetes: a mediational approach. *Psychosom Med* 67:195–199, 2005

Lustman PJ, Anderson RJ, Freedland KE, de Groot M, Carney RM, Clouse RE: Depression and poor glycemic control: a meta-analytic review of the literature. *Diabetes Care* 23:934–942, 2000a

Lustman PJ, Freedland KE, Griffith LS, Clouse RE: Fluoxetine for depression in diabetes: a randomized double-blind placebo-controlled trial. *Diabetes Care* 23:618–623, 2000b

Lustman PJ, Griffith LS, Freedland KE, Kissel SS, Clouse RE: Cognitive behavior therapy for depression in type 2 diabetes mellitus: a randomized, controlled trial. *Ann Intern Med* 129:613–621, 1998

Lustman PJ, Clouse RE, Griffith LS, Carney RM, Freedland KE: Screening for depression in diabetes using the Beck Depression Inventory. *Psychosom Med* 59:24–31, 1997a

Lustman PJ Griffith LS, Clouse RE, Freedland KE, Eisen SA, Rubin EH, Carney RM, McGill JB: Effects of nortriptyline on depression and glycemic control in diabetes: results of a double-blind, placebo-controlled trial. *Psychosom Med* 59:241–250, 1997b

Lustman PJ, Griffith LS, Freedland KE, Clouse RE: The course of major depression in diabetes. *Gen Hosp Psychiatry* 19:138–143, 1997c

Lustman PJ, Griffith LS, Clouse RE: Depression in adults with diabetes. Results of 5-yr follow-up study. *Diabetes Care* 11:605–612, 1988

Lustman PJ, Harper GW, Griffith LS, Clouse RE: Use of the Diagnostic Interview Schedule in patients with diabetes mellitus. *J Nerv Ment Dis* 174:743–746, 1986

McCollum M, Ellis SL. Regensteiner JG, Zhang W, Sullivan PW: Minor depression and health status among US adults with diabetes mellitus. *Am J Manag Care* 13:65–72, 2007

Nichols L, Barton PL, Glazner J, McCollum M: Diabetes, minor depression and health care utilization and expenditures: a retrospective database study. *Cost Effectiveness and Resource Allocation* 5(4), 2007.

Paile-Hyvarinen M, Wahlbeck K, Eriksson JG: Quality of life and metabolic status in mildly depressed women with type 2 diabetes treated with paroxetine: a single-blind randomised placebo controlled trial. *BMC Family Practice* 4(7), 2003

Peyrot M, Rubin RR: Persistence of depressive symptoms in diabetic adults. *Diabetes Care* 22:448–452, 1999

Polonsky WH, Fisher L. Earles J, Dudl RJ, Lees J, Mullan J, Jackson RA: Assessing psychosocial distress in diabetes. *Diabetes Care* 28:626–631, 2005

Pouwer F, Beekman ATF, Nijpels G, Dekker JM, Snoek FJ, Kostense PJ, Heine RJ, Deeg DJH: Rates and risks for co-morbid depression in patients with type 2

diabetes mellitus: results from a community-based study. *Diabetologia* 46:892–898, 2003

Radloff L: The CES-D scale: a self-report depression scale for research in the general population. *Applied Psychological Measurement* 1:385–401, 1977

Robins L, Wing J, Wittchen HU, Helzer JE, Babor TF, Burke J, Farmer A, Jablenski A, Pickens R, Regier DA, et al.: The Composite International Diagnostic Interview: an epidemiologic instrument suitable for use in conjunction with different diagnostic systems in different cultures. *Arch Gen Psychiatry* 45:1069–1077, 1988

Roy A, Roy M: Depressive symptoms in African-American type I diabetics. *Depression and Anxiety* 13:28–31, 2001

Sacco WP, Yanover T: Diabetes and depression: the role of social support and medical symptoms. *J Behav Med* 29:523–531, 2007

Saydah SH, Brancati FL, Golden SH, Fradkin J, Harris MI: Depressive symptoms and the risk of type 2 diabetes mellitus in a US sample. *Diabetes/Metabolism Research and Reviews* 19:202–208, 2003

Shaban MC, Fosbury J, Kerr D, Cavan DA: The prevalence of depression and anxiety in adults with type 1 diabetes. *Diabet Med* 23:1381–1384, 2006

Simon GE, Katon WJ, Lin EHB, Rutter C, Manning WG, Von Korff M, Ciechanowski P, Ludman EJ, Young BA: Cost-effectiveness of systematic depression treatment among people with diabetes mellitus. *Arch Gen Psychiatry* 64:65–72, 2007

Spitzer R, Williams JBW, Gibbon M, First MB: The Structured Clinical Interview for DSM-III-R (SCID) - I: history, rationale, and description. *Arch Gen Psychiatry* 49:624–629, 1992

Stewart SM, Rao U, Emslie GJ, Klein D, White PC: Depressive symptoms predict hospitalization for adolescents with type 1 diabetes mellitus. *Pediatrics* 115:1315–1319, 2005

Trief PM, Morin PC, Izquierdo R, Teresi JA, Eimicke JP, Goland R, Starren J, Shea S, Weinstock RS: Depression and glycemic control in elderly ethnically diverse patients with diabetes. *Diabetes Care* 29:830–835, 2006

Vickers KS, Nies MA, Patten CA, Dierkhising R, Smith SA: Patients with diabetes and depression may need additional support for exercise. *Am J Health Behav* 30:353–362, 2006

Vileikyte L, Leventhal H, Gonzale J, Peyrot M, Rubin R, Ulbrecht J, Garrow A, Waterman C, Cavanagh P, Boulton A: Diabetic peripheral neuropathy and depressive symptoms. *Diabetes Care* 28:2378–2383, 2005

Von Korff M, Katon W, Lin EHB, Simon G, Ciechanowski P, Ludman E, Oliver M, Rutter C, Young B: Work disability among individuals with diabetes. *Diabetes Care* 28:1326–1332, 2005

Wagner J, Abbott G: Depression and depression care in diabetes: relationship to perceived discrimination in African Americans. *Diabetes Care* 30:364–366, 2007a

Wagner JA, Tennen H: History of major depressive disorder and diabetes outcomes in diet- and tablet-treated post-menopausal women: a case control study. *Diabet Med* 24:211–216, 2007b

Wagner J, Tsimikas J, Abbott G, de Groot M, Heapy A: Racial and ethnic differences in diabetic patient-reported depression symptoms, diagnosis, and treatment. *Diabetes Research and Clinical Practice* 75:119–122, 2006

Welch GW, Jacobson AM, Polonsky WH: The Problem Areas in Diabetes scale: an evaluation of its clinical utility. *Diabetes Care* 20:760–766, 1997

Williams JBW, Gibbon M, First MB, Spitzer RL, Davies M, Borus J, Howes MJ, Kane J, Pope HG Jr, Rounsaville B, Wittchen H-U: The Structured Clinical Interview for DSM-III-R (SCID) - II: multisite test-retest reliability. *Arch Gen Psychiatry* 49:630–636, 1992

Williams MM, Clouse RE, Nix BD, Rubin EH, Sayuk GS, McGill JB, Gelenberg AJ, Ciechanowski PS, Hirsch IB, Lustman PJ: Efficacy of sertraline in prevention of depression recurrence in older versus younger adults with diabetes. *Diabetes Care* 30:801–806, 2007

Zhang X, Norris SL, Gregg EW, Cheng YJ, Beckles G, Kahn HS: Depressive symptoms and mortality among persons with and without diabetes. *Am J Epidemiol* 161:652–660, 2005

Zhao W, Chen Y, Lin M, Sigal RJ: Association between diabetes and depression: sex and age differences. *Public Health* 120:696–704, 2006

第二章
进食障碍和饮食行为失调

Deborah Young –Hyman，PhD，CDE

进食障碍和饮食行为失调的定义

美国精神病学会（APA）心理健康诊断手册（《精神疾病的诊断和统计手册》DSM-IV-TR2000 年）把饮食行为失调定义为限制热量摄入，过度锻炼，使用泻药和其他药物的排空肠道方式，暴饮暴食及糖尿病患者有意减少或遗漏使用胰岛素的行为。DEB 的认知，包括对体重和体型的关注，有助于诊断标准的形成。ED 的主要诊断类别能够反映行为类型，包括厌食症、暴食症和其他不进行特殊说明的进食障碍。ED vs DEB 的诊断是依据行为和认知的频率。通过自我报告或访谈记录的行为和认知达到频率界值，才能达到诊断（ED）的水平。低频的行为和认知则考虑是亚临床（DEB）症状。两者虽然行为不同，但共同的特征是人们渴望控制体重和改变外表，其行为和认知干扰了其他日常生活并且很极端。对于体型的担忧导致了适应不良的体重管理行为。一般人群的行为标准适用于有额外胰岛素处理行为（遗漏或减少）的糖尿病患者。

糖尿病患者：一个脆弱的群体

1 型和 2 型糖尿病患者超重和肥胖的比率会升高。在寻求减重的健康个体及 1 型糖尿病（T1D），特别是年轻女性，体重状态与 DEB 有很大的关联。尽管存在 T2D 患者关注体重指数升高和暴食的比率增加的证据，但在 T2D 患者中与体重、体重担忧、ED 和 DEB 发展相关的证据是不足的。

饮食节制，食品关注（如糖类监测和限制）、分量的控制，通过选择性的食物摄入来控制血糖，规划性的锻炼是糖尿病治疗的组成部分，是实现良好的血糖控制的基石。当这些治疗行为应用不合理，如快速减重、执行过度、干扰日常生活和（或）导致危害健康时，这些治疗行为就会发展为 DEB。

正在进行的糖尿病治疗会把患者暴露于一种会触发 DEB 发生的情况中。这些包括：因为向家人成员报告/监测食物摄入量、体育活动和血糖而感觉丧失自主权；需要卫生保健提供者监督和问责来保持健康和体重；治疗方案的后遗症如对进食态度的改变；由于自我和身体概念的改变而增加脆弱感和失控感；以及开启胰岛素治疗后的体重增加。排除其他心理、家庭、社会的影响，坚持治疗可能是糖尿病患者易患 DEB 的危险因素。

虽然关于 DEB 是否与 T1D 患者长期较差的代谢控制有关还存在疑问，但已证明可诊断的 ED 和行为类别为亚临床 DEB 的存在与并发症的增加相关：视网膜病变、神经病变、暂时的脂质异常、糖尿病酮症酸中毒的住院率增加和短期较差的代谢控制。横断面研究表明增高的 HbA1C 与可诊断的 ED、亚临床 DEB 及故意的胰岛素治疗遗漏有关。DEB 与 T2D 并发症之间的关联还没有被广泛地研究。T2D 患者拒绝开始胰岛素治疗（社会心理的胰岛素抵抗力）可能部分是由于担心体重增加，但这只是轶事，还没有经过系统的测试。

当患者增加、体重减轻和（或）血糖控制恶化[包括重度低血糖和（或）酮症酸中毒]不能用疾病进程、管理改变、药物或胰岛素治疗方案、监控的减肥计划、明显的不依从性或精神疾病来解释时，尤其是年轻女性应进行 DEB 评估。

可诊断的 ED 和亚临床 DEB 的患病率

可诊断的 ED 在糖尿病人群中的患病率较低。与健康对照者相比，T1D 人群中可诊断的 ED 和 DEB 的患病率有不同的评估范围。患 T1D 的青少年和年轻女性的评估范围是 3.8%～31%。一些研究发现了与普通人群相似的比例，或者更高的比例，但是评估方法是不同的。

亚临床 DEB 在美国和文化西化的人群都正在增加，可能与强调消瘦

的理想观念和对超重/肥胖的关注有关。因为节食行为较普遍及耻于自我
报告 DEB 的行为，亚临床 DEB 的患病率可能被低估。一个比较流行的
看法是，当考虑把故意减少胰岛素剂量或漏用胰岛素作为清除行为来
控制体重时，那么 DEB 患病率的增加与糖尿病的诊断有关，尤其是 T1D
患者中的女性和青春期少女。然而，最近的一项使用以人群为基础的
健康对照样本的研究没有显示可诊断的 ED 患病率的升高与糖尿病人
群有关。

　　暴食行为和胰岛素遗漏为在 T1D 患者中最常报道的 DEB，而热量
限制/约束和暴食在 T2D 女性中最常报道。糖尿病男孩的 DEB 患病率比
女性要低得多，但可能会增加。少数民族的 T2D 患病率更高可能与增加
的 DEB 患病率相关，但这种关系尚未被证实。比较 DEB 在 1 型和 2 型
糖尿病患者中发生的研究表明两者的发病率相似；然而，行为类型并不
相同。"以瘦为美的驱动"和"对身体不满意"在 T2D 患者中更常见。
故意遗漏胰岛素（导致糖尿）在 T1D 患者中更常见。

　　在试图减肥的超重年轻女性中，有 T1D 和未患糖尿病，体重状态是
DEB 强力的预测因素。研究 BMI 的报告指出，T1D 人群 BMI 已经明显
高于健康对照组，平均 BMI 高于正常范围。体重的评估，独立的诊断，
可能本身就会预测较高的 DEB 患病率。然而，很少有研究在年龄、性别
和体重相匹配的情况下研究糖尿病组与健康对照组的 EDB 患病率。当
BMI 相匹配受试者被用来进行 T2D 超重和肥胖者与寻求减肥的非糖尿
病人群和一个非临床肥胖样本比较时，全体人群都被诊断了低水平的暴
食症（所有组＜5%）。然而，肥胖糖尿病患者 ED 检查中得分最低，但
在约束量表中得分最高。约束量表中分数更高是由于治疗行为。虽然有
强有力的文件表明使用 DSM 标准考虑亚临床 DEB 行为，如暴食、清除
（定义为故意胰岛素遗漏）和热量限制在糖尿病患者中比较常见，但还不
知道这些报告反映了多少基于糖尿病管理方案依从性的认知。

　　体重增加是良好血糖控制的结果，可能成为体重担忧的驱动因素，
也是成功治疗的一个不良反应。虽然推测在这一群体中 DEB 与增高的
BMI 水平相关，但只有一个研究对糖尿病人群（1 型和 2 型糖尿病，男
性和女性，年龄范围 18～65 岁）的体重状态进行了分层研究。3%正常
体重或低于正常体重的女性现患 DEB，而 6.8%的超重女性和 10.3%的肥

胖女性报道有 DEB。这些患病率与具有同等 BMI 的寻求减肥的样本类似。控制体重的需要与达到良好的血糖控制之间可能存在冲突（在 1 型和 2 型糖尿病患者中都存在）。特别是，年轻女性和青少年女性特意为了控制体重而遗漏胰岛素使用。改善血糖控制的恐惧是"因为我将增加体重"，并且糖尿病特定的心理痛苦预示了胰岛素故意遗漏。虽然医学营养治疗的其中一个目标（MNT）是防止体重增加，然而继发于胰岛素治疗成功的体重增加发生时，并不经常使用监督体重管理项目。

糖尿病人群中 ED 和 DEB 的病因：精神病症状，方案依从性（或不依从）或生理失调

ED 和 DEB 的主要危险因素（非糖尿病的人群）是体重和体型的担忧，早期饮食问题和节食，其他形式的精神病理学的存在，性虐待和其他不良的生活经历和较低自我价值感。除了体重忧虑和抑郁，糖尿病人群中的这些危险因素与 DEB 发生之间的关系没有得到重视。

确定 DEB 的发生是归因于糖尿病及其管理是复杂的，因为缺乏对同时发生的精神病症状，疾病的社会心理调整和糖尿病管理方案的后遗症的评估研究。Bryden 等追踪了 1 型糖尿病青少年和年轻人的 BMI 及对体重和体型的担忧；因为男性和女性都变得超重，所以 DEB 增加。然而，没有评估独立于体重问题的基线和持续的心理状态。相比之下，Pollock 等对新诊断为 T1D 的男孩和女孩（年龄 8～13 岁）进行了随访，随访时间是从诊断日直到第 14 年。评估了 DEB 的存在，医疗方案依从性和精神症状，包括体重问题。研究发现了可诊断的 ED（使用 DSM-III）的低发生率（3.8%），然而"有饮食问题的青少年患精神障碍的可能性是其余病人的 9 倍"。最近的一项研究发现，T1D 女性发生胰岛素限制与体重增加的恐惧和自我管理方案问题相关。与糖尿病护理相关的特有的饮食行为问题，看上去像是与精神疾病高发及疾病调控差相关的普遍的不依从症群中的一部分。

两项研究证明了精神病发病率与 2 型糖尿病患者 DEB 有关，不受体重状态约束。其中一项研究表明，更多的超重和肥胖患者有可能诊断为

ED，并且 ED 患者明显有更多的焦虑障碍和更倾向于患抑郁症。第二项研究表明，DEB 与神经病理学密切相关，如抑郁、自卑，一般的精神病理学但不是体重。鉴于已经知道情感障碍（特别是抑郁症）和糖尿病存在共病情况，以及在健康人群中情感障碍和 DEB 的共病情况，DEB 可能成为较差的心理调整和（或）较差的疾病适应众多原因中的一个，这与肥胖和 T2D 患者存在共患有关。

　　触发的行为和特殊的 DEB 病症嵌入糖尿病治疗方案。缺乏成功的 MNT 会使患者在饮食行为和血糖方面感到失控感。饮食行为的失控感，关注食物和热量限制是 DSM-Ⅳ-TR 对厌食症、暴食症不做其他特殊说明的 ED 的诊断标准。暴食症的主要标准包括主观自我评价在短时间内反复吃大量的食物，绝对比大多数人在类似情况下吃得多。糖尿病患者做出这种主观判断（食物量大或过多）可能是由于未能遵守 MNT 处方，特别是在低血糖治疗的背景下。其他可能性存在于错误地坚持 DEB 行为。因为热量限制是治疗处方的一部分，与适当的食物摄入相关的不准确判定可能发生在下列情况中：糖类计算，血糖水平降低，症状原因的误判，或与运动有关的营养摄入过度。

　　糖尿病患者饥饿和饱腹感的激素失调的证据表明控制食物摄入和随之而来的血糖水平是很困难的。而且，胰岛素的非生理剂量影响食欲调节。激素失调（包括内源性胰岛素和胰淀素分泌）、肠促胰岛素生产的失调有助于肠道代谢，疾病的并发症如胃轻瘫和血糖水平的波动，特别是低血糖，可能促使脆弱的患者采用不良体重管理策略（如胰岛素操作）来控制饥饿和相关的体重增加。

ED 和 EDB 的测量

　　迄今为止，大多数研究使用普通人群中标准化的测量工具来确定糖尿病患者的 ED 和 DEB。问卷包括但不局限于饮食态度测试（EAT）-40 和 EAT-26、进食障碍清单（EDI-3）、暴食症测试-修订（BULIT-R）和进食障碍检查，这些以访谈形式进行。评估工具包括态度和行为中嵌入的糖尿病治疗方案。例如，BULIT-R 项目（"你觉得你能够控制你摄入的食物量吗？"及"当我不饿时我吃很多食物"）可以参考糖尿病护理方案

（前者是饮食限制的处方，后者是饮食计划的处方），胰岛素的糖类比率，和（或）低水平血糖的治疗。当使用健康人群标准化的问卷时，由于诊断饮食失调的态度与 DEB 和部分糖尿病治疗处方的项目重叠，1 型糖尿病和 2 型糖尿病患者的分数可能升高。当在非糖尿病人群中使用标准化的问卷调查或访谈技术时，建议进行问题修改来陈述行为意图，包括胰岛素操作。一些研究已经扩展了 EDE 和 SCID 访谈形式涵盖这些问题。

发现了两个例外的问卷：糖尿病饮食问题调查（DEPS），由 Antisded、Laffel 和 Anderson 创建并由 Markowitz 等细化，以及 AHEAD（评估青少年糖尿病患者的健康和饮食）调查。这两个问卷都包括了专门以减少体重为目的的胰岛素调整问题，都设立了关于糖尿病管理的问题和因治疗引起的血糖控制和体重增加的问题。然而，两者在临床人群的 ED 独立诊断上都没有得到验证。一项证实调查问卷有效性的研究评估了糖尿病管理背景下的饥饿和饱腹感，糖尿病治疗和饱腹感量表（DTSS-20）表明 T1D 患者在感觉饱胀、饥饿和（或）饮食摄入失控时经常体验矛盾的临床情况（与血糖的控制水平、日常的 MNT 和胰岛素剂量相关）。推测，缺乏合适的饥饿和饱腹感提示与激素失调有关（参见关于食欲的生理失调的部分）。

为了确定 ED 的诊断或记录亚临床 DEB，糖尿病人群全面的评估应包括对疾病适应的评估、整体心理状态的评估、体重和体型担忧的评估、关于胰岛素使用的不适应或减肥的医疗方案的特殊问题的评估，以及在血糖控制水平的背景与饥饿和饱腹相关的本体感觉提示的可靠性。

当前研究成果的局限性

DEB 与糖尿病相关性的研究空白包括：①在遵从医疗方案和适应疾病的情况下评估 DEB；②了解胰岛素和药物剂量对饥饿感和饱腹感的影响；③饮食处方/医学营养治疗作为信息/态度的潜在来源导致对食物摄入的失控感；④需要适当的对照组，如防止增重或减重的健康体重匹配人群、少数民族对照组和其他影响体重/代谢的慢性疾病组；⑤不完整的心理表征样本；⑥歧视与不服从相关的先存/逐步发展的精神病理；⑦需要使用糖尿病特定的评估工具的。

以往对糖尿病人群中 DEB 患病率的研究没有系统地阐述以下问题：方案强度、采取方案决策的责任，卫生保健提供者对血糖和体重结果的预期及与医疗管理有关的饮食认知。糖尿病治疗知识或方案依从性对 DEB 患病率的贡献还不确定。很少有研究从诊断之初就监控患者的心理症状（尤其是抑郁症）、DEB、体重增加或防止体重增加的方案调整与糖尿病的关系或年代。对成年女性的研究没有考虑使用激素避孕或激素替代疗法（HRT），这可能会导致过度的体重增加和食欲增加。最后，到目前为止，没有研究同时评估激素和肠促胰岛素的生理标志物对饥饿和饱腹失调及糖尿病管理背景下的 DEB 症状的影响。

筛查和管理建议

DEB 作为一个严重的和潜在威胁生命的糖尿病共患病被人们接受，尽管关于它的诊断和流行还存在争议。还没有发现已发表的关于糖尿病人群的 DEB 或 ED 治疗的随机对照干预试验。因此筛选建议来自于现存文献，治疗建议采取的是健康人群的 DEB 干预。

如果怀疑 DEB，应该执行如下筛查

1. 使用糖尿病特定的测量工具来区分指示方案依从性 vs DEB 的行为来控制体重，不考虑血糖控制目标。

2. 评估整体心理适应以确定行为是否指示 DEB，精神疾病和（或）对诊断较差的适应及治疗方案的要求（不服从）。当无法解释血糖控制不佳、体重增加和（或）体重减轻的发生时，已知有精神疾病的患者应筛查 DEB。

3. 评估胰岛素和其他药物剂量/总量及低血糖的发作作为缺乏饱腹感和（或）食物摄入的失控感的潜在原因。评估提示食物需要或血糖水平背景下的治疗（用药物）的内在提示的准确性。

4. 评估膳食处方和信息（MNT）对与摄食相关的态度和行为的潜在影响，包括食物关注、暴食及真实的或主观的饮食约束的自我评估（ADA 2007）。

5. 评估患者达到良好的血糖控制的期望: 社会心理适应, 生活质量, 饮食行为和体重的代价是什么。

如果筛查提示DEB,应该执行正式的评估和管理:

1. 参考社会心理/精神疾病的评估。一旦通过问卷调查和访谈确定了ED/DEB,应该向熟悉糖尿病医疗管理和 DEB 治疗的精神护理专家处转诊。

2. 当 DEB 治疗开始时, 治疗专家及患者接受治疗时的社会支持网中的关键人物(儿童和青少年的父母,成人的伴侣或亲密的家庭/社区成员)应该被纳入糖尿病管理团队。

3. 根据症状的严重程度,应考虑药物(抗抑郁和抗焦虑)和住院治疗。

4. 常规监测 DEB 症状, 医疗管理访问也是持续的治疗过程的一部分, 这样的糖尿病护理方案可以适当调整。仔细评估糖尿病行为护理的贡献, 知识, 行为意图, 应该进行血糖和体重的目标。合并糖尿病的治疗人员的 DEB 治疗计划有助于确保处方方案行为可以根据需要调整。

5. 非糖尿病的人群中使用认知行为疗法、人际关系治疗和综合认知疗法与辅助药物治疗来解决重大精神症状是公认的治疗方法,应该提供给那些有糖尿病的患者。基于成功的干预方法, 治疗可以单独一名患者或一组患者, 由一名训练有素且熟悉 DEB 和糖尿病的专业人员(通常为行为训练的心理学家、社会工作者或营养师)给予治疗。

6. 措施应针对具体适应不良行为(如操纵胰岛素或药物遗漏), 以确保健康, 应该对身体形象、自尊、自主权、人际关系和疾病的自我效能感认知, 特别是血糖和体重的控制, 根据症状报告, 改善心理健康。推荐在用于普遍人群的程序上添加自我行为管理, 特别强调糖尿病团队管理在维持血糖控制中的背景作用。如果代谢紊乱(严重的低血糖和酮症酸中毒)发现与 DEB 共患, 代谢紊乱必须首先通过医疗管理稳定。

参 考 文 献

Abrams J: Lifestyle changes most often suggested for weight complaints: special report: annual pill survey. *Contracept Technol Update* 13:154–156, 1992

Ackard DM, Vik N, Neumark-Sztainer D, Schmitz KH, Hannan P, Jacobs DR Jr: Disordered eating and body dissatisfaction in adolescents with type 1 diabetes and a population-based comparison sample: comparative prevalence and clinical implications. *Pediatr Diabetes* 9:312–319, 2008

Affenito SG, Adams CH: Are eating disorders more prevalent in females with type 1 diabetes mellitus when the impact of insulin omission is considered? *Nutr Rev* 59:179–182, 2001

Affenito SG, Backstrand JR, Welch GW, Lammi-Keefe CJ, Rodriguez NR, Adams CH: Subclinical and clinical eating disorders in IDDM negatively affect metabolic control. *Diabetes Care* 20:182–184, 1997a

Affenito SG, Lammi-Keefe CJ, Vogal S, Backstand JR, Welch GW, Adams CH: Women with insulin-dependent diabetes mellitus (IDDM) complicated by eating disorders are at risk for exacerbated alterations in lipid metabolism. *Eur J Clin Nutr* 51:462–466, 1997b

Alice Hsu YY, Chen BH, Huang MC, Lin SJ, Lin MF: Disturbed eating behaviors in Taiwanese adolescents with type 1 diabetes mellitus: a comparative study. *Pediatr Diabetes* 10:74–81, 2009

American Diabetes Association: Standards of medical care in diabetes: 2007. *Diabetes Care* 30 (Suppl. 1):S4–S41, 2007

American Diabetes Association Task Force for Writing Nutrition Principles and Recommendations for the Management of Diabetes and Related Complications: American Diabetes Association position statement: evidence-based nutrition principles and recommendations for the treatment and prevention of diabetes and related complications. *J Am Diet Assoc* 102:109–118, 2002

American Psychiatric Association: Eating disorders. In *Diagnostic and Statistical Manual of Mental Disorders, DSM-IV-TR*. 4th ed. Washington, DC, American Psychiatric Association, 2000, p. 583-597

Anderson BJ, Vangsness L, Connell A, Butler D, Goebel-Fabbri A, Laffel LM: Family conflict, adherence, and glycaemic control in youth with short duration type 1 diabetes. *Diabet Med* 19:635–642, 2002

Anderson RJ, Freedland KE, Clouse RE, Lustman PJ: The prevalence of comorbid depression in adults with diabetes: a meta-analysis. *Diabetes Care* 24:1069–1078, 2001

Antisdel JE, Laffel LMB, Anderson B: Improved detection of eating problems in women with type 1 diabetes using a newly developed survey (abstract). *Diabetes* 50 (Suppl. 1):A47, 2001

Arriaza CA, Mann T: Ethnic differences in eating disorder symptoms among college students: the confounding role of body mass index. *J Am Coll Health* 49:309–315, 2001

Bantle JP, Wylie-Rosett J, Albright AL, Apovian CM, Clark NG, Franz MJ, Hoogwerf BJ, Lichtenstein AH, Mayer-Davis E, Mooradian AD, Wheeler ML: Nutrition recommendations and interventions for diabetes–2006: a position statement of the American Diabetes Association. *Diabetes Care* 29:2140–2157, 2006

Battaglia MR, Alemzadeh R, Katte H, Hall PL, Perlmuter LC: Brief report: disordered eating and psychosocial factors in adolescent females with type 1 diabetes mellitus. *J Pediatr Psychol* 31:552–556, 2006

Biggs MM, Basco MR, Patterson G, Raskin P: Insulin withholding for weight control in women with diabetes. *Diabetes Care* 17:1186–1189, 1994

Bryden KS, Neil A, Mayou RA, Peveler RC, Fairburn CG, Dunger DB: Eating habits, body weight, and insulin misuse: a longitudinal study of teenagers and young adults with type 1 diabetes. *Diabetes Care* 22:1956–1960, 1999

Bubb JA Pontious SL: Weight loss from inappropriate insulin manipulation: an eating disorder variant in an adolescent with insulin-dependent diabetes mellitus. *Diabetes Educ* 17:29–32, 1991

Colton P, Olmsted M, Daneman D, Rydall A, Rodin G: Disturbed eating behavior and eating disorders in preteen and early teenage girls with type 1 diabetes: a case-controlled study. *Diabetes Care* 27:1654–1659, 2004

Colton P, Rodin GM, Olmsted MP, Daneman D: Eating disturbances in young women with type 1 diabetes mellitus: mechanisms and consequences. *Psychiatric Annals* 29:213–218, 1999

Cooper Z, Cooper PJ, Fairburn CG: The validity of the eating disorder examination and its subscales. *Br J Psychiatry* 154:807–812, 1989

Criego A, Crow S, Goebel-Fabbri AE, Kendall D, Parkin CG: Eating disorders and diabetes screening and detection. *Diabetes Spectrum* 22:143–146, 2009

Crow S, Keel PK, Kendall D: Eating disorders and insulin-dependent diabetes mellitus. *Psychosomatics* 39:233–243, 1998

Daneman D, Rodin G, Jones J, Colton P, Rydall A, Maharaj S, Olmsted M: Eating disorders in adolescent girls and young adult women with type 1 diabetes. *Diabetes Spectrum* 15:83–105, 2002

Daneman D, Olmsted M, Rydall A, Maharaj S, Rodin G: Eating disorders in young women with type 1 diabetes. *Hormone Research* 50 (Suppl. 1):79–86, 1998

Davis S, Alonso MD: Hypoglycaemia as a barrier to glycemic control. *J Diabetes Complications* 18:60–68, 2004

Davis SN, Renda SM: Psychological insulin resistance: overcoming barriers to starting insulin therapy. *Diabetes Educ* 32 (Suppl 4):146S–152S, 2006

de Man Lapidoth J, Ghaderi A, Norring C: Eating disorders and disordered eating among patients seeking non-surgical weight-loss treatment in Sweden. *Eat Behav* 7:15–26, 2006

de Zwaan M, Pyle RL, Mitchell JE: Pharmacological treatment of anorexia nervosa, bulimia nervosa, and binge eating disorder. In *Handbook of Eating Disorders and Obesity*. Thompson JK, Ed. Hoboken, NJ, John Wiley & Sons, 2004, p. 186–217

Decaluwe V, Braet C: Prevalence of binge-eating disorder in obese children and adolescents seeking weight-loss treatment. *Int J Obes Relat Metab Disord* 27:404–409, 2003

Dupre J: Glycaemic effects of incretins in type 1 diabetes mellitus: a concise review, with emphasis on studies in humans. *Regul Pept* 128:149–157, 2005

Engstrom I, Kroon M, Arvidsson C-G, Segnestam K, Snellman K, Aman J: Eating disorders in adolescent girls with insulin-dependent diabetes mellitus: a population-based case-control study. *Acta Paediatr* 88:175–180, 1999

Erkolahti RK, Ilonen T, Saarijarvi S: Self-image of adolescents with diabetes mellitus type-I and rheumatoid arthritis. *Nord J Psychiatry* 57:309–312, 2003

Fairburn CG, Peveler RC, Davies B, Mann JI, Mayou RA: Eating disorders in young adults with insulin dependent diabetes mellitus: a controlled study. *BMJ* 303:17–20, 1991

Gallo MF, Lopez LM, Grimes DA, Schulz KF, Helmerhorst FM: Combination contraceptives: effects on weight. *Cochrane Database Syst Rev* CD003987, 2006

Gallo MF, Grimes DA, Schulz KF, Helmerhorst FM: Combination estrogen-progestin contraceptives and body weight: systematic review of randomized controlled trials. *Obstet Gynecol* 103:359–373, 2004

Garner DM: *Eating Disorder Inventory-3 Professional Manual*. Lutz, FL, Psychological Assessment Resources, 2004

Garner DM, Olmsted MP, Bohr Y, Garfinkle PE: The Eating Attitudes Test: psychometric features and clinical correlates. *Psychol Med* 12:871–878, 1982

Garner DM, Garfinkel PE: The Eating Attitudes Test: an index of the symptoms of anorexia nervosa. *Psychol Med* 9:273–279, 1979

Goebel-Fabbri A, Anderson BJ, Fikkan J, Franko DL, Pearson K, Weinger K: Improvement and emergence of insulin restriction in women with type 1 diabetes. *Diabetes Care* 34:545–550, 2011

Goebel-Fabbri A: Disturbed eating behaviors and eating disorders in type 1 diabetes: clinical significance and treatment recommendations. *Curr Diab Rep* 9:133–139, 2009

Goebel-Fabbri A, Fikkan J, Franko DL, Pearson K, Anderson BJ, Weinger K: Insulin restriction and associated morbidity and mortality in women with type 1 diabetes. *Diabetes Care* 31:415–419, 2008

Hay LC, Wilmshurst EG, Fulcher G: Unrecognized hypo- and hyperglycemia in well-controlled patients with type 2 diabetes mellitus: the results of continuous glucose monitoring. *Diabetes Technol Ther* 5:19–26, 2003

Herpertz S, Albus C, Kielmann R, Hagemann-Patt H, Lichtblau K, Köhle K, Mann K, Senf W: Comorbidity of diabetes mellitus and eating disorders: a follow-up study. *J Psychosom Res* 51:673–678, 2001

Herpertz S, Albus C, Lichtblau K, Köhle K, Mann K, Senf W: Relationship of weight and eating disorders in type 2 diabetic patients: a multicenter study. *Int J Eat Disord* 28:68–77, 2000

Herpertz S, Albus C, Wagener R, Kocnar M, Wagner R, Henning A, Best F, Foerster H, Schulze Schleppinghoff B, Thomas W, Köhle K, Mann K, Senf W: Comorbidity of diabetes and eating disorders. Does diabetes control reflect disturbed eating behavior? *Diabetes Care* 21:1110–1116, 1998a

Herpertz S, Wagener R, Albus C, Kocnar M, Wanger R, Best F, Schulze Schleppinghoff B, Filz H, Forster K, Thomas W, Mann K, Kohle K, Senf W: Diabetes mellitus and eating disorders: a multicenter study on the comorbidity of the two diseases. *J Psychosom Res* 44:503–515, 1998b

Higgins SC, Gueorguiev M, Korbonits M: Ghrelin, the peripheral hunger hormone. *Ann Med* 39:116–136, 2007

Hockey S, Brown LJ, Lunt H: Prevalence of insulin self manipulation in young women with insulin dependent diabetes. *N Z Med J* 106:474–476, 1993

Hudson JI, Hudson MS, Wentworth SM: Self-induced glycosuria: a novel method of purging in bulimia. *JAMA* 249:2501, 1983

Jacobi C, Hayward C, de Zwaan M, Kraemer HC, Agras WS: Coming to terms with risk factors for eating disorders: application of risk terminology and suggestions for a general taxonomy. *Psychol Bull* 130:19–65, 2004

Johnson SB, Perwien AR, Silverstein JH: Response to hypo- and hyperglycemia in adolescents with type I diabetes. *J Pediatr Psychol* 25:171–178, 2000

Jones J, Lawson ML, Daneman D, Olmsted MP, Rodin G: Eating disorders in adolescent females with and without type 1 diabetes: cross sectional study. *BMJ* 320:1563–1566, 2006

Kelly SD, Howe CJ, Hendler JP, Lipman TH: Disordered eating behaviors in youth with type 1 diabetes. *Diabetes Educ* 31:572–583, 2005

Khan Y, Montgomery AM: Eating attitudes in young females with diabetes: insulin omission identifies a vulnerable subgroup. *Br J Med Psychol* 69(Pt 4):343–353, 1996

Klingensmith GJ, Ed: *Intensive Diabetes Management.* 3rd ed. Alexandria, VA, American Diabetes Association, 2003, p. 160

Koda JE, Fineman M, Rink TJ, Dailey GE, Muchmore DB, Linarelli LG: Amylin concentrations and glucose control. *Lancet* 339:1179–1180, 1992

Kruger DF, Gatcomb PM, Owen SK: Clinical implications of amylin and amylin deficiency. *Diabetes Educ* 25:389–397, 1999

Larger F: Weight gain and insulin treatment. *Diabetes & Metabolism* 31(4 Pt 2):4S51–4S56, 2005

Liu L, Lawrence JM, Davis C, Liese AD, Pettitt DJ, Pihoker C, Dabelea D, Hamman R, Waitzfelder B, Kahn HS: Prevalence of overweight and obesity in youth with diabetes in USA: the SEARCH for Diabetes in Youth Study. *Pediatric Diabetes* 10:1399–1405, 2009

Mannucci E, Tesi F, Ricca V, Pierazzuoli E, Barciulli E, Moretti S, Di Bernardo M, Travaglini R, Carrara S, Zucchi T, Placidi GF, Rotella CM: Eating behavior in obese patients with and without type 2 diabetes mellitus. *Int J Obes Relat Metab Disord* 26:848–853, 2002

Markowitz J, Butler DA, Volkening LK, Antisdel JE, Anderson BJ, Laffel LM: Brief screening tool for disordered eating in diabetes: internal consistency and external validity in a contemporary sample of pediatric patients with type 1 diabetes. *Diabetes* 33:495–500, 2010

Meltzer LJ, Johnson SB, Prine JM, Banks RA, Desrosiers PM, Silverstein JH: Disordered eating, body mass, and glycemic control in adolescents with type 1 diabetes. *Diabetes Care* 24:678–682, 2001

Nathan D, Delahanty L: *Beating Diabetes.* Boston, McGraw-Hill, 2005

Neumark-Sztainer D, Patterson J, Mellin A, Ackard DM, Utter J, Story M, Sockalosky J: Weight control practices and disordered eating behaviors among adolescent females and males with type 1 diabetes: associations with sociodemographics, weight concerns, familial factors, and metabolic outcomes. *Diabetes Care* 25:1289–1296, 2002a

Neumark-Sztainer D, Story M, Hannan PJ, Perry CL, Irving LM: Weight-related concerns and behaviors among overweight and nonoverweight adolescents: implications for preventing weight-related disorders. *Arch Pediatr Adolesc Med* 156:171–178, 2002b

Papelbaum M, Appolinário JC, Moreira Rde O, Ellinger VC, Kupfer R, Coutinho WF: Prevalence of eating disorders and psychiatric comorbidity in a clinical sample of type 2 diabetes mellitus patients. *Rev Bras Psiquiatr* 27:135–138, 2005

Parkman H, Hasler H, Fisher R: American Gastroenterological Association technical review on the diagnosis and treatment of gastroparesis. *Gastroenterology* 127: 1592–1622, 2004

Peterson CB, Wonderlich SA, Mitchell JE, Crow SJ: Integrative cognitive therapy for bulimia nervosa. In *Handbook of Eating Disorders and Obesity.* Thompson JK, Ed. Hoboken, NJ, John Wiley & Sons, 2004, p. 245–262

Peveler RC, Bryden KS, Neil HA, Fairburn CG, Mayou RA, Dunger DB, Turner HM: The relationship of disordered eating habits and attitudes to clinical outcomes in young adult females with type 1 diabetes. *Diabetes Care* 28:84–88, 2005

Peveler RC, Fairburn CG, Boller I, Dunger D: Eating disorders in adolescents with IDDM: a controlled study. *Diabetes Care* 15:1356–1360, 1992

Pike KM, Devlin MJ, Loeb C: Cognitive-behavioral therapy in the treatment of anorexia nervosa, bulimia nervosa, and binge eating disorder. In *Handbook of Eating Disorders and Obesity.* Thompson JK, Ed. Hoboken, NJ, John Wiley & Sons, 2004, p. 130–162

Pinhas-Hamiel O, Standiford D, Hamiel D, Dolan LM, Cohen R, Zeitler PS: The type 2 family: a setting for development and treatment of adolescent type 2 diabetes mellitus. *Arch Pediatr Adolesc Med* 153:1063–1067, 1999

Pollock M, Kovacs M, Charron-Prochownik D: Eating disorders and maladaptive dietary/insulin management among youths with childhood-onset insulin-dependent diabetes mellitus. *J Am Acad Child Adolesc Psychiatry* 34:291–296, 1995

Pollock-BarZiv SM, Davis C: Personality factors and disordered eating in young women with type 1 diabetes mellitus. *Psychosomatics* 46:11–18, 2005

Polonsky WH: *Diabetes Burnout: What to Do When You Can't Take It Anymore.* Alexandria, VA, American Diabetes Association, 1999, p. 348

Polonsky WH, Anderson BJ, Lohrer PA, Aponte JE, Jacobson AM, Cole CF: Insulin omission in women with IDDM. *Diabetes Care* 17:1178–1185, 1994

Rodin G, Olmsted MP, Rydall AC, Maharaj SI, Colton PA, Jones JM, Biancucci LA, Daneman D: Eating disorders in young women with type 1 diabetes mellitus. *J Psychosom Res* 53:943–949, 2002

Rodin GM, DanemanD: Eating disorders and IDDM. A problematic association. *Diabetes Care* 15:1402–1412, 1992

Rodin G, Craven J, Littlefield C, Murray M, Daneman D: Eating disorders and intentional insulin treatment in adolescent females with diabetes. *Psychosomatics* 32:171–176, 1991

Rodin GM, Johnson LE, Garfinkel PE, Daneman D, Kenshole AB: Eating disorders in female adolescents with insulin dependent diabetes mellitus. *Int J Psychiatry Med* 16:49–57, 1986–1987

Rydall AC, Rodin GM, Olmsted MP, Devenyi RG, Daneman D: Disordered eating behavior and microvascular complications in young women with insulin-dependent diabetes mellitus.[See comment.] *N Engl J Med* 336:1849–1854, 1997

Sherwood NE, Neumark-Sztainer D: Internalization of the sociocultural ideal: weight-related attitudes and dieting behaviors among young adolescent girls. *Am J Health Promot* 15:228–231, 2001

Shisslak CM, Mays MZ, Crago M, Jirsak JK, Taitano K, Cagno C: Eating and weight control behaviors among middle school girls in relationship to body weight and ethnicity. *J Adolesc Health* 38:631–633, 2006

Steel JM, Lloyd GG, Young RJ, MacIntyre CC: Changes in eating attitudes during the first year of treatment for diabetes. *J Psychosom Res* 34:313–318, 1990

Steel JM, Young RJ, Lloyd GG, MacIntyre CC: Abnormal eating attitudes in young insulin-dependent diabetics. *Br J Psychiatry* 155:515–521, 1989

Steel JM, Young RJ, Lloyd GG, Clarke B: Clinically apparent eating disorders in young diabetic women: associations with painful neuropathy and other complications. *Br Med J (Clin Res Ed)* 294(6576):859–862, 1987

Stice E: Risk and maintenance factors for eating pathology: a meta-analytic review. *Psychol Bull* 128:825–848, 2002

Stice E, Bearman SK: Body-image and eating disturbances prospectively predict increases in depressive symptoms in adolescent girls: a growth curve analysis. *Dev Psychol* 37:597–607, 2001

Stice E, Hayward C, Cameron RP, Killen JD, Taylor CB: Body-image and eating disturbances predict onset of depression among female adolescents: a longitudinal study. *J Abnorm Psychol* 109:438–444, 2000

Stice E, Agras WS, Hammer LD: Risk factors for the emergence of childhood eating disturbances: a five-year prospective study. *Int J Eat Disord* 25:375–387, 1999

Striegel-Moore RH, Nicholson TJ, Tamborlane WV: Prevalence of eating disorder symptoms in preadolescent and adolescent girls with IDDM. *Diabetes Care* 15:1361–1368, 1992

Surgenor L, Horn J, Hudson SM: Links between psychological sense of control and disturbed eating behavior in women with diabetes mellitus: implications for predictors of metabolic control. *J Psychosom Res* 52:121–128, 2002

Svensson M, Engstrom I, Aman J: Higher drive for thinness in adolescent males with insulin-dependent diabetes mellitus compared with healthy controls. *Acta Paediatr* 92:114–117, 2003

Tantleff-Dunn S, Gokee-LaRose J, Peterson RD: Interpersonal psychotherapy for the treatment of anorexia nervosa, bulimia nervosa, and binge eating disorder. In *Handbook of Eating Disorders and Obesity.* Thompson JK, Ed. Hoboken, NJ, John Wiley & Sons, 2004, p. 163–187

Telch CF, Stice E: Psychiatric comorbidity in women with binge eating disorder: prevalence rates from a non-treatment-seeking sample. *J Consult Clin Psychol* 66:768–776, 1998

Thelen MH, Farmer J, Wonderlich S, Smith M: A revision of the bulimia test: the BULIT-R. *Psychological Assessment* 3:119–124, 1991

Varnado PJ, Williamson DA, Bentz BG, Ryan DH, Rhodes SK, O'Neil PM, Sebastian SB, Barker SE: Prevalence of binge eating disorder in obese adults seeking weight loss treatment. *Eat Weight Disord* 2:117–124, 1997

Wilfley D, Friedman MA, Dounchis JZ, Stein RI, Welch RR, Ball SA: Comorbid psychopathology in binge eating disorder: relation to eating disorder severity at baseline and following treatment. *J Consult Clin Psychol* 68:641–649, 2000

Wing R, Nowalk MP, Marcus MD, Keoske R, Finegold D: Subclinical eating disorders and glycemic control in adolescents with type 1 diabetes. *Diabetes Care* 9:162–167, 1986

Wolman C, Resnick MD, Harris LJ, Blum RW: Emotional well-being among adolescents with and without chronic conditions. *J Adolesc Health* 15:199–204, 1994

Young-Hyman D, Davis C, Looney S, Grigsby C, Peterson C: Development of the diabetes treatment and satiety scale (DTSS-20). *Diabetes* 60 (Suppl. 1):A218, 2011a

Young-Hyman D, Laffel L, Markowitz J, Norman J, Muir A, Lindsley K: Evaluating eating disorder risk (EDR) in T1D youth transitioning to insulin pump (CSII) therapy (Rx). *Diabetes* 60 (Suppl. 1):A226, 2011b

Young-Hyman D, Laffel L, Markowitz J, Norman J, Muir A, Lindsley K: Evaluating eating disorder risk at time of teen T1D diagnosis (DX). *Diabetes* 60 (Suppl. 1):A229, 2011c

Young-Hyman D, Davis C: Disordered eating behavior in individuals with diabetes: importance of context, classification and evaluation. *Diabetes Care* 33:683–689, 2010

Young-Hyman D: Eating Disorders. In *Diagnostic and Statistical Manual of Mental Disorders, DSM-IV-TR.* 4th ed. Washington, DC, American Psychiatric Association, 2000, p. 583–597

第三章

低 血 糖 症

Linda Gonder-Frederick，PhD，Daniel J. Cox，PhD，ABPP，
Harsimran Singh，PhD，and Jaclyn A. Shepard，PsyD

低血糖症的问题：定义和流行病学

　　低血糖反应是最常见的糖尿病急性并发症，大多数不可避免，特别是使用胰岛素的患者。低血糖症可根据生物学和症状进行定义。生物学定义为任何＜3.9 mmol/L（70 mg/dl）的血糖水平就认为是低血糖症。然而，把所有血糖水平＜70 mg/dl 与症状学定义等同看待是个误区。症状上，低血糖症根据中枢神经系统的影响来定义。糖尿病控制和并发症试验（DCCT）把低血糖症分为 3 个等级：轻度、中度、重度。轻度低血糖症是以由拮抗激素和轻度神经低血糖症引起的症状为特征，没有显著的认知功能障碍，进食糖类物质后可快速缓解；中度低血糖症可能出现日常功能障碍，但是个人保留了识别症状和起始治疗的执行能力。

　　当轻度或中度低血糖反应不能被及时地识别或治疗，那么重度低血糖症（SH）即会发生。重度低血糖症，由于认知损害、意识不清或突然发作，严重的神经低血糖症妨碍自我治疗的能力。重度低血糖反应本身很危险，特别是当没有其他人在身边提供紧急救助，或当患者进行潜在危险活动（如开车）时。重度低血糖症引发的死亡率，虽然不常发生，但确实存在，统计占 1 型糖尿病患者死亡率的 2%～4%。这些死亡有些与夜间低血糖相关，导致所谓"床上死亡"现象的发生。

　　没有确切的低血糖症发生频率的数据，但是估计 1 型糖尿病患者平均每周发作 2 次，大多数是轻度或中度。对于重度低血糖症，各项研究的流行病学评估有很大的不同。DCCT 中，重度低血糖症在强化胰岛素治疗组中 65%的患者每年至少发生 1 次，平均每 100 名患者每年发作 61.2 次。其他前瞻性研究报道发作频率范围为每 100 人每年 4.8～19 次。然

而，流行率不能准确反映事实，大多数发作集中在少数重度低血糖症频发和复发患者子群中。无论是对成人还是儿童，80%～100%的低血糖反应发生在 20%～33%的患者中。在儿童和成人中，重度低血糖症并不是总发生在白天，50%或以上的发作发生在夜间。

一些研究报道 2 型糖尿病中存在更低的低血糖症发生率，特别是当患者应用全套治疗方案时，包括仅应用饮食治疗和低剂量口服药物治疗。低血糖症在 2 型糖尿病诊断后的最初几年中通常很少发生，推测是由于拮抗激素机制未受损。然而，在开始使用胰岛素后，低血糖症（包括重度低血糖症）在 1 型和 2 型糖尿病患者中的发生率基本相当。口服磺脲类药物也很大程度增加了 2 型糖尿病患者的低血糖症发生。

低血糖症对身体和情绪健康的影响

低血糖症的实际影响可从患者个人生活到他们的工作和社会关系，伴随生活质量的潜在消极后果。低血糖反应显著地与消极后果相关，包括不愉悦的症状、潜在的尴尬和不便。由重度低血糖症所致的身体损伤的流行病学研究较罕见，然而，临床经验显示低血糖症很常见。最近的回顾性和前瞻性调查显示一个子群发生低血糖相关的驾驶小事故和车祸的风险更高。

1 型糖尿病人群，急性低血糖症可能导致多种认知区域受损，包括即刻和视觉记忆、延迟记忆、前瞻记忆、视觉运动和空间感。对于频发的重度低血糖反应也可能对大脑和认知功能产生长期消极影响已有关注，然而，这一领域的研究产生了不同结果。这些模棱两可的结果可能部分由于糖尿病发病年龄的样本差异。研究调查了 SH 和它与认知功能损害的关系，以及 SH 可能对 1 型糖尿病低龄儿童发育中的大脑的破坏作用比大龄儿童或成人更大。5 岁或 6 岁前诊断的 1 型糖尿病儿童或青少年比那些更晚诊断的人显示出更差的认知功能。在高龄的 2 型糖尿病人群中，越来越多的证据显示 SH 的发生与随后的痴呆高风险相关，但这可能是多种因素结合的结果，包括慢性高血糖症和低血糖症。

反复低血糖和 SH 也对糖尿病患者和其他重要的社会心理功能、健康状况、整体生活质量有消极影响。成年糖尿病患者，有证据显示 SH

进展的问题与慢性情绪改变、幸福感和能级减少、无助感、焦虑和沮丧相关，并且他们可能有情感障碍的风险。针对健康花费和由生产力下降导致的间接损失来看，SH 的治疗和管理对患者和保健系统也是较沉重的经济负担。

与低血糖相关的不愉快症状和经历可能引起糖尿病患者严重焦虑和其他严重情况，这些可能导致低血糖恐惧（FOH）。高水平的 FOH 可能损坏 1 型糖尿病儿童家庭的生活质量，并且当孩子经历低血糖发作或昏迷时，父母可能表现出相当大的恐惧。高 FOH 可能反过来影响 1 型糖尿病儿童的血糖控制，因为父母可能鼓励比临床期望值更高的血糖水平来规避未来事件的发生。经历过 SH 复发的患者配偶，他们不仅有高水平的 FOH，还有更多的睡眠障碍（由夜间低血糖症的焦虑引起）和婚姻冲突。尽管大量研究调查 FOH，但还是很难经验性地记录它对糖尿病管理的影响。然而，一些科研证据和许多临床证据显示，1 型糖尿病和胰岛素治疗的 2 型糖尿病患者的高水平 FOH 及 1 型糖尿病年轻患者的父母，都有助于维持较高血糖水平的治疗行为。研究数据也显示 FOH 是不能适应胰岛素剂量最常见的原因，因为低血糖症是胰岛素强化治疗最恐惧的并发症。FOH 也是 1 型和 2 型糖尿病患者锻炼的主要障碍。

低血糖症的危险因素

所有的糖尿病低血糖反应都是由于过量的胰岛素或与食物摄入和体育运动相关的其他降血糖药物导致的。社会心理学上，一些因素如更高的胰岛素敏感性、较高的血糖多变性、肾功能损伤及一些延缓胃排空的药物，都可增加低血糖症风险。大量的研究显示血糖控制和降低 HbA1C（如更多的胰岛素强化治疗）的变量，导致青年和成人低血糖症风险增加。一些研究试图超越这些广义关系，明确低血糖反应快速、离散的前兆。这项研究显示糖尿病管理在低血糖风险中起着重要作用，在 1 型和 2 型糖尿病患者中，75%或更多的低血糖反应是行为诱发的。对于青年和成人，大量的低血糖反应归因于减少食物摄入（包括错过正餐）和增加体育活动。最近一项 84 名儿童和青少年的回顾性研究发现大多数的 SH 反应发生在进餐（糖类）延迟时，紧随其后的是强烈的体育运动和过量的胰岛素注射。另一项包括超过 1300 位的 1 型和 2 型糖尿病成年患者的回顾性研究把每日锻炼确定为 SH 的主要因素。超出预期的剧烈活动也是突出的常见因素。

临床经验显示许多患者只是初步理解食物和运动对血糖水平的影响。临床医师不能假设患者及其护理者了解更多的低血糖症复杂的行为危险因素，例如，高脂饮食，可导致延迟的和（或）被抑制的血糖反应；或延长中度体育活动的时间，这可能比短暂的剧烈锻炼利用更多的葡萄糖。不适当的决定和行为导致低血糖，也可能发生在对自己糖尿病管理不坚持或不谨慎的患者身上，包括漏餐或加餐，或是在计算餐量时未计算糖类含量。精神状态导致的失常行为也能极大地增加患者风险，特别是以厌食或暴饮暴食为特征的饮食行为紊乱。

对于一些患者，频繁和反复的低血糖反应可能与情绪或认知的问题相关，这些问题促使决策和判断失误，或者处理低血糖的风险性行为。患者可能轻视或者忽视潜在的低血糖反应的严重性，享受家人护理和关心的附带效益，或者认为延迟治疗是与糖尿病进行有力斗争的一种"获胜"形式。

另一个没有研究但是很重要的危险因素是患者的认知：信念、态度及对低血糖症的判断和治疗。临床上常遇到一些患者，他们认为自己在低血糖水平（如<54mg/dl）功能运转良好，或低血糖是血糖控制良好的必要部分。这些信念和态度可能导致患者在治疗低血糖时保有更低的个人血糖临界值，或者延迟治疗，这些都更大程度地增加了风险。

一些患者也进行高血糖的过度治疗，或者有时称为糖尿病"微管理"，经常导致胰岛素过量注射或"堆积"。这些患者可能对糖尿病管理过度谨慎，并且过于积极地避免高血糖和远期并发症。然而，对高血糖的过度焦虑可能引起适应不良并导致避免高血糖的极端行为（如增加胰岛素剂量），这可能增加低血糖反应。

当更多轻度或中度的低血糖反应不能被足够快速或充分地识别和治疗，SH 反应就会发生。SH 发生的可能性已被描述为一种生物心理学行为模型，这是试图整合复杂的生理、心理、行为进程，从而决定危险水平。这一模型的第一步是轻度或中度低血糖症发生，这就激发了必然的生理反应，包括激素反馈调节和神经低血糖症。接着，这些导致了肾上腺素分泌和神经低血糖症状，而后患者发觉和识别这些症状，从而在观念上做出合适的决定和自我治疗以避免 SH。

　　然而，当低血糖症状没有发生、识别或给予及时的行为治疗时，那么潜在的 SH 将不能避免，这通常发生在有低血糖相关自主调节失常（HAAF）的患者。患有 HAAF 的患者，频繁的低血糖反应导致低血糖负反馈调节缺陷（肾上腺素）且低血糖意识（HA）减少。在低血糖发生时，这能导致血糖下降的更低，并且直到血糖水平非常低才能产生预警症状，这就极大地增加了严重神经性低血糖症的可能性和精神困扰，因而可能阻止及时的自我治疗。HA 减低和 SH 风险的关系在 1 型和 2 型糖尿病患者中已很好地被证明，据估计多达 60% 的 SH 反应与预警症状无关。大约 25% 的 1 型糖尿病患者出现不同程度的 HA 减低。

　　促使 HAAF、HA 减低和 SH 风险的因素包括低血糖反应频发、强化胰岛素治疗、过低的 HbA1C 水平、过长的糖尿病病程、体育锻炼、抑制夜间的负反馈和饮酒。吸烟是 SH 的另一风险因素，尽管在是否与 HAAF 相关这一点上并不清楚。即使未患 HAAF 和 HA 减低，患者可能也无法察觉低血糖的早期预警症状。一些现场研究发现 1 型糖尿病的成人和儿童可能无法识别低于 70mg/dl（3.9mmol/L）一半以上的血糖水平。另一项前瞻性现场研究对近期有或无 SH 病史的 1 型糖尿病成人进行了 6 个多月的随访。这一研究重做了 HAAF 相关因素（如 HA 减低、低血糖频发）和 SH 风险的关系；然而，高风险组患者也表现出认知和行为的差异。特别是，有 SH 病史的患者在低血糖时显示出更多的认知损害，并且倾向于用食物而不是快速反应的糖类物质来治疗低血糖反应。

　　已证实，父母在察觉孩子低血糖的能力方面很差。促使父母和孩子不能察觉低血糖症的因素包括关注和知觉过程，对低血糖症状不准确的观念，和对非低血糖相关引起的症状的错误认定。情绪压力也可能有消极影响，例如，有抑郁症状的学龄期儿童显示出更差的低血糖觉察。

　　年龄是 SH 的一个主要因素，高龄患者和低龄儿童风险最高。肾功能不全和（或）药物增加了高龄患者的风险，而且血糖控制差的高龄患者更多发低血糖反应。1 型糖尿病青春期患者比成人患者风险更高，6 岁以下的儿童比 6 岁以上的儿童风险高。一项前瞻性研究证实了大龄儿童中精神疾病和高 SH 风险之间的关系，另一项研究对青春期有情绪障碍和家庭问题的患者进行了调查，他们有暗中蓄意注射胰岛素过量的行为。最近一项对 1000 多名的 1 型和 2 型糖尿病成人患者的研究发现抑郁是 SH 的一个危险因素。在高龄患者中，认知障碍和痴呆也显著增加 SH 风险。较低的社会经济地位（SES）组的成人有更高的风险，包括那些食用不安全食品和由于无力购买食物而遭受饥饿的患者。对于儿童和青春期的患者，保险额不足显著地增加了风险。

减少 SH 风险的干预

减少低血糖频率和（或）改善及时察觉和治疗低血糖反应的任何干预都会有效减少 SH 风险。减少低血糖频率和 SH 的干预也通常会减少 FOH。减少 SH 风险的重要基础是为患者提供足够的糖尿病教育，理解胰岛素、食物、身体锻炼的失衡如何产生，并且避免这种失衡的方法。因为有限的人力资源，这种类型的患者教育和培训（尤其是教育患者注意 HA）不可能实施，尽管这是糖尿病自我管理教育（DSME）的推荐部分。一些作者甚至认为当患者向强化胰岛素治疗过渡时，欠缺的患者教育是患者经历低血糖症增加的一个主要原因。除了低血糖症预防以外，患者还需要恰当的低血糖反应治疗、快速反应和适当避免 SH 重要性方面的教育。这种教育应当涉及低血糖的症状学培训，包括症状的生理基础及其对充分自我治疗能力的影响。

当患者出现 SH 相关问题时，干预的首要目标通常是胰岛素治疗方案。大量研究显示长效胰岛素类似物减少 1 型和 2 型糖尿病患者日间和夜间低血糖发生率。许多研究也显示持续的皮下胰岛素注入（CSII）或胰岛素泵治疗显著减少成人和儿童的低血糖发生频率和 SH 风险。然而，两项针对这篇文献的近期 Meta 分析指出 CSII 不总是减少低血糖症。胰岛素的其他改变可能也被指出，例如，锻炼时中断基础胰岛素剂量可能显著减少儿童低血糖症。尝试多种不同的胰岛素治疗方案但仍持续有严重 SH 问题的患者可考虑进行外科移植。然而，这种手术有明显的术中和术后并发症，对大多数患者来说，胰腺细胞移植并不能导致长期的胰岛素非依赖。并且，尽管胰腺细胞移植后血糖调节的负反馈和症状得到改善，但是肾上腺素反应（低血糖症的信号）的强度仍可受损。

除了减少低血糖反应的发生频率，干预可集中提高发现低血糖的能力。有研究致力于开发增加低血糖意识的药物，但这些药物目前还不可用。一些研究发现，如果患者能在仅仅几周的时间内严格避免血糖水平＜70mg/dl（3.9mmol/L），激素负反馈和肾上腺素预警症状就能及时修复。不幸的是，没有大样本临床试验来评估这种干预，从而确定哪一部分患者可能对治疗有反应，或者哪类支持项目是患者获得成功所需的。另外，只有一项长期随访研究调查了是否单一的治疗项目（3个月的医师监督来避免低血糖）能够产生持久的效果。

随着最近糖尿病管理技术的进步，持续血糖监测（CGM）被越来越多地应用于低血糖症的觉察和减少。当血糖趋势显示低血糖症即将发生时CGM能给患者提供示警。一项早期的随机试验显示1型糖尿病患者和需要胰岛素治疗的2型糖尿病患者佩戴3个连续72小时的持续血糖监测仪，与使用传统血糖监测的患者相比，能显著改善血糖波动。特别是，那些使用持续血糖监测仪的患者减少了21%的低血糖时间，增加了26%的时间在目标血糖范围。更多的近期临床试验集中研究长期持续使用持续血糖监测仪对低血糖症风险的影响。一项近期研究表明，1型成人和青年糖尿病患者进行CGM 26周，较使用自我血糖监测（SMBG）的对照组相比，低血糖症发生的时间显著变短，正常血糖的时间显著变长。尽管这些结果是有前景的，但其他研究表明CGM不能有效地减少所有患者的低血糖症。青少年糖尿病基金会（JDRF）研究结果发现任一年龄组的CGM与SMBG（6个月）相比，在低血糖症时间或SH频率上没有显著的统计学差异。然而，这项研究中的成人能达到更好的血糖控制且没有增加低血糖风险。传感器增强型胰岛素泵（SAP）治疗，整合了CGM使用和胰岛素泵治疗，这是闭环式控制系统（或"人工胰腺"）发展的第一步，是最新的糖尿病技术旨在降低高血糖的同时避免低血糖症。许多研究，包括两项大型临床试验[SAP治疗减低HbA1C（STAR3）；胰岛素泵传感治疗控制HbA1C（SWITCH）]，都正在评估SAP治疗对成人糖尿病患者的可行性和效果，最近对1型糖尿病青年的研究也在进行中。早期的发现已经表明了其对成人和儿童代谢控制的有益效果，包括改善HbA1C，不增加低血糖症。其可能对糖尿病管理产生一种消极影响，即由于血糖反馈延迟而导致过度治疗低血糖症。然而，当介绍这一技术时，这种时间滞后应当在它的使用章节中说明（参见第十一章）。

因为糖尿病管理行为在低血糖症和 SH 中起着重要作用，所以行为干预能有效减少风险并不令人吃惊。行为干预得到的最科学的研究，是血糖意识训练（BGAT），设计旨在提高患者识别症状和识别低血糖信号其他线索的能力，并且预估治疗因素的效果，如胰岛素、食物和关于血糖水平高的体育活动。BGAT 是一项有组织、有指南的训练项目，它整合了糖尿病教育、自我监测和自我评估策略及个人糖尿病管理行为的评估。一篇近期的文章回顾了美国和欧洲的 15 项 BGAT 研究，显示干预有许多治疗益处，如提高低血糖症觉察，减少低血糖和 SH 的发生频率并且减少 FOH。在初期强化胰岛素治疗后完成 BGAT 的患者表明，保留了负反馈的完整性，避免了典型的与糖尿病控制提高相关的低血糖频率的增加。

尽管有证据显示 BGAT 的有效性，但它没有得到广泛的宣传。这是一项高强度和高要求的训练项目，存在偿还问题，并且没有足量的接受过培训且有经验的专业护理人员来提供 BGAT。为使其更广泛地使用，BGAT 从网上传输转化为家庭 BGAT，并且鼓励初期的测试。一项类似的心理行为干预也使用这样的策略，例如，血糖症状日记和血糖水平的精确评估，它已经在德国对照试验中被开发和测试。对这项干预进行长期随访发现实验组 SH 发生率显著降低并且没有 HbA1C 的升高。

低强度行为干预可能有效也具有令人信服的证据，故建议应该在开发、测试和宣传这类项目上做出更多的努力。例如，特别的设计结构化门诊患者教育是为了教会患者低血糖症的病因、影响和治疗，从而能够阻止与强化胰岛素方案相关风险的增加。另一项干预结合了心理教育的病例管理方法，减少了 60% 的 SH 反应。Norway 研究也非常鼓舞人心，研究显示大量患者教育材料（录像带和手册）的发布减少了 1 型糖尿病儿童的 SH 反应且无需以代谢控制为条件。这项随机对照研究在超过 24 个月的时间里随访了 200 多位儿童患者，发现实验干预组的 SH 反应从 45% 减少至 24%。

这些相对简单的干预（以教学法为重点）的成功结果，表明不充分的患者教育是一种未被认识但非常重要的 SH 风险因素。一些教育和行为干预的积极结果，结合许多患者发现的这些困难，显示已证明有效地减少 SH 风险的项目在糖尿病护理中没有执行。由于个人和医疗健康系统中低血糖症的重大经济负担，这些研究似乎是物有所值的。鉴于其对糖尿病患者生活质量、情感幸福、身体安全和健康上的影响，低血糖问题还没有得到它应有的重视，并且减少发生率的干预也无法充分应用。很明显，前面的问题需要更多的努力，包括研究、临床护理、电子医疗和糖尿病宣传，需要朝着寻找有效实施干预的方向努力，来解决糖尿病低血糖的问题。

护理建议

1. 在 1 型和 2 型糖尿病患者中低血糖症很常见，并且应该在每一次门诊谈话中对患者进行评估以明确他们是否有这方面的问题。如果有这些问题，应当执行更详细的评估来明确是否需要进行患者教育或其他干预，遵照由 Cradock and Frier 提供的全面的低血糖症干预的范例。通常，患者不愿意与专业护理人员讨论 SH 反应，因为他们害怕会被限制参加某些特定的活动和（或）职业。

2. FOH 很常见，并且应当在患者和家庭成员中定期进行评估，包括糖尿病儿童的父母，特别是伴有抑郁或 SH 反应的心理创伤的人。当患者呈现出慢性高 BG 水平，那么应该考虑高水平 FOH 的可能性。

3. 在低血糖评估的临床访视中，应该确定与低血糖反应相关的糖尿病管理行为（例如，错过餐点，增加体育运动，多变的工作行程改变胰岛素剂量方案）的潜在问题，从而指导患者咨询/教育。

4. 表现出与增加低血糖反应相关的危险行为的患者，与临床上重大的情感或认知问题相关，这些人将受益于糖尿病管理和行为干预专家的心理治疗或咨询。

5. 需要评估低血糖症及其治疗的观念以明确可增加风险的态度和行为。一些问题可能有助于评估，包括"血糖低至多少时你才认为需要升高血糖"及"糖低至多少时才影响你的思考和功能"。

6. 当关注高血糖似乎有助于增加低血糖事件发生时，临床医师可能考虑糖尿病教育者的额外教育课程，以及护理方案的改变，来鼓励更多的监测及患者 MNT 改进的补偿策略。

7. 鉴于激素负反馈和症状临界值可以随着时间改变，低血糖认知/觉察应当在每次临床访视中评估。对未报告传统低血糖意识障碍的患者进行识别低血糖症能力的评估，因为这些患者甚至无法察觉 50%以上的低血糖反应。识别低血糖的能力也应当在儿童糖尿病患者及其父母中进行评估，因为研究显示较差的识别低血糖的能力可能是 SH 的危险因素。

8. 有精神或认知问题共病的患者也和那些经济地位较低组一样，由于其较高的危险水平，可能需要保证更密切的监测 SH 相关问题。

9. 理论上，所有患者应当接受低血糖症的全面教育，包括它的病因、对认知功能的影响和立即治疗的必要性。对于低血糖症反复发作的患者组，这一教育应当是临床护理的持续部分。应该提供关于 HAAF 的教育，以及频发轻度低血糖反应对反馈调节和识别预警症状能力的影响的教育，用转变行为改变策略的方式留意现有信息。另外，当医师不能提供后续服务时，关于发生率和鉴别的常规筛查可能需要与易得到的治疗资源（如印刷或网页来源的信息）、建议相结合。

10. 患者在临床访视中应当评估轻度低血糖反应的发生频率，因为这些是 HAAF 和 SH 的危险因素。应该为每周发作一次以上的患者提供关于轻度低血糖症频发对症状和激素反应的影响的教育，并且，应当和患者讨论随访治疗方案的可能性，这一方案旨在避免这些低血糖事件，从而改善负反馈调节。

11. CGM 或 SAP 治疗应当考虑在下列患者中应用：由于低血糖意识障碍所致的反复 SH、夜间低血糖问题、高水平 FOH、低血糖妨碍生活质量，以及独居的患者。鉴于这些治疗技术的复杂性，考虑使用 CGM 或 SAP 治疗的患者应当从糖尿病教育者那里接受全面而系统的培训。

12. 在 BGAT 和 BGATHome（如 BG 认知日记）中使用的一些策略，在已出版并被健康护理者使用，包括心理学家、糖尿病教育者、护士和临床医师。建议将这些策略作为干预资源，特别当专业培训者不在当地时。

参 考 文 献

Alemzadeh R, Berhe T, Wyatt DT: Flexible insulin therapy with glargine insulin improved glycemic control and reduced severe hypoglycemia among pre-school-aged children with type 1 diabetes mellitus. *Pediatrics* 115:1320–1324, 2005

Allen C, LeCaire T, Palta M, Daniels K, Meredith M, D'Alession DJ: Risk factors for frequent and severe hypoglycemia in type 1 diabetes. *Diabetes Care* 24:1878–1881, 2001

Allen KV, Frier BM: Nocturnal hypoglycemia: clinical manifestations and thera-peutic strategies toward prevention. *Endocr Prac* 9:530–543, 2003

Amiel SA: Hypoglycemia: from the laboratory to the clinic. *Diabetes Care* 32:1364–1371, 2009

Avogaro AJ, Bristow D, Bier DM, Cobelli C, Toffolo G: Stable-label intravenous glucose tolerance test minimal model. *Diabetes* 38:1048–1055, 1989

Banarer S, Cryer PE: Hypoglycemia in type 2 diabetes. *Med Clin North Am* 88:1107–1116, 2004

Barnard K, Thomas S, Royle P, Noyes K, Waugh N: Fear of hypoglycaemia in parents of young children with type 1 diabetes: a systematic review. *BMC Pedi-atr* 10:50, 2010

Battelino T, Phillip M, Bratina N, Nimri R, Oskarsson P, Bolinder J: Effect of continuous glucose monitoring on hypoglycemia in type 1 diabetes. *Diabetes Care* 34:795–800, 2011

Bjørgaas M, Sand T, Gimse R: Quantitative EEG in type 1 diabetic children with and without episodes of severe hypoglycemia: a controlled, blind study. *Acta Neurol Scand* 93:398–402, 1996

Block JM, Buckingham B: Use of real-time continuous glucose monitoring tech-nology in children and adolescents. *Diabetes Spectr* 21:84–90, 2008

Bode BW, Tamborlane WV, Davidson PC: Insulin pump therapy in the 21st cen-tury: strategies for successful use in adults, adolescents, and children with dia-betes. *Postgrad Med* 111:69–77, 2002

Bognetti E, Brunelli A, Meschi F, Viscardi M, Bonfanti R, Chiumello G: Fre-quency and correlates of severe hypoglycaemia in children and adolescents with diabetes mellitus. *Eur J Pediatr* 156:589–591, 1997

Boileau P, Aboumrad B, Bougnères P: Recurrent comas due to secret self-admin-istration of insulin in adolescents with type 1 diabetes. *Diabetes Care* 29:430–431, 2006

Boland E, Monsod T, Delucia M, Brandt CA, Fernando S, Tamborlane WV: Lim-itations of conventional methods of self-monitoring of blood glucose: lessons learned from 3 days of continuous glucose sensing in pediatric patients with type 1 diabetes. *Diabetes Care* 24:1858–1862, 2001

Boland EA, Grey M, Oesterle A, Fredrickson L, Tamborlane WV: Continuous subcutaneous insulin infusion: a new way to lower risk of severe hypoglyce-mia, improve metabolic control, and enhance coping in adolescents with type 1 diabetes. *Diabetes Care* 22:1779–1784, 1999

Brauser D: Elderly dementia patients at serious risk for hypoglycemia. Paper pre-sented at the annual meeting of the American Association for Geriatric Psy-chiatry (AAGP), San Antonio, TX, Abstract NR-20, March 2011

Brazeau A-S, Rabasa-Lhoret R, Strychar I, Mircescu H: Barriers to physical activ-ity among patients with type 1 diabetes. *Diabetes Care* 31:2108–2109, 2008

Brito-Sanfiel M, Diago-Cabezudo JI, Calderon A: Economic impact of hypogly-cemia on healthcare in Spain. *Expert Rev Pharmacoecon Outcomes Res* 10:649–660, 2010

Brunelle RL, Llewelyn J, Anderson JH Jr, Gale EAM, Koivisto VA: Meta-analysis of the effect of insulin lispro on severe hypoglycemia in patients with type 1 diabetes. *Diabetes Care* 21:1726–1731, 1998

Bulsara MK, Holman CD, Davis EA, Jones TW: The impact of a decade of chang-ing treatment on rates of severe hypoglycemia in a population-based cohort of children with type 1 diabetes. *Diabetes Care* 27:2293–2298, 2004

Buse JB, Dailey G, Ahmann AA, Bergenstal RM, Green JB, Peoples T, Tanenberg RJ, Yang Q: Baseline predictors of A1C reduction in adults using sensor-aug-mented pump therapy or multiple daily injection therapy: the STAR 3 experi-ence. *Diabetes Technol Ther* 13:601–606, 2011

Chelliah A, Burge MR: Hypoglycemia in elderly patients with diabetes mellitus: causes and strategies for prevention. *Drugs Aging* 21:511–530, 2004

Chico A, Vidal-Rios P, Subira M, Novials A: The continuous glucose monitoring system is useful for detecting unrecognized hypoglycemias in patients with type 1 and type 2 diabetes but is not better than frequent capillary glucose measurements for improving metabolic control. *Diabetes Care* 26:1153–1157, 2003

Clarke WL, Cox DJ, Gonder-Frederick LA, Julian D, Kovatchev B, Young-Hyman D: The biopsychobehavioral model of risk of severe hypoglycemia II: self-management behaviors. *Diabetes Care* 22:580–584, 1999

Clarke WL, Gonder-Frederick LA, Snyder AL, Cox DJ: Maternal fear of hypo-glycemia in their children with insulin dependent diabetes mellitus. *J Pediatr Endocrinol Metab* 11:189–194, 1998

Clarke WL, Cox DJ, Gonder-Frederick LA, Julian D, Schlundt D, Polonsky W: Reduced awareness of hypoglycemia in adults with IDDM: a prospective study of hypoglycemic frequency and associated symptoms. *Diabetes Care* 18:517–522, 1995

Colquitt JL, Green C, Sidhu MK, Hartwell D, Waugh N: Clinical and cost-effec-tiveness of continuous subcutaneous insulin infusion for diabetes. *Health Tech-nol Assess* 8:1–171, 2004

Conget I, Battelino T, Giménez M, Gough H, Castañeda J, Bolinder J; SWITCH Study Group: The SWITCH study (sensing with insulin pump therapy to control HbA(1c)): design and methods of a randomized controlled crossover trial on sensor-augmented insulin pump efficacy in type 1 diabetes suboptimally controlled with pump therapy. *Diabetes Technol Ther* 13:49–54, 2011

Cosmescu A, Felea D, Mătăsaru S: [Severe hypoglycemia in children and adoles-cents suffering from type 1 diabetes mellitus]. *Rev Med Chir Soc Med Nat Iasi* 112:955–958, 2008

Cox DJ, Ritterband L, Magee J, Clarke W, Gonder-Frederick L: Blood glucose awareness training delivered over the internet. *Diabetes Care* 31:1527–1528, 2008

Cox DJ, Gonder-Frederick L, Ritterband L, Patel K, Schachinger H, Fehm-Wolf-sdorf G, Hermanns N, Snoek F, Zrebiec J, Polonksy W, Schlundt D, Kovatchev B, Clarke WL: Blood glucose awareness training: what is it, where is it, and where is it going? *Diabetes Spectr* 19:43–49, 2006a

Cox DJ, Kovatchev B, Vandecar K, Gonder-Frederick L, Ritterband L, Clarke W: Hypoglycemia preceding fatal car collisions. *Diabetes Care* 29:467–468, 2006b

Cox DJ, Penberthy JK, Zrebiec J, Weinger K, Aikens JE, Frier BM, Stetson B, DeGroot M, Trief P, Schaechinger H, Hermanns N, Gonder-Frederick L, Clarke WL: Incidence of driving mishaps and their correlates among drivers with diabetes. *Diabetes Care* 26:2329–2334, 2003

Cox DJ, Gonder-Frederick L, McCall A, Kovatchev B, Clarke WL: The effects of glucose fluctuation on cognitive function and QOL: the functional costs of hypoglycaemia and hyperglycaemia among adults with type 1 or type 2 diabe-tes. *Int J Clin Pract Suppl* 129:20–26, 2002

Cox DJ, Gonder-Frederick L, Kovatchev B, Young-Hyman D, Donner TW, Julian DM, Clarke W: Biopsychobehavioral model of severe hypoglycemia II: under-standing the risk of severe hypoglycemia. *Diabetes Care* 22:2018–2025, 1999

Cox DJ, Gonder-Frederick L, Antoun B, Clarke WL, Cryer P: Psychobehavioral metabolic parameters of severe hypoglycemic episodes. *Diabetes Care* 13:458–459, 1990

Cox DJ, Gonder-Frederick L, Lee JH, Julian DM, Carter WR, Clarke WL: Effects and correlates of blood glucose awareness training among patients with IDDM. *Diabetes Care* 12:313–318, 1989

Cox DJ, Irvine A, Gonder-Frederick L, Nowacek G, Butterfield J: Fear of hypo-glycemia: quantification, validation, and utilization. *Diabetes Care* 10:617–621, 1987

Cradock S, Frier B: Determining the risk of hypoglycaemia people with type 2 diabetes: an approach for clinical practice. *Br J Diabetes Vasc Dis* 10:44–46, 2010

Cranston I, Lomas J, Maran A, Macdonald I, Amiel SA: Restoration of hypogly-caemia awareness in patients with long-duration insulin-dependent diabetes. *Lancet* 344:283–287, 1994

Cryer PE: Diverse causes of hypoglycemia-associated autonomic failure in diabe-tes. *N Engl J Med* 350:2272–2279, 2004

Cryer PE, Davis SN, Shamoon H: Hypoglycemia in diabetes. *Diabetes Care* 26:1902–1912, 2003

Cryer PE: Hypoglycaemia: the limiting factor in the glycaemic management of type I and type II diabetes. *Diabetologia* 45:937–948, 2002

Dagogo-Jack S: Hypoglycemia in type 1 diabetes mellitus: pathophysiology and prevention. *Treat Endocrinol* 3:91–103, 2004

Dagogo-Jack S, Fanelli CG, Cryer PE: Durable reversal of hypoglycemia unawareness in type 1 diabetes. *Diabetes Care* 22:866–867, 1999

Davis CL, Delamater AM, Shaw KH, La Greca AM, Edison MS, Perez-Rodriguez JE, Nemery R: Parenting styles, regimen adherence, and glycemic control in 4- to 10-year-old children with diabetes. *J Pediatr Psychol* 26:123–129, 2001

Davis EA, Keating B, Byrne G, Russell M, Jones TW: Hypoglycemia: incidence and clinical predictors in a large population-based sample of children and ado-lescents with IDDM. *Diabetes Care* 20:22–25, 1997

Davis RE, Morrissey M, Peters JR, Wittrup-Jensen K, Kennedy-Martin T, Currie CJ: Impact of hypoglycaemia on quality of life and productivity in type 1 and type 2 diabetes. *Curr Med Res Opin* 21:1477–1483, 2005

Davis S, Alonso MD: Hypoglycemia as a barrier to glycemic control. *J Diabetes Complications* 18:60–68, 2004

Deary IJ, Sommerfield AJ, McAulay V, Frier B: Moderate hypoglycaemia obliter-ates working memory in humans with and without insulin treated diabetes. *J Neurol Neurosurg Psychiatry* 74:278–279, 2003

Diabetes Control and Complications Trial Research Group: Long-term effect of diabetes and its treatment on cognitive function. *N Engl J Med* 356:1842–1852, 2007

Diabetes Control and Complications Trial Research Group: Hypoglycemia in the Diabetes Control and Complications Trial. *Diabetes* 46:271–286, 1997

Diabetes Control and Complications Trial Research Group: Resource utilization and costs of care in the Diabetes Control and Complications Trial. *Diabetes Care* 18:1468–1478, 1995

Diabetes Control and Complications Trial Research Group: Effect of intensive diabetes treatment on the development and progression of long-term complications in adolescents with insulin-dependent diabetes mellitus: Diabetes Control and Complications Trial. *J Pediatr* 125:177–188, 1994

Diabetes Control and Complications Trial Research Group: Epidemiology of severe hypoglycemia in the Diabetes Control and Complications Trial. *Am J Med* 90:450–459, 1991

Draelos MT, Jacobson AM, Weinger K, Widom B, Ryan CM, Finkelstein DM, Simonson DC: Cognitive function in patients with insulin-dependent diabetes mellitus during hyperglycemia and hypoglycemia. *Am J Med* 98:135–144, 1995

Ewing FM, Deary IJ, McCrimmon RJ, Strachan MWJ, Frier BM: Effect of acute hypoglycaemia on visual information processing in adults with type 1 diabetes mellitus. *Physiol Behav* 64:653–660, 1998

Fanelli C, Pampanelli S, Epifano L, Rambotti AM, Ciofetta M, Modarelli F, Di Vincenzo A, Annibale B, Lepore M, Lalli C: Relative roles of insulin and hypoglycaemia on induction of neuroendocrine responses to, symptoms of, and deterioration of cognitive function in hypoglycaemia in male and female humans. *Diabetologia* 37:797–807, 1994

Fisher LK, Halvorson M: Future developments in insulin pump therapy: progression from continuous subcutaneous insulin infusion to a sensor-pump system. *Diabetes Educ* 32 (Suppl. 1):47S–52S, 2006

Friedrich LV, Dougherty R: Fatal hypoglycemia associated with levofloxacin. *Pharmacother* 24:1807–1812, 2004

Frier BM: How hypoglycaemia can affect the life of a person with diabetes. *Diabetes Metab Res Rev* 24:87–92, 2008

Garg S, Zisser H, Schwartz S, Bailey T, Kaplan R, Ellis S, Jovanovic L: Improvement in glycemic excursions with a transcutaneous, real-time continuous glucose sensor: a randomized controlled trial. *Diabetes Care* 29:44–50, 2006

Geddes J, Wright RJ, Zammitt NN, Deary IJ, Frier B: An evaluation of methods of assessing impaired awareness of hypoglycemia in type 1 diabetes. *Diabetes Care* 30:1868–1870, 2007

Gold AE, Frier BM, MacLeod KM, Deary IJ: A structural equation model for predictors of severe hypoglycaemia in patients with insulin-dependent diabetes mellitus. *Diabet Med* 14:309–315, 1997

Gold AE, Deary IJ, Jones RW, O'Hare JP, Reckless JPD, Frier BM: Severe deterioration in cognitive function and personality in five patients with long-standing diabetes: a complication of diabetes or a consequence of treatment? *Diabet Med* 11:499–505, 1994

Gonder-Frederick L, Schmidt K, Vajda K, Greear M, Singh H, Shepard J, Cox D: Psychometric properties of the Hypoglycemia Fear Survey-II for adults with type 1 diabetes mellitus. *Diabetes Care* 34:801–806, 2011

Gonder-Frederick L, Zrebiec J, Bauchowitz A, Lee J, Cox D, Kovatchev B, Ritterband L, Clarke W: Detection of hypoglycemia by children with type 1 diabetes 6 to 11 years of age and their parents: a field study. *Pediatrics* 121:e489–e495, 2008

Gonder-Frederick L, Cox DJ, Clarke W: Helping patients understand, recognize, and avoid hypoglycemia. In *Practical Psychology for Diabetes Clinicians*. Anderson BJ, Rubin RR, Eds. Alexandria, VA, American Diabetes Association, 2002, p. 113–124

Gonder-Frederick L, Cox DJ, Clarke W, Julian D: Blood glucose awareness training. In *Psychology in Diabetes Care*. Snoek F, Skinner TC, Eds. London, John Wiley and Sons, 2000, p. 169–206

Gonder-Frederick L, Cox DJ, Kovatchev B, Julian D, Clarke W: The psychosocial impact of severe hypoglycemic episodes on spouses of patients with IDDM. *Diabetes Care* 20:1543–1546, 1997a

Gonder-Frederick L, Cox DJ, Kovatchev B, Schlundt D, Clarke W: A biopsychobehavioral model of risk of severe hypoglycemia. *Diabetes Care* 20:661–669, 1997b

Graveling AJ, Frier B: Risks of marathon running and hypoglycaemia in type 1 diabetes. *Diabet Med* 27:585–588, 2010

Griffith R, Tengnah C: Legal basis for standards of driving with diabetes. *Br J Community Nurs* 16:19–22, 2011

Haugstvedt A, Wentzel-Larsen T, Graue M, Søvik O, Rokne B: Fear of hypoglycaemia in mothers and fathers of children with type 1 diabetes is associated with poor glycaemic control and parental emotional distress: a population-based study. *Diabet Med* 27:72–78, 2010

Heller SR: Minimizing hypoglycemia while maintaining glycemic control in diabetes. *Diabetes* 57:3177–3183, 2008

Hetderson JN, Allen KV, Deary IJ, Frier BM: Hypoglycaemia in insulin-treated type 2 diabetes: frequency, symptoms and impaired awareness. *Diabet Med* 20:1016–1021, 2003

Hepburn DA, Patrick AW, Eadington DW, Ewing DJ, Frier B: Unawareness of hypoglycaemia in insulin-treated diabetic patients: prevalence and relationship to autonomic neuropathy. *Diabet Med* 7:711–717, 1990

Hermanides J, Nørgaard K, Bruttomesso D, Mathieu C, Frid A, Dayan CM, Diem P, Fermon C, Wentholt IM, Hoekstra JB, Devries JH: Sensor-augmented pump therapy lowers HbA(1c) in suboptimally controlled type 1 diabetes: a randomized controlled trial. *Diabet Med*. doi: 10.1111/j.1464-5491.2011.03256.x

Hermanns N, Kulzer B, Krichbaum M, Kubiak T, Haak T: Long-term effect of an education program (HyPOS) on the incidence of severe hypoglycemia in patients with type 1 diabetes. *Diabetes Care* 33:e36, 2010

Hermanns N, Kulzer B, Krichbaum M, Kubiak T, Haak T: Affective and anxiety disorders in a German sample of diabetic patients: prevalence, comorbidity and risk factors. *Diabet Med* 22:293–300, 2005

Hermanns N, Kubiak T, Kulzer B, Haak T: Emotional induced changes during experimentally induced hypoglycaemia in type 1 diabetes. *Biol Psychol* 63:15–44, 2003

Hershey T, Lillie R, Sadler M, White NH: Severe hypoglycemia and long-term spatial memory in children with type 1 diabetes mellitus: a retrospective study. *J Int Netorpsychol Soc* 9:740–750, 2003

Hirai FE, Moss SE, Klein BEK, Klein R: Severe hypoglycemia and smoking in a long-term type 1 diabetic population: Wisconsin Epidemiologic Study of Diabetic Retinopathy. *Diabetes Care* 30:1437–1441, 2007

Hirsch IB: Insulin analogues. *N Engl J Med* 352:174–183, 2005

Holmes CS, Koepke KM, Thompson RG, Gyves PW, Weydert JA: Verbal fluency and naming performance in type 1 diabetes at different blood glucose concentrations. *Diabetes Care* 7:454–459, 1984

Holstein A, Egberts E-H: Risk of hypoglycaemia with oral antidiabetic agents in patients with type 2 diabetes. *Exp Clin Endocrinol Diabetes* 111:405–414, 2003

Home P, Bartley P, Russell-Jones D, Hanaire-Brouton H, Heeg J-E, Abrams P, Landin-Olsson M, Hylleberg B, Lang H, Draeger E; Study to Evaluate the Administration of Detemir Insulin Efficacy, Safety and Suitability (STEADINESS) Study Group: Insulin detemir offers improved glycemic control compared with NPH insulin in people with type 1 diabetes: a randomized clinical trial. *Diabetes Care* 27:1081–1087, 2004

Honkasalo MT, Elonheimo OM, Sane T: Severe hypoglycemia in drug-treated diabetic patients needs attention: a population-based study. *Scand J Prim Health Care*. doi: 10.3109/02813432.2011.580090

Jaser SS, Whittemore R, Ambrosino JM, Lindemann E, Grey M: Coping and psychosocial adjustment in mothers of young children with type 1 diabetes. *Child Health Care* 38:91–106, 2009

Jeha GS, Karaviti LP, Anderson B, Smith EO, Donaldson S, McGirk T, Haymond MW: Continuous glucose monitoring and the reality of metabolic control in preschool children with type 1 diabetes. *Diabetes Care* 27:2881–2886, 2004

Jørgensen HV, Pedersen-Bjergaard U, Rasmussen AK, Borch-Johnsen K: The impact of severe hypoglycemia and impaired awareness of hypoglycemia on relatives of patients with type 1 diabetes. *Diabetes Care* 26:1106–1109, 2003

Juvenile Diabetes Research Foundation Continuous Glucose Monitoring Study Group, Tamborlane WV, Beck RW, Bode BW, Buckingham B, Chase HP, Clemons R, Fiallo-Scharer R, et al.: Continuous glucose monitoring and intensive treatment of type 1 diabetes. *N Engl J Med* 359:1464–1476, 2008

Katakura M, Naka M, Kondo T, Nishii N, Komatsu M, Sato Y, Yamauchi K, Hiramatsu K, Ikeda M, Aizawa T, Hashizume K: Prospective analysis of mortality, morbidity, and risk factors in elderly diabetic subjects: Nagano study. *Diabetes Care* 26:638–644, 2003

Kerr D, Macdonald IA, Heller SR, Tattersall RB: Alcohol causes hypoglycaemic unawareness in healthy volunteers and patients with type 1 (insulin-dependent) diabetes. *Diabetologia* 33:216–221, 1990

Kinsley BT, Weinger K, Bajaj M, Levy CJ, Simonson DC, Quigley M, Cox DJ, Jacobson AM: Blood glucose awareness training and epinephrine responses to hypoglycemia during intensive treatment in type 1 diabetes. *Diabetes Care* 22:1022–1028, 1999

Kordonouri O, Pankowska E, Rami B, Kapellen T, Coutant R, Hartmann R, Lange K, Knip M, Danne T: Sensor-augmented pump therapy from the diagnosis of childhood type 1 diabetes: results of the Paediatric Onset Study (ONSET) after 12 months of treatment. *Diabetologia* 53:2487–2495, 2010

Kubiak T, Hermanns N, Schreckling H-J, Kulzer B, Haak T: Evaluation of a self-management-based patient education program for the treatment and prevention of hypoglycemia-related problems in type 1 diabetes. *Patient Educ Couns* 60:228–234, 2006

Kubiak T, Hermanns N, Schreckling H-J, Kulzer B, Haak T: Assessment of hypoglycaemia awareness using continuous glucose monitoring. *Diabet Med* 21:487–490, 2004

Laiteerapong N, Karter AJ, Liu JY, Moffet HH, Sudore R, Schillinger D, John PM, Huang ES: Correlates of quality-of-life in older adults with diabetes: the Diabetes and Aging Study. doi: 10.2337/dc10-2424

Leese GP, Wang J, Broomhall J, Kelly P, Marsden A, Morrison W, Frier BM, Morris A: Frequency of severe hypoglycemia requiring emergency treatment in type 1 and type 2 diabetes: a population-based study of health service resource use. *Diabetes Care* 26:1176–1180, 2003

Leiter LA, Yale J-F, Chiasson J-L, Harris SB, Kleinstiver P, Sauriol L: Assessment of the impact of fear of hypoglycemic episodes on glycemic and hypoglycemic management. *Can J Diabetes* 29:186–192, 2005

Linkeschova R, Raoul M, Bott U, Berger M, Sprauĺ M: Less severe hypoglycaemia, better metabolic control, and improved quality of life in type 1 diabetes mellitus with continuous subcutaneous insulin infusion (CSII) therapy: an observational study of 100 consecutive patients followed for a mean of 2 years. *Diabet Med* 19:746–751, 2002

Litton J, Rice A, Friedman N, Oden J, Lee MM, Freemark M: Insulin pump therapy in toddlers and preschool children with type 1 diabetes mellitus. *J Pediatr* 141:490–495, 2002

Lundkvist J, Berne C, Bolinder B, Jönsson L: The economic and quality of life impact of hypoglycaemia. *Eur J Health Econ* 6:197–202, 2005

McCrimmon RJ, Frier BM: Hypoglycaemia, the most feared complication of insulin therapy. *Diabetes Metab* 20:503–512, 1994

Meloche RM: Transplantation for the treatment of type 1 diabetes. *World J Gastroenterol* 13:6347–6355, 2007

Mühlhauser I, Berger M: Diabetes education and insulin therapy: when will they ever learn? *J Intern Med* 233:321–326, 1993

Munshi MN, Segal AR, Suhl E, Staum F., Desrochers L., Sternthal A, Giusti J, McCarthy R, Lee Y, Bonsignore P, Weinger K: Frequent hypoglycemia among elderly patients with poor glycemic control. *Arch Intern Med* 171:362–364, 2011

Murata GH, Duckworth WC, Shah JH, Wendel CS, Mohler MJ, Hoffman RM: Hypoglycemia in stable, insulin-treated veterans with type 2 diabetes: a retrospective study of 1662 episodes. *J Diabetes Complications* 19:10–17, 2005

Murata GH, Hoffman RM, Shah JH, Wendel CS, Duckworth WC: A probabilistic model for predicting hypoglycemia in type 2 diabetes mellitus. *Arch Intern Med* 164:1445–1450, 2004

Myers VH, Boyer BA, Herbert JD, Barakat LP, Scheiner G: Fear of hypoglycemia and self-reported posttraumatic stress in adults with type 1 diabetes treated by intensive regimens. *J Clin Psychol Med Settings* 14:11–21, 2007

Nordfeldt S, Johansson C, Carlsson E, Hammersjo J-A: Persistent effects of a pedagogical device targeted at prevention of severe hypoglycaemia: a randomized, controlled study. *Acta Paediatr* 94:1395–1401, 2005a

Nordfeldt S, Ludvigsson J: Fear and other disturbances of severe hypoglycaemia in children and adolescents with type 1 diabetes mellitus. *J Pediatr Endocrinol Metab* 18:83–91, 2005b

Nordfeldt S, Johansson C, Carlsson E, Hammersjo J-A: Prevention of severe hypoglycaemia in type I diabetes: a randomised controlled population study. *Arch Dis Child* 88:240–245, 2003

Patton SR, Dolan LM, Henry R, Powers SW: Fear of hypoglycemia in parents of young children with type 1 diabetes mellitus. *J Clin Psychol Med Settings* 15:252–259, 2008

Perros P, Frier BM: The long-term sequelae of severe hypoglycemia on the brain in insulin-dependent diabetes mellitus. *Horm Metab Res* 29:197–202, 1997

Pettersson B, Rosenqvist U, Deleskog A, Journath G, Wändell P: Self-reported experience of hypoglycaemia among adults with type 2 diabetes mellitus (Exhype). *Diabetes Res Clin Pract* 92:19–25, 2011

Plank J, Kohler G, Rakovac I, Semlitsch BM, Horvath K, Bock G, Kraly B, Pieber TR: Long-term evaluation of a structured outpatient education programme for intensified insulin therapy in patients with type 1 diabetes: a 12-year follow-up. *Diabetologia* 47:1370–1375, 2004

Rami B, Nachbaur E, Waldhoer T, Schober E: Continuous subcutaneous insulin infusion in toddlers. *Eur J Pediatr* 162:721–722, 2003

Ratner RE, Hirsch IB, Neifing JL, Garg SK, Mecca TE, Wilson C, on behalf of the U.S. Study Group of Insulin Glargine in Type 1 Diabetes: Less hypoglycemia with insulin glargine in intensive insulin therapy for type 1 diabetes. *Diabetes Care* 23:639–643, 2000

Reach G, Zerrouki A, Leclercq D, d'Ivernois J-F: Adjusting insulin doses: from knowledge to decision. *Patient Educ Couns* 56:98–103, 2005

Reviriego J, Gomis R, Marañés JP, Ricart W, Hudson P, Sacristán JA: Cost of severe hypoglycaemia in patients with type 1 diabetes in Spain and the cost-effectiveness of insulin lispro compared with regular human insulin in preventing severe hypoglycaemia. *Int J Clin Pract* 62:1026–1032, 2008

Rewers A, Chase HP, Mackenzie T, Walravens P, Roback M, Rewers M, Hamman RF, Klingensmith G: Predictors of acute complications in children with type 1 diabetes. *JAMA* 287:2511–2518, 2002

Richardson T, Weiss M, Thomas P, Kerr D: Day after the night before: influence of evening alcohol on risk of hypoglycemia in patients with type 1 diabetes. *Diabetes Care* 28:1801–1802, 2005

Rickels MR, Schutta MH, Mueller R, Kapoor S, Markmann JF, Naji A, Teff KL: Glycemic thresholds for activation of counterregulatory hormone and symptom responses in islet transplant recipients. *J Clin Endocrinol Metab* 92:873–879, 2007

Ritholz M: Is continuous glucose monitoring for everyone? Consideration of psychosocial factors. *Diabetes Spectr* 21:287–289, 2008

Rosenstock J, Dailey G, Massi-Benedetti M, Fritsche A, Lin Z, Salzman A: Reduced hypoglycemia risk with insulin glargine: a meta-analysis comparing insulin glargine with human NPH insulin in type 2 diabetes. *Diabetes Care* 28:950–955, 2005

Ryan C: Does moderately severe hypoglycemia cause cognitive dysfunction in children? *Pediatric Diabetes* 5:59–62, 2004

Ryan C: Neurobehavioral complications of type 1 diabetes: examination of possible risk factors. *Diabetes Care* 11:86–93, 1988

Ryan C, Vega A, Drash A: Cognitive deficits in adolescents who developed diabetes early in life. *Pediatrics* 75:921–927, 1985

Samann A, Mühlhauser I, Bender R, Kloos C, Muller UA: Glycaemic control and severe hypoglycaemia following training in flexible, intensive insulin therapy to enable dietary freedom in people with type 1 diabetes: a prospective implementation study. *Diabetologia* 48:1965–1970, 2005

Sandoval DA, Guy DL, Richardson MA, Ertl AC, Davis SN: Effects of low and moderate antecedent exercise on counterregulatory responses to subsequent hypoglycemia in type 1 diabetes. *Diabetes* 53:1798–1806, 2004

Scaramuzza AE, Iafusco D, Rabbone I, Bonfanti R, Lombardo F, Schiaffini R,

Buono P, Toni S, Cherubini V, Zuccotti GV; Diabetes Study Group of the Italian Society of Paediatric Endocrinology and Diabetology: Use of integrated real-time continuous glucose monitoring/insulin pump system in children and adolescents with type 1 diabetes: a 3-year follow-up study. *Diabetes Technol Ther* 13:99–103, 2011

Schultes B, Jauch-Chara K, Gais S, Hallschmid M, Reiprich E, Kern W, Oltmanns KM, Peters A, Fehm HL, Born J: Defective awakening response to nocturnal hypoglycemia in patients with type 1 diabetes mellitus. *PLoS Med* 4:e69, 2007

Seligman HK, Davis TC, Schillinger D, Wolf MS: Food insecurity is associated with hypoglycemia and poor diabetes self-management in a low-income sample with diabetes. *J Health Care Poor Underserved* 21:1227–1233, 2010

Shahar J: Helping your patients become active. *Diabetes Spectr* 21:59–62, 2008

Shapiro AM, Ricordi C, Hering BJ, Auchincloss H, Lindblad R, Roberston RP, Secchi A, et al.: International trial of the Edmonton protocol for islet transplantation. *N Engl J Med* 355:1318–1330, 2006

Singh H, Gonder-Frederick L, Shepard J, Cox DJ: Hypoglycemia-related cognitive dysfunction and its consequences in diabetes. *Int Diabetes Monit* 22:238–242, 2010

Slover RH, Welsh JB, Criego A, Weinzimer SA, Willi SM, Wood MA, Tamborlane WV: Effectiveness of sensor-augmented pump therapy in children and adolescents with type 1 diabetes in the STAR 3 study. *Pediatr Diabetes*. doi: 10.1111/j.1399-5448.2011.00793.x

Sommerfield AJ, Deary IKJ, McAulay V, Frier BM: Moderate hypoglycemia impairs multiple memory functions in healthy adults. *Neuropsychology* 17:125–132, 2003

Sovik O, Thordarsen H: Dead in bed syndrome in young diabetic patients. *Diabetes Care* 22 (Suppl. 2):B40–B42, 1999

Stahl M, Berger W, Schachinger H, Cox D: Spouse's worries concerning diabetic partner's possible hypoglycemia. *Diabet Med* 15:619–620, 1998

Steppel JH, Horton FS: Beta-cell failure in the pathogenesis of type 2 diabetes mellitus. *Curr Diab Rep* 4:169–175, 2004

Strachan MWJ, Reynolds RM, Marioni RE, Rice JF: Cognitive function, dementia and type 2 diabetes mellitus in the elderly. *Nat Rev Endocrinol* 7:108–114, 2011

Strachan MWJ, Deary IJ, Ewing FM, Frier BM: Recovery of cognitive function and mood after severe hypoglycemia in adults with insulin-treated diabetes. *Diabetes Care* 23:305–312, 2000

Svoren BM, Butler D, Levine B-S, Anderson BJ, Laffel LM: Reducing acute adverse outcomes in youths with type 1 diabetes: a randomized, controlled trial. *Pediatrics* 112:914–922, 2003

Swade TF, Emanuele NV: Alcohol and diabetes. *Compr Ther* 23:135–140, 1997

Tansey MJ, Tsalikian E, Beck RW, Mauras N, Buckingham BA, Weinzimer SA, Janz KF, et al., on behalf of The Diabetes Research in Children Network (DirecNet) Study Group: The effects of aerobic exercise on glucose and counterregulatory hormone concentrations in children with type 1 diabetes. *Diabetes Care* 29:20–25, 2006

Weissberg-Benchell J, Antisdel-Lomaglio J, Seshadri R: Insulin pump therapy: a meta-analysis. *Diabetes Care* 26:1079–1087, 2003

Whitmer RA, Karter AJ, Yaffe K, Quesenberry CP, Selby JV: Hypoglycemic episodes and risk of dementia in older patients with type 2 diabetes mellitus. *JAMA* 301:1565–1572, 2009

Wild D, von Maltzahn R, Brohan E, Christensen T, Clauson P, Gonder-Frederick L: A critical review of the literature on fear of hypoglycemia in diabetes: implications for diabetes management and patient education. *Patient Educ Couns* 68:10–15, 2007

Williams SA, Pollack MF, Dibonaventura M: Effects of hypoglycemia on health-related quality of life, treatment satisfaction and healthcare resource utilization in patients with type 2 diabetes mellitus. *Diabetes Res Clin Pract* 91:363–370, 2011

Wirsén A, Tallroth G, Lindgren M, Agardh C-D: Neuropsychological performance differs between type 1 diabetic and normal men during insulin-induced hypoglycemia. *Diabet Med* 9:156–165, 1992

Wolpert HA: Use of continuous glucose monitoring in the detection and prevention of hypoglycemia. *J Diabetes Sci Technol* 1:146–150, 2007

Workgroup on Hypoglycemia, American Diabetes Association: Defining and reporting hypoglycemia in diabetes: a report from the American Diabetes Association Workgroup on Hypoglycemia. *Diabetes Care* 28:1245–1249, 2005

Wredling R, Levander S, Adamson U, Lins P-E: Permanent neuropsychological impairment after recurrent episodes of severe hypoglycemia in man. *Diabetologia* 33:152–157, 1990

Yki-Jarvinen H, Dressler A, Ziemen M, on behalf of the HOE 901/3002 Study Group: Less nocturnal hypoglycemia and better post-dinner glucose control with bedtime insulin glargine compared with bedtime NPH insulin during insulin combination therapy in type 2 diabetes. *Diabetes Care* 23:1130–1136, 2000

Young-Hyman DL, Davis CL: Disordered eating behavior in individuals with diabetes: importance of context, evaluation, and classification. *Diabetes Care* 33:683–689, 2010

Zammitt N, Frier BM: Hypoglycemia in type 2 diabetes: pathophysiology, frequency, and effects of different treatment modalities. *Diabetes Care* 28:2948–2961, 2005

第四章
1 型糖尿病儿童的认知障碍

Clarissa S. Holmes，PhD

针对青少年糖尿病患者认知状况的研究在 20 世纪下半叶开始变得越来越多且其复杂性日益增加。与神经影像学技术的结合使人们更好地了解其生理机制及新的认知模型。虽然对神经影像学检查结果的讨论超出了本章的范围，但读者可以参考一些近期发表的综述。尽管在了解青少年患者中糖尿病和认知状况、家庭差异和人口因素（如社会阶层状态）之间的关系方面取得了一些研究成果，仍存在一些基本因素可解释显著的个体认知差异，与普通人群的研究结果是一致的。

智力表现

1 型糖尿病（T1D）的儿童一般具有平均或高于平均水平的智力（IQ>85）。与普通人群一样，T1D 儿童智力测试结果均值为 100，标准差为 15，存在个人和家庭差异。虽然 T1D 儿童的整体智商水平在平均范围内，但比没有糖尿病的儿童稍微低 3 分。尽管这是科研兴趣点，但如此量级的一组差异并没有临床意义。

韦氏量表是学校最常用的能力测试。有不同的版本可供选择：对于不到 7 岁的儿童有韦氏学龄前儿童智力测验量表（WPPSI-Ⅲ），6～16 岁学龄儿童可选用韦氏儿童智力测验量表-Ⅳ（WISC-Ⅳ），大于 16 岁的青少年可选用韦氏成人智力测验量表（WAIS-Ⅳ）。也有其他量表，但很少使用，如考夫曼儿童成套评价测验第二版（K-ABC-Ⅱ）和鉴别能力量表第二版（DAS-Ⅱ）。

学习障碍

对于大多数患有糖尿病的儿童来说，其学习成绩在年级平均水平或与其智商相一致。然而有 5%的孩子在阅读、数学、写作上有障碍，成绩低于年龄、学校教育和智力水平的预期值。患有糖尿病的儿童，特别是具有疾病危险因素的儿童，学习上较容易发生问题。

成绩评估与学习障碍

学习障碍的诊断标准，依当地教育和学区的不同而有差异。不过，由美国精神医学学会（2000 年）出版的精神疾病诊断与统计手册Ⅳ（DSMⅣ）包括以下内容：学习成绩的平均智力水平大体上低于智商、年龄或学校教育。通常存在认知障碍和神经心理问题（即注意力、记忆力、学习处理问题）。语言能力、执行力/规划力、注意力、视觉空间功能、记忆力和学习力，以及感官能力通常用发育神经心理学评估第二版（NEPSY-Ⅱ）进行评估。处理能力如记忆可用特殊方法进行评估，如韦克斯勒记忆量表第三版（WMS-Ⅲ）、记忆与学习的广泛评估第二版（WRAML-Ⅱ）和儿童记忆量表（CMS）。通常来说，这些特定的神经心理学测试只能由学校外经过专门培训的神经心理学家来管理。特殊课堂辅助的标准通常需要达到一个"临床界值"，一般用于在个人管理成绩测试中的表现低于 IQ 预期值 15 分以上（1~2 个标准差）的患者。在大多数学校广泛应用的成绩测试为伍德科克–约翰逊认知能力测验（WJ-Ⅲ-ACH）、广泛能力评估第四版（WRAT-4）、Wecbsler 个人能力测试–第三版（WIAT-Ⅲ）。像这种 IQ 测试，通常都是提供标准化的分数，即 100 分的平均分和 15 分的标准差。对大多数的儿童糖尿病患者来说，学习障碍可能是"亚临床"和低于正式诊断所需的严重水平。医疗保险通常覆盖心理教育评估的费用，这种评估应由专业人员完成。当地学校心理学家提供了另一种免费的选择，但是这种选择可能需要较长的候诊时间。家长可以在精神卫生机构找有执照的私人心理学家或临床心理学家来进行评估。对于正式诊断为学习障碍的儿童，需要每三年重新评估一次学习状态。

辅导服务

20 世纪 90 年代早期研究记载，儿童糖尿病学校课堂辅助的发生率较高。对于幼儿，尤其是不足 5 岁的儿童修改了医疗管理建议，旨在避免严重低血糖发作导致的癫痫或神志不清。在过去的 10 年里，很少有青年糖尿病特殊课堂辅助的研究，并且已有的研究也相互矛盾。因此，早期的研究不再能准确地反映当前的特殊课堂辅助的发生率。

1974 年通过的残疾儿童法案（PL 94–142），现在被称为残疾人教育法（IDEA），强制要求所有州给有残障情况的儿童提供最低限免费公共教育（FAPE），例如，特殊的教育与学习需要，可以得到联邦资助。服务的界限可能基于智力低下或边界值，以及个人管理智商值与伴随认知处理困难的成绩测试间的显著差异，如临床上显著的记忆问题。如果符合这些标准，可以提供相应的服务和个人教育计划（IEP）配制。个人教育计划为教室里的孩子记录特定服务或提供膳宿。只有那些临床诊断有学习障碍的糖尿病儿童才有资格获得这些重点服务。关于残疾人教育法更多信息，请访问：www.ed.gov/offices/OSERS/OSEP 或通过 ADA 访问 http://www.diabetes.org/living-with-diabetes /parents- and-kids/diabetes-care-at-school/written-care-plans。

大多数糖尿病儿童通过 1973 年残疾人教育法获得大范围但不太集中的教育服务和住宿的资格。该法禁止对"残疾"个人的歧视，其中包括临时残疾，如断腿。根据该法案第 504 条，有医疗状况的学生可以得到膳宿，像其他学生一样参加课内和课外活动。正式学习障碍的诊断并不能接受教育住宿及 504 计划。通常来说，504 计划是根据糖尿病医疗管理计划（DMMP）或医嘱开出推荐以学校为基础的医疗保健计划的处方。该 DMMP 是一种个性化的健康计划（IHP），由学校护士记录，指定做什么，何地，何时，由何人提供的糖尿病护理。这个健康计划只在学校提供医疗服务而没有教育住宿。504 计划为糖尿病相关住宿教育提供书面指导且受到联邦法律保护。普通服务和例外条款可能包括存储和管理胰岛素和血糖监测设备（或由学校提供），以及允许学生在教室携带和吃零食。为了适应日常就医允许频繁缺课请假，特殊时间上厕所或前往饮水机取水。接受联邦资金的私立学校也必须对这些学生相关的请求负责。教师、心理学家、学校护士或校长可以组织 504 会面。会面之前，家长可以写信，解释自己孩子的糖尿病相关的需求，以及他们如何能更好地适应学校。如果有必要，医生可以写信，解释特殊的医疗需求。更多有关 504 计划的信息可以访问 http：//www.isbe.net/spec-ed/pdfs/ parent_guide/ch15-section_504.pdf 或通过美国糖尿病协会访问 http：//www. diabetes.org /living- with-diabetes/parents-and-kids/d iabetes-care-at-school/ written-care-plans。

学习障碍相关的神经心理技能

尽管一般都具有平均智商，但亚组儿童可以在特定的认知处理问题上或神经心理学问题上诸如视觉空间或记忆能力障碍方面，在较高的风险。临床上，学习障碍的定义为低于平均智力水平 15 分以上（1～2 个标准差）。如下问题已在糖尿病儿童的亚组进行了描述，个人可能会或不会受到影响。

慢性疾病相关的发现

疾病早期（定义为小于 5 年，也有些人定义为小于 7 年）与最重要的技能破坏相关，与其他组相比，糖尿病儿童相在精神处理速度、词语记忆和学习上得分都是最低的（低 4～6 分）。如此巨大的差异可以在学校的表现上反映出来，在情绪沮丧时及与其他较强的技能比较表现出相对劣势时，这种差异可以被患儿自己察觉。晚发病儿童的分数在非言语/视觉空间技能、视觉记忆和学习能力、学习成绩方面仅轻微下降（2～3分）。然而，但是这种差异会随着病程的延长变得更大，与病程较长且早期发病的成年人相比最大差异可达 7 分。

相比于 5 年以下的短病程，长病程（超过 5 年，但在儿童人群通常小于 8 年或 9 年）与空间和视觉/感知觉技能轻度降低（2～3 分）有关。横断面和队列研究表明，在糖尿病确诊两年内，语言记忆和词汇量增长方面均会下降。

反复的重度低血糖和慢性高血糖

重度低血糖导致癫痫发作或意识丧失在不同年龄对大脑可能有不同的影响，对 5 岁或 6 岁以下的儿童的视觉空间和发散思维能力有更大的影响。对于年龄较大的儿童，对于重度低血糖是否影响语言记忆存在争议，如果有影响，那么这个血糖阈值是多少。在临床上，有害的持续影响可能只见于多次重度低血糖发作（如大于 5 次），或见于孩子大脑发育的敏感期（即 5 岁以下）。在葡萄糖代谢的另一方面，反复/持久的高血糖或较差的代谢控制（HbA1C 水平大于 9%）的患者与那些代谢控制较好者相比，其普通词汇智力显著降低（下降 7 分）。和代谢控制较好的儿童相比，其视觉和语言学习能力更差且成绩不及格。学龄前的儿童，如果长期高血糖（体现为更高的 HbA1C 水平），就会出现一般认知能力下降，接受语言能力下降和精细运动速度减慢。对于年龄稍大的学龄儿童，较差的慢性代谢控制与注意力不足和学习成绩下降有关。较差的代谢控制可与先前的每一个疾病危险因素相互作用并产生放大效应。

急性疾病相关的发现

除了这些一般的慢性认知的影响，急性、暂时性认知障碍也被证明与糖尿病有关。急性轻度低血糖症（血糖水平>50 mg/dl 且<90 mg/dl）与高级执行功能（注意力、计划、复杂的决策）短暂下降和中断相关，也与语言流畅、记忆、行动速度下降有关。准确性通常是完整的。在课堂上，有低血糖症的孩子接受新信息会有一些障碍。孩子可能会出现嗜睡或昏睡。反应速度和其他认知功能很难持续一堂课 45 分钟的时间。尽管没有证据表明血糖水平不稳会增加注意力缺乏的发生率，但有报道指出糖尿病和多动症有关。临床上，伴随轻度低血糖症出现的注意力问题与忽略的注意力缺陷症的亚型相一致，但如果它继发于低血糖症，则不应该被诊断，可它仍是一个隐性医疗问题。在血糖波动稳定时（尤其是低血糖症），由注意力缺陷症引起的注意力不集中亚型会被准确诊断。涉及癫痫或意识丧失的急性短暂低血糖是"严重"的事件，应根据重症低血糖症复发的相应指南进行处理。

与低血糖相比，急性高血糖（血糖值大于 300 mg/dl）在儿童中研究相对更少，但有初步证据显示其语言记忆和词汇成绩轻度下降，认知功能速度减低，这与急性低血糖的影响类似。

评估神经心理状态

神经心理状态及相关学科的评估应遵循公认的准则，以此来确定需要学术援助的孩子，需要对其进行记忆与其他神经心理相关的特别测试。虽然测试可以通过任何有执照的心理医生进行，但是由受过训练的神经心理学家或从事糖尿病患儿工作的专业人士进行测试，结果会更准确。神经心理障碍往往与特定学科领域，如阅读或数学学习障碍相伴发生。联邦和各种州政府会每三年为确诊患有学习障碍的重新测试并更发新证。采用的测试指南同样也适用于有亚临床学习问题的人群。一般来说，如果孩子的学习障碍干扰了日常生活或课堂表现，就应该送交儿科医生或儿童心理学家。这项建议包括始终无法完成某一学科的孩子，记忆或认知处理技能存在障碍的孩子。老师或家长使用心理教育筛查可帮助确定问题产生的原因。阅读、数学和写作能力的筛查测试可以由教育专家进行。如果发现有问题，接着应该进行全面的测试来确定是否具有提供辅助学校服务的资格。医疗保险往往覆盖由专业人士执行的心理教育评估的费用。当地学校心理学家可以提供另一种免费的选择，尽管这种选择可能需要较长的候诊时间。

评估的注意事项

对于儿童糖尿病患者来说，排除或识别出医学上比较常见的相关问题，如缺课、较差的血糖控制和血糖波动是很重要的，所有这些都可能与学习成绩下降及记忆和注意力问题相关。

在心理评估时，心理医生首先应该确定患儿能够完成血糖测试和处理低血糖发作。孩子在评估时应该携带血糖仪，最好准备一些果汁、点心，以防低血糖发作。在心理测试开始前应该快速检测血糖，以确保孩子最大限度地处于最佳状态。即使是轻度的低血糖症（血糖水平＞60

mg/dl 且＜90 mg/dl ），对心理测试表现和成绩也会产生不利影响。如果是中度或重度低血糖症（血糖水平小于 50mg/dl），心理测试应改天进行，以便有时间恢复最佳的认知状态。然而，如果在评估过程中怀疑出现轻度低血糖，应该暂停评估，用孩子自带的血糖仪检测血糖，并立即进食。花生酱饼干和果汁为测试提供了很好的补给。在食用 15 克的糖类和 15 分钟的等待之后，患儿再重新测试血糖水平来确认血糖正常，然后心理测试可以继续进行。

学习障碍的治疗

对学习障碍的治疗建议应考虑孩子潜在的认知优势和劣势，以及受影响的知识领域。传统意义上，如果存在学习问题，可以通过促进延迟技能获得（如注意力缺乏）的补救策略来治疗，或使用针对剩余能力的补偿策略及促进最佳技能（优势强化）使用的环境策略来治疗。通常运用联合技术，但大多数的治疗文献已经表明青少年糖尿病患者并没有典型的明显神经障碍。虽然这些策略反映了当今的思想，但是缺乏治疗有效性的经验验证。当前并没有关于青年糖尿病方面的研究。因此，这些治疗建议是根据一般学习障碍孩子的治疗建议而提出的，并不是专门针对儿童糖尿病患者提出的。

干预建议

1. **问题的规避**　临床经验表明，最好是发扬"优势"，而不是补救"软肋"。例如，空间感弱可以通过给予口头指引，而不是书写、绘制地图或采用发音对应视觉词的阅读方法来弥补。

2. **辅助学习设备**　采用辅助学习设备对于解决问题是有益的。例如，对于单纯记忆问题，使用计算器可以弥补数学记忆困难并为实践与认知学习提供了机会。

3. **降低心理运动功效**　可以在测试中不定时或增加测试时间。

4. **避免羞辱孩子**　所有的人都有优缺点，诊断有学习障碍的糖尿病孩子可能与正常孩子只差一点点。

5. **帮助孩子、家庭和学术机构**　了解由于血糖波动造成的短暂认知缺陷和诊断为学习困难患儿之间的差异。

6. **自我尊重困难可能会存在**　如果持续存在这种情况或比较严重，应当向学校辅导员或经过培训的治疗师寻求心理学治疗，尝试安抚并让患儿肯定自我、了解自我。由于糖尿病的原因患儿已经产生自我意识的改变，这可能会增加其自我价值感降低的倾向性（参见第十四章）。

预防或最小化认知困难

广大青年糖尿病患者没有明显的临床或亚临床学习障碍。但是，在血糖浓度发生变化时可以在课堂上出现短暂的记忆障碍、注意力障碍和心理运动功效降低，随之而产生的挫败感会影响学习成绩。长期队列研究表明，青少年糖尿病患者与非糖尿病对照组相比在中学阶段有比较高的辍学率，这一发现值得关注。

疾病的护理与记忆状态有关。即使在平均范围内的单纯记忆也更多地与日常血糖监测相关，这种相关独立于智商的强大效应和社会阶级地位的影响。一些策略似乎真的可以避免日常护理的减少和学习困难，这些策略可最大程度地降低暂时性血糖波动及其对记忆和注意力的继发变化。同样的，长期血糖控制不佳（以 HbA1C 作为提示），会导致学习成绩下降。在某些情况下，这种关联独立于社会阶层，大脑慢性代谢环境的正常化可能有助于避免认知困难，避免学习成绩下降。

糖尿病控制和并发症试验（DCCT）与糖尿病干预和并发症流行病学研究（EDIC）表明，青少年时期参与以上两项研究，在 18.5 年的学习过程中保持良好的血糖控制，随访到中年时只有轻微的心理运动功效减低。不管是"自我管理能力"或糖尿病知识，频繁的血糖监测和就餐/吃零食及胰岛素强化治疗方案，这些努力可使血糖水平恢复正常。

重要的是，"忘记"执行特定的治疗行为，如血糖监测，是在各种儿科治疗方案和青年治疗方案中常见的自我管理依从性问题。忘记自我管理的行为应该实事求是地处理，因为这非常普遍。而不是假设他们无依从性或认知处理缺陷，健康护理人员能够识别行为模式或环境模式（即周围不断出现"遗忘行为"的示例),来最大化地促进自我管理行为发生的环境和行为改变。或者,存在另一种解释,表明此种行为不是字面上的遗忘,也有可能是因为尴尬或不方便(参见第十四章)。相比之下,影响学习成绩的记忆问题(如很难记住数学公式)应仔细监测,并考虑进行心理教育评估的可能。

已经证明早期发病和高血糖与儿童和青少年的认知能力较差有相关性。然而,这个人群学习障碍的主要推动力是社会经济环境和智力。糖尿病儿童认知缺陷和一般人群有相同的诊断水平。很少有研究对代谢引发的问题、不依从医疗方案的行为、认知障碍这三者进行区分。目前还没有对儿童糖尿病患者的学习或记忆问题进行系统干预的测试。因此,普遍接受的方法包括缺陷全面评估,补偿学习策略和辅助设备等。一旦发现孩子的学习障碍,建议对他们进行系统的重新评估。临床专家推荐以下策略以促进疾病护理行为,从而更好地控制血糖。

1. **评估** 当遗忘行为成为疾病管理的障碍,治疗应针对缘由,尽可能区分出特定疾病的神经认知后遗症(如低血糖发作期间失忆)、不依从性、认知缺陷或学习障碍,或疾病本身导致的心理调整能力差(如抑郁症),这些都可反映在不服从自我管理行为上。如果行为缺陷与疾病有关,如血糖控制差,那么应告知其医疗管理团队并同时告知补救方案。

2. **辅助人员** 患儿的家庭成员如果掌握较多的疾病治疗知识,那么就可以最大限度地减少记忆和其他认知需求,并且帮助维持更好的疾病管理。这通常需要父母或看护人花更多的时间来监督患儿的自我管理行为。如果父母与患儿的关系变得紧张,医疗服务人员可以提供有益的帮助。

3. **辅助记忆设备** 对于某些问题,采用辅助记忆设备是有益的。例如,对于忘记检查血糖,可以利用手表报警来提醒测血糖,也可以利用带警铃的电话或建立固定的套路,如总是吃东西前检查血糖,这样有助于将常规的疾病管理任务整合到日常生活中。

参 考 文 献

American Psychiatric Association: *Diagnostic and Statistical Manual of Mental Disorders*. 4th Ed. (DSM-IV). Washington, DC, American Psychiatric Association, 2000

Bade-White PA, Obrzut JE: The neurocognitive effects of type 1 diabetes mellitus in children and young adults with and without hypoglycemia. *Journal of Developmental and Physical Disabilities* 21:425–440, 2009

Cohen MJ: *Children's Memory Scale*. San Antonio, TX, The Psychological Corporation, 1997

Crawford SG, Kaplan BJ, Field, LL: Absence of an association between insulin-dependent diabetes mellitus and developmental learning difficulties. *Hereditas* 122:73–78, 1995

Donnelly JE, Donnelly WJ, Thong YH: Parental perceptions and attitudes toward asthma and its treatment: a controlled study. *Social Science and Medicine* 24:431–437, 1987

Elliott CD: *Differential Ability Scales*. 2nd Ed. San Antonio, TX, Harcourt Assessment, 2007

Ferguson SC, Blane A, Wardlaw J, Frier BM, Perros P, McCrimmon RJ, Deary IJ: Influence of an early-onset age of type 1 diabetes on cerebral structure and cognitive function. *Diabetes Care* 28:1431–1437, 2005

Gaudieri PA, Greer TF, Chen R, Holmes CS: Cognitive function in children with type 1 diabetes. *Diabetes Care* 31:1892–1897, 2008

Gonder-Frederick LA, Zrebeic JF, Bauchowitz AU, Ritterband LM, Magee JC, Cox DJ, Clarke WL: Cognitive function is disrupted by both hypo- and hyperglycemia in school-aged children with type 1 diabetes: a field study. *Diabetes Care* 32:1001–1006, 2009.

Hagan JW, Barclay CR, Anderson BJ, Freeman DJ, Segal SS, Bacon G, Goldstein GW: Intellective functioning and strategy use in children with insulin-dependent diabetes mellitus. *Child Development* 61:1714–1727, 1990

Hannonen R, Tupola S, Ahonen T, Riikonen R: Neurocognitive functioning in children with type-1 diabetes with and without episodes of severe hypoglycemia. *Developmental Medicine & Child Neurology* 45:262–268, 2003

Hershey T, Lillie R, Sadler M, White NH: Severe hypoglycemia and long-term spatial memory in children with type 1 diabetes mellitus: a retrospective study. *Journal of the International Neuropsychological Society*, 9:740–750, 2003

Hershey T, Bhargava N, Sadler M, White NH, Craft S: Conventional versus intensive diabetes therapy in children with type 1 diabetes. *Diabetes Care* 22:1318–1324, 1999

Holmes CS, Morgan KL, Powell PW: Neuropsychological sequelae of type 1 and type 2 diabetes. In *Handbook of Medical Neuropsychology: Applications of Cognitive Neuroscience*. Armstrong CL, Morrow L, Eds. New York, Springer, 2010, p. 415–430

Holmes CS, Chen RS, Streisand R, Marschall D, Soutor SA, Swift E, Cant C: Predictors of youth diabetes care behaviors and metabolic control: a structural equation modeling approach. *Journal of Pediatric Psychology* 31:770–784, 2006

Holmes CS, Dunlap WS, Chen RS, Cornwell JM: Gender differences in the learning status of diabetic children. *Journal of Consulting and Clinical Psychology* 60:698–704, 1992

Kanne SM, Grissom MO, Farmer JE: Interventions for children with neuropsychological disorders. In *Pediatric Neuropsychology: Research, Theory, and Practice*. Yeates KW, Ris MD, Taylor HG, Pennington BR, Eds. New York, Guilford Press, 2010

Kaufman FR, Epport K, Engilman R, Halvorson M: Neurocognitive functioning in children diagnosed with diabetes before age 10 years. *Journal of Diabetes and Its Complications* 13:31–38, 1999

Kaufman AS, Kaufman NL: *Kaufman Assessment Battery for Children*. 2nd ed. Circle Pines, MN, American Guidance Service, 2004

Korkman M, Kirk U, Kemp S: *A Developmental Neuropsychological Assessment*. 2nd ed. San Antonio, TX, The Psychological Corporation, 2007

Kovacs M, Ryan C, Obrosky DS: Verbal intellectual and visual memory performance of youths with childhood-onset insulin-dependent diabetes mellitus. *Journal of Pediatric Psychology* 19:475–483, 1994

Lezak MD, Howieson DB, Loring DW: *Neuropsychological Assessment*. 4th ed. New York, Oxford University Press, 2001

Lin A, Northam EA, Rankins D, Werther GA, Cameron FJ: Neuropsychological profiles of young people with type 1 diabetes 12 yr after disease onset. *Pediatric Diabetes* 11:235–243, 2010

McCarthy AM, Lindgren S, Mengeling MA, Tsalikian E, Engvall JC: Effects of diabetes on learning in children. *Pediatrics* 109:1–10, 2002

Meyers KEC, Thomson PD, Weiland H: Noncompliance in children and adolescents after renal transplantation. *Transplantation* 62:186–189, 1996

Modi AC, Quittner AL: Barriers to treatment adherence for children with cystic fibrosis and asthma: what gets in the way? *Journal of Pediatric Psychology* 31:846–858, 2006

Musen G: Cognition and brain imagining in type 1 diabetes. *Current Diabetes Rep* 8:132–137, 2008a

Musen G, Jacobson AM, Ryan CM, Cleary PA, Waberski BH, et al.: Impact of diabetes and its treatment on cognitive function among adolescents who participated in the Diabetes Control and Complications Trial. *Diabetes Care* 31:1933–1938, 2008b

Northam EA, Lin A: Hypoglycaemia in childhood onset type 1 diabetes: part villain, but not the only one. *Pediatric Diabetes* 11:134–141, 2010

Northam EA, Anderson PJ, Jacobs R, Hughes M, Warner GL, Werther GA: Neuropsychological profiles of children with type 1 diabetes 6 years after disease onset. *Diabetes Care* 24:1541–1546, 2001

Overstreet S, Holmes CS, Dunlap WP, Frentz J: Sociodemographic risk factors to disease control in children with diabetes. *Diabetic Medicine* 14:153–157, 1997a

Overstreet S, Holmes CS, Dunlap WP, Frentz J: Sociodemographic risk factors to intellectual and academic functioning in children with diabetes. *Intelligence* 24:367–380, 1997b

Patino-Fernandez AM, Dellamater AM, Applegate EB, Brady E, Eidson M, Nemery R, Gonzalez-Mendoza L, Richton S: Neurocognitive functioning in preschool-age children with type 1 diabetes mellitus. *Pediatric Diabetes* 11:424–430, 2010

Perantie DC, Lim A, Wu A, Weaver P, et al.: Effects of prior hypoglycemia and hyperglycemia on cognition in children with type 1 diabetes mellitus. *Pediatric Diabetes* 9:87–95, 2008

Raskin SA: Current approaches to cognitive rehabilitation. In *Handbook of Medical Neuropsychology*. Armstrong CL, Morrow L, Eds. New York, Springer, 2010

Reich JN, Kaspar C, Puczynski MS, Puczynski S, Cleland J, Dellángela K, Emanuele MA: Effect of hypoglycemic episode on neuropsychological functioning in diabetic children. *Journal of Clinical and Experimental Neuropsychology* 12:613–626, 1990

Rovet JF, Ehrlich RM, Czuchta D: Intellectual characteristics of diabetic children at diagnosis and one year later. *Journal of Pediatric Psychology* 15:775–788, 1990

Rovet JF, Ehrlich RM, Hoppe M: Specific intellectual deficits in children with early onset diabetes mellitus. *Child Development* 59:226–234, 1988

Ryan CM, Atchison J, Puczynski S, Puczynski M, Arslanian S, Becker D: Mild hypoglycemia associated with deterioration of mental efficiency in children with insulin-dependent diabetes mellitus. *Journal of Pediatrics* 117:32–38, 1990

Ryan CM, Vega A, Drash A: Cognitive deficits in adolescents who developed diabetes early in life. *Pediatrics* 75:921–927, 1985

Sattler JM: *Assessment of Children: Cognitive Applications*. 4th ed. New York, Sattler, 2001

Sheslow D, Adams W: *Wide Range Assessment of Memory and Learning*. 2nd ed. Wilmington, DE, Wide Range, 2003

Silverstein J, Klingensmith G, Copeland K, Plotnick L, Kaufman F, Laffel L, Deeb L, Grey M, Anderson B, Holzmeister LA, Clark N: Care of children and adolescents with type 1 diabetes: a statement of the American Diabetes Association. *Diabetes Care* 28:186–212, 2005

Soutor S, Chen RS, Streisand R, Kaplowitz P, Holmes CS: Memory matters: developmental differences in predictors of chronic disease care behaviors. *Journal of Pediatric Psychology* 29:493–505, 2004

Wechsler D: *Wechsler Individual Achievement Test*. 3rd ed. San Antonio, TX, NCS Pearson, 2009

Wechsler D: *Wechsler Adult Intelligence Scale*. 4th ed. San Antonio, TX, Harcourt Assessment, 2008

Wechsler D: *Wechsler Intelligence Scale for Children*. 4th ed. San Antonio, TX, Harcourt Assessment, 2003

Wechsler D: *Wechsler Primary and Preschool Scale of Intelligence*. 4th ed. San Antonio, TX, Harcourt Assessment, 2002

Wechsler D: *Wechsler Memory Scale*. 3rd ed. San Antonio, TX, Harcourt Assessment, 1997

Wilkinson GS, Robertson GJ: *Wide Range Achievement Test*. 4th ed. Lutz, FL, Psychological Assessment Resources, 2006

Woodcock RW, McGrew KS, Mather N: *Woodcock-Johnson III Tests of Achievement*. Itasca, IL, Riverside Publishing, 2001

第五章
成人糖尿病患者的神经认知功能障碍

Christopher M. Ryan，PhD

50 多年前通过对 16 名儿童期罹患糖尿病且血糖控制不佳的青年和中年人进行大脑尸检，人们首次发现糖尿病对认知功能有影响，其特征为中枢神经系统的功能和结构受损。生前这些患者表现出精神损害和（或）神经异常，并且都有严重的微血管和大血管合并症，包括失明、肾功能不全及冠心病。尸检的神经病理学表现为弥漫性分布的脱髓鞘病变，其病理变化在脑神经和视交叉尤其明显，原因是由于灰质、基底节的胶质细胞增生产生大量白质束，同时有全脑血管的显著变化。这曾经被认为是"糖尿病脑病"的证据，因为脑病理变化的程度似乎与糖尿病相关的视网膜和肾脏并发症的严重程度有关，并且与其他神经系统疾病完全不同。

自 1965 年以来，有大量研究系统评价了儿童和成人糖尿病患者的大脑功能和结构，但没有人描述 Reske-Nielsen 和他的同事在病例研究中提到的广泛性神经病理学异常。因为他们研究的这些患者在 20 世纪三四十年代时患糖尿病，那时的疾病管理质量非常差，所以人们认为这些病例有历史偏差，不能准确反映当今患者所呈现的中枢神经改变的类型。然而，这些早期的观察提供了一种"原理论证"，即在某些情况下，糖尿病可以显著地影响脑的完整性。

最近的研究表明，虽然脑功能障碍确实与糖尿病相关，但它的影响程度在大多数情况下是轻微的，并且其临床表现略有差别，这取决于患者是 1 型还是 2 型糖尿病。本章借鉴了神经心理学、电生理学、脑血管学、神经影像学和神经代谢评估来确定成人糖尿病相关的"神经认知表型"。

鉴于证据等级的重要性，令人沮丧的是与认知结果有关的随机临床试验并不多[如糖尿病控制和并发症试验/糖尿病干预和并发症的流行病学研究组（DCCT/EDIC）]，荟萃分析的研究也集中在成人糖尿病，尽管文章本身很优秀，但是这方面的文献很少。本章所涉及的大部分研究均符合 B 级证据：均为设计良好的描述性队列研究、运用多种方法评估认知功能（或其他恰当的方法衡量脑功能或结构）、受试者的代谢和生物学状态、统计学上相匹配的非糖尿病对照组及充足的统计学数据来探究"适度"效应的大小，如标准化效应值≥0.4。尽管存在研究人群、结果测量参数和统计方法的差异，但这些研究却得出了比较一致的结论。

成人 1 型糖尿病患者

认知表现

成人 T1D 研究表明较长的糖尿病病史（通常是 20～30 年），以及临床上重要的并发症会影响认知和大脑结构。如果某研究检查大群组的糖尿病成人——不考虑并发症或其他疾病相关的特征，该研究会发现这些成人认知障碍的程度与在青少年糖尿病患者中观察到的结果相似。当与非糖尿病成人相比，糖尿病成人智力、注意力、精神运动速度、认知灵活性和视觉感知能力会更差。表 5-1 是从 33 个病例/对照研究（患者年龄限制在 18～50 岁）的 Meta 分析中总结出的结果，阐明了糖尿病相关认知障碍的受限功能有哪些。很显然，不是所有的认知领域受到同等程度的影响，其语言能力、学习和记忆能力表现正常。

该研究，以及近期其他的研究结果，提出了四个要点：第一，糖尿病相关的认知障碍的程度较小，效应值范围是 0.3～0.8 个标准差。第二，学习和记忆能力，既往被认为早期脑功能障碍最敏感的区域，尽管他们有 20 年以上的糖尿病病史，但这些患者完全不受影响，第三，这种缺陷模式类似于儿童 1 型糖尿病的报道，因为几乎所有成人的 1 型糖尿病都是从儿童或青少年时期诊断的。因此在缺乏整个生命历程的前瞻性研究的情况下，要确定认知改变是从什么年龄段首次出现的，是非常具有挑战性的。第四，成人糖尿病患者的测试表现显然较差，包括可变智力、注意力、认知灵活性、精神运动速度和视知觉，这些测试都要求快速反应。另一个观察得出的结论是，精神迟缓可能是与 T1D 相关的基本缺陷，这不仅出现在成人中，也出现在患 T1D 的幼儿和儿童中。

表 5-1　1 型糖尿病成人的认知特点

区域	效应值	显著性（P）	总人数	研究数
整体认知	0.40	＜0.001	660	16
智力				
■ 固化智力	0.80	＜0.01	276	5
■ 可变智力	0.50	＜0.01	168	4
语言	0.05	NS	144	4
注意力				
■ 视觉	0.40	＜0.001	195	5
■ 持续性	0.30	＜0.01	217	3
学习和记忆				
■ 工作记忆	0.10	NS	244	8
■ 语言学习	0.20	NS	204	5
■ 语言延迟记忆	0.30	NS	157	3
■ 视觉学习	0.10	NS	187	5
■ 视觉延迟记忆	0.10	NS	157	4
精神运动速度	0.60	＜0.05	368	8
认知灵活性	0.50	＜0.001	364	9
视知觉	0.40	＜0.001	202	5

依据已发表的论文进行 Meta 分析。每个认知域的标准化效应值（Cohen's *d*）反映了糖尿病患者与非糖尿病患者的差别。

1 型糖尿病老年患者表现出更多的受限模式或认知功能障碍，但影响更小。关于该问题的单一研究表明，在一个认知领域（信息处理速度，$d=0.34$），糖尿病患者显然比同龄（大约 61 岁）非糖尿病人群表现得更差。这些可能反映了某种事实，即糖尿病组倾向于在成年早期诊断认知功能障碍，而不是儿童时期，或非糖尿病对照组患高血压和动脉粥样硬化这些疾病也可能干扰认知功能，这些都是合理的解释但是没有得到证明。

电生理特性

若能证明糖尿病与减慢的脑电波活动有关[用脑电图（EEG），儿童和成人的感觉和相关诱发电位技术进行测试]，那么其结果就与认知功能减慢的证据相一致。在血糖正常，静息状态下进行研究时，年轻人表现出快脑电波（α，β，γ）活动降低且在大脑颞区最为明显，慢脑电波（δ 和 θ）在额叶区域活动增加。这与代谢控制程度或重症低血糖病史无关，而与个体受试者有关，更大程度的慢波活动与较慢的周围神经传导速度有关。后一种关系与糖尿病可引起周围神经病变和"中枢神经病变"的观点是一致的。如果神经减缓（外周和中枢）是糖尿病的重要表现，人们则期待找到 EEG 减慢的程度与认知减慢之间的关联。不幸的是，这项研究或其他研究在相同的研究对象中都没有系统地进行定量测量。

脑血管结果

脑血流量（CBF）在 T1D 成年人中是改变的，灌注程度减少和增加均可在额叶和额颞叶脑区频繁出现。在一项大型研究中，糖尿病组中 82% 的中年人，在一个或多个兴趣区域出现灌注不足的证据，而对照受试者只有 10%；同样，58% 的糖尿病受试者表现出高灌注，而对照组只有 20%。这些由单光子发射计算机化断层显像（SPECT）获得的结果，发现基本上所有脑区都出现了脑灌注的变化，影响最大的区域是小脑、额叶和额颞区。这些受试者均无显著的心血管疾病，但许多人有视网膜病变，从而得出结论即脑灌注改变的发生与糖尿病微血管并发症相关。

该观点的额外支持来自于一个较小的研究，用正电子发射计算机化断层显像（PET）测量有或无周围神经病变的糖尿病患者的脑葡萄糖利用率。区域脑代谢率显著降低只见于那些有并发症的患者。这些研究结果，和脑血管反应的研究数据一样，支持糖尿病引起脑微血管病理学改变（尤其是脑中阻力小动脉）的观点。尽管未经证实，但其潜在的病理生理学机制很可能与那些糖尿病微血管并发症的发展机制相似或完全一致。遗憾的是，这些脑血管改变的程度与认知改变的关系至今未在糖尿病人群中进行研究。然而，对其他患者人群（如脑卒中）的研究表明脑血管的改变，尤其是灌注不足，对认知功能有显著的影响。

脑结构异常

复杂的神经影像研究很少包含大样本的 1 型糖尿病成人患者，但现存的研究已经反复证明患者存在轻度的结构性变化，特别是在皮质灰质。在迄今为止最大规模的研究中，对 1 型糖尿病的成人患者和 36 名健康对照者进行了磁共振成像（MRI）评估，该技术用基于体素的形态（VBM）学分析测量脑密度，它是一种行之有效的半自动定量方法。糖尿病组表现为多个脑区域的灰质密度降低，包括左后扣带、左颞脑回及右侧海马旁回。这些测量值比健康对照组低 4%～5%，并且与 HbA1C 值相关，但与认知功能测试分数或低血糖症复发无关。因为该研究排除了临床上有显著增殖性糖尿病视网膜病变的患者，故很难得出结构变化和微血管病之间可能存在关系的强有力结论，尽管两次分析表明大脑密度测量和亚临床视网膜病变严重程度之间的关系具有显著的统计学意义。一个较小的病例对照研究为血管并发症和大脑结构之间的关系提供了强力支持，这项研究明确的包含晚期增值性糖尿病视网膜病的患者，并与未患微血管病变的糖尿病患者进行了对比。视网膜病变患者在额叶脑回，枕叶及小脑的灰质密度显著减少，这与 HbA1C 值、糖尿病病程、诊断年龄或血压无关。

白质的变化似乎更难以判断——至少在传统的神经影像技术与临床评价系统一起使用时无法评估。然而，扩散张量成像（DTI）程序的开发和改进可以识别病程长的 T1D 中年患者脑中白质微小结构异常。DTI是一种神经成像技术，依据水分子在组织中扩散的方向进行制图。当水分子通过屏障（如细胞膜、纤维、髓鞘）受限时，向一个方向的扩散速率会加快；"各向异性扩散"程度的分析显示水分子更倾向于向白质这样有固定排列顺序的组织扩散。在他们开创性的研究中，Kodl 等对 25 名代谢控制良好的糖尿病成人和人口统计学上相似的非糖尿病患者进行了对比，发现一些完整性异常的白质束，尤其是后放射冠和视放射区域，与某些疾病相关的参数有关，包括较长的糖尿病病程和较高的 HbA1C值。此外，正如预期的我们对脑-行为关系的理解一样，这些结构异常的大小与认知任务的表现（需要视觉空间分析和手眼协调）之间有很强的相关性。虽然二次分析指出，这种影响往往在有微血管并发症的糖尿病患者中更大，但是研究样本太小，且并发症的严重程度也有限。鉴于在糖尿病患者中特征性地发现了白质异常可能是神经迟缓的原因，在以后的研究中更广泛地使用 DTI 技术是非常有意义的。

神经化学异常

目前已经注意到 1 型糖尿病青少年和成人患者中均有脑化学变化。质子磁共振波谱（1H-MRS）已经证实，在一个大样本的糖尿病成年人群中，糖尿病患者和非糖尿病患者在大脑的葡萄糖水平和重要神经递质水平上有显著差异。总体来讲，糖尿病组（123 人）的前额叶葡萄糖浓度为 89%，比健康非糖尿病对照组（38 人）高。此外，持久的血糖控制与前额叶的葡萄糖值存在线性关系。与对照组相比，脑神经递质水平[复合测量谷氨酸、谷氨酰胺和 γ-氨基丁酸（GLX）]高了 9%，并且再次验证了 HbA1C 值与 GLX 值之间存在剂量–反应关系。在这组糖尿病患者中认知表现也显著受损，有三个区域影响最大，即记忆功能、执行功能和精神运动速度。

谷氨酸通常是兴奋性神经递质，但过量时容易在细胞外间隙积聚，对神经元产生兴奋性毒性作用。如果这种状态随后导致神经元坏死，人们希望找到认知功能障碍和 GLX 水平之间的关系。这项研究正好表明：较高水平的 GLX 与较差的记忆和执行功能的表现密切相关。虽然，在研究了所有糖尿病患者后，未发现大脑的葡萄糖水平与认知表现之间有可靠的统计学关系，但二次分析结果表明，通过对比血糖控制较好组与较差组（HbA1C＞8%），在血糖控制较差的亚组中，其较高的大脑葡萄糖水平与神经运动速度减慢有关。在控制较差的亚组中脑内葡萄糖较高的水平与反应下降有关。这一系列研究结果证明了磁共振波谱分析的价值，并且说明了糖尿病在一定程度上可以影响脑葡萄糖、神经代谢和认知。

在一群有微血管并发症的中年患者中，磁共振波谱分析也可成功揭示神经元坏死和脱髓鞘的存在。与健康对照组相比，有视网膜病变的患者有更高水平的胆碱标记化合物（胆碱——髓磷脂代谢和其他细胞磷脂的标记物），在白质和丘脑最明显。肌醇（肌醇——神经胶质增生或激活的标志）在白质中也有所升高，而血糖水平在所有脑区均升高。长期代谢控制较差与代表神经元完整性的两种标记物——N-乙酰天冬氨酸和谷氨酸呈负相关，同样也与脑白质的胆碱呈负相关。这些发现已成为解释轴突损伤、脱髓鞘和其他神经病理学的证据，也是微血管变化（继发于慢性高血糖症）介导神经胶质过细胞增生的证据。这与一项早期研究的阴性数据相一致，这项研究没发现脑代谢异常是因为它把有显著微血管并发症的患者明确排除在外。

生物医学风险因素

1 型糖尿病成人患者表现出独特的神经认知表型。在语言智能、注意力、精神运动速度和认知灵活性上，他们比非糖尿病同龄人表现更差，但在学习和记忆上表现正常。其他的脑功能变化包括神经传输速度显著减慢，由 EEG 和跨多个脑区域的其他技术测定，以及脑血流异常变化，表现为一些脑区显著灌注不足而其他脑区灌注过度。脑结构也受到影响，表现为多个脑区的灰质密度轻微减少（−5%），以及白质完整性的改变，尤其是连接一个皮质区与另一个皮质或皮质下区的长轴突的改变。神经化学物质的改变也存在：大脑的葡萄糖水平升高，提示神经元、轴突和支持神经胶质细胞受损的某些代谢产物也升高。

较早的研究已经把这些表现归结于中度、重度低血糖症反复发作的结果。这种解释与动物实验数据和临床病历报告相一致，表明长期的低血糖（长时间内血糖＜1.5mmol/L）可诱导多个脑区的皮质改变，包括额叶和颞叶皮质及基底节、海马和脑干。近期着眼于中度低血糖的反复发作的研究，未能找到认知（或其他脑的完整性的测试）与一次或多次低血糖事件发生的可靠关联。例如，包含 1114 名受试者的 DCCT / EDIC 认知随访研究数据显示，在 18.5 年的随访中，经历一次或多次严重低血糖发作与随着时间推移所表现的 8 个认知域的改变无关。另一方面，有较差的代谢控制（HbA1C＞8.8%）病史的患者，随着时间的推移确实表现出显著的下降，但只表现对神经运动速度有要求的任务上。同样，一项对已发表论文进行系统的 Meta 分析的数据也未发现低血糖反复发作与认知测试的表现有任何关系。不幸的是，研究低血糖和神经认知结果之间的关系的困难在于定量低血糖发作的数目和严重程度是具有挑战性的。几乎所有的研究，除了 DCCT，被迫依赖医疗记录数据（极不完整），或对早年发生事件的个人回忆（极不可靠）。因此，不可能完全忽视中度、重度低血糖在一定程度上对神经认知表现有影响，尽管更大规模、更近期的研究对此进行了仔细的调查，但还是未能发现令人信服的支持这一观点的证据。另一方面，大量的研究（使用测试大脑完整性的各种方法）已经发现，微血管并发症和慢性高血糖症的其他指标很大程度地增加了神经认知功能障碍的风险。

在一个早期的纵向研究中，对 1 型糖尿病青年和中年患者进行了 7 年多的随访，并与一群健康的非糖尿病同龄患者进行对比。在随访期间患者发生了认知改变，但他们只限于单一区域，即神经运动速度的改变，并且局限于那些在临床上有显著微血管并发症的患者（如增殖性糖尿病视网膜病变），或者在随访期间诊断了临床显著并发症的患者。那些在任何时间点都没有并发症的患者，其病情不会随时间恶化。采取多变量的方式来确定可能使精神运动速度下降的生物医学变量，这些研究人员发现，在基线水平就存在微血管并发症的患者占变量的 12%，新发展的微血管和大血管并发症各自占了额外的 17% 和 7%，收缩压和糖尿病病程都分别占了 8%～9%。

那些纵向研究结果与 1 型糖尿病青年的横断面数据一致。不仅背景性糖尿病视网膜病变的存在是认知功能障碍的预测因子（尤其是在可变智力、注意力、集中力和信息处理速度方面），而且这些早期的微血管改变也与小局灶性白质异常有关，在基底节部位最明显，此区域已经确定对跨多个皮质和皮质下大脑区域的信息传递和组织至关重要。

对 DCCT / EDIC 认知研究的近期分析也为微血管病变和认知之间的联系提供了令人信服的证据。在 18.5 年的随访期间，复杂的统计模型确定了 5 个变量来独立预测精神运动速度下降：年龄，低学历，终身 HbA1C 值较高和两个临床上显著的微血管并发症，即增殖性糖尿病视网膜病变和肾脏并发症的存在。此外，早期大血管病变（颈动脉中层管壁增厚）的标志与迟缓表现只有一点关系，但在最后的统计模型里，高血压、高胆固醇血症或腰围这些因素与认知结果无关。这项工作表明，微血管疾病是其他方面健康的 T1D 中年患者认知功能障碍突出的危险因素。事实上，那些关系的关联度很小，充其量可能反映 DCCT / EDIC 参与者相对较好的代谢控制和（或）血糖监测，以及他们得到了很好的健康管理。

几乎所有把认知与糖尿病患者微血管并发症联系起来的大型研究，都认为视网膜病变是其最强的生物医学预测指标。有趣的是，对非糖尿病的中年人的研究也发现，视网膜微动脉瘤的存在可能将认知损害的风险增加一倍。这在记忆、精神运动速度和所谓的额叶测试方面最为明显。多个研究已经反复证明视网膜微血管异常也增加脑萎缩和亚临床脑梗死的风险——特别是当血压也升高的时候。这些调查结果，连同视网膜和脑供血之间确定的结构同源性表明，视网膜微血管异常可作为脑微血管病的替代标记。因此，使用数字化眼底摄影不仅可以提供视网膜血管完整性的信息，也可对脑微循环进行无创性评估。我们可以想象代谢控制不佳的糖尿病成人患者将要发生的一系列事件。慢性高血糖致微血管病变，如果它影响大脑微血管结构的程度达到其影响视网膜和肾脏的程度，降低的脑血流和由此诱发的脑灌注不足可通过降低葡萄糖及其他营养物质对脑组织的传递效率来引起脑部异常的发展。

不幸的是，这种模式并不能解释为什么糖尿病患者，特别是那些在儿童期确诊的患者，在确诊的 2 年内就开始出现神经认知功能障碍，甚至比开始出现亚临床微血管并发症的时间早。其他一系列的代谢过程，尚未完全确定，也可能围绕诊断时间陆续发生，也可能通过这样一种方式影响脑发育，即像糖尿病微血管病变那样增加糖尿病患者对后续脑损害的敏感性。

成人 2 型糖尿病患者

认知表现

关于 2 型糖尿病（T2D）患者的早期研究是为了验证糖尿病引起老化过程加速的假设。由于记忆改变是正常衰老的最早表现之一，那些集中于学习和记忆能力的早期研究发现，T2D 老年人患者在学习新信息并保留一段时间（30 分钟以上）的能力确实大大受损。从那时起这些基本看法就已经被复制和扩展，而现在清楚的是，相对于年龄匹配的非糖尿病成人，T2D 患者对要求神经运动速度，执行功能和解决问题的能力，以及学习和记忆的测试都表现较差。效应值在最好的情况下也较小——Cohen's 效应值通常为 0.25～0.5 个标准差，与 T1D 成人患者的研究报告类似。学习和记忆障碍的存在是 1 型和 2 型糖尿病成人患者认知特点最明显的区别。

回顾这一主题的大量文献中，在影响最大的认知区域方面及组间影响程度方面，各种研究存在较大程度的变异性。在某种程度上，这可能反映了人口老龄化的异质性：这些研究招募的老年人可能有显著不同的教育经历，也可能有其他疾病存在的情况（如高血压、血管疾病、超重/肥胖），情绪（如抑郁症）、代谢紊乱（如胰岛素抵抗或高胰岛素血症）和已知会影响认知测试表现的遗传特征[（如载脂蛋白 E4 抗体（apo E4）]。因此，更多近期的研究把这些类型的混杂变量考虑在内，并且一致发现糖尿病老年人的认知功能测试与未患糖尿病者只有轻微的不同。这一现象在三项研究的数据中得到了很好的例证，这三项研究招募了不同类型的研究对象（表 5-2）。

表 5-2　三项研究中糖尿病-非糖尿病对照组的三个认知领域的效应值

	研究 1：平均年龄 50 岁	研究 2：平均年龄 66 岁	研究 3：平均年龄 73 岁	3 个研究的均值
处理速度	0.50	0.37	0.43	0.43
执行功能	0.45	0.25	0.37	0.36
学习/记忆	0.23	0.16	0.37	0.25

研究 1 总共包含了 100 名研究对象；研究 2 总共包含了 106 名研究对象；研究 3 总共包含了 136 名研究对象。

研究 1 集中在中年人（年龄范围：34～65 岁，平均 50 岁），从糖尿病研究注册表中招募了 50 人同时从他们的非糖尿病朋友或家人中招募了 50 人。研究 2 的数据来自全科医生办公室的 68 名老年糖尿病患者（年龄范围：56～80 岁，平均 66 岁）和 38 名未患糖尿病者，他们彼此是朋友、家人或熟人；测试分成两个时间点，前后间隔 4 年。研究 3 从内科招募了 92 名高龄（年龄范围：大于 60 岁，平均 73）的 2 型糖尿病患者，作为对照的是 44 名同龄的健康配偶或是有背部疼痛和周围神经疾病的门诊患者。三项研究的所有受试者都完成了基本医疗评估，并且进行了相同的用以评估三大认知区域的神经认知测试：信息处理、执行功能，以及学习和记忆。表 5-2 显示，同一认知域内，糖尿病和非糖尿病受试者的表现明显不同，这取决于研究对象的人口学和生物医学特性。然而，在这些不同的群体，某些区域始终比其他区域对糖尿病的影响更为敏感，处理速度受到的影响最强烈（$d=0.43$），其次是执行功能（$d=0.36$）。学习和记忆能力似乎受影响最小（平均 $d=0.2$ S），但这可能反映了一个事实,即这些技能受到其他生物医学并发症的强烈影响,特别是高血压——通常与 T2D 有关联。的确,在学习/记忆域有最大统计学意义的研究,对高血压进行后续统计调整后却没有统计学差异。

在这些横断面研究中,由于较长的糖尿病病程和较差的代谢控制是最一致的与较差的认知表现相关的两个变量,人们可能会期望看到糖尿病患者认知功能相对于对照受试者,在纵向随访研究下降更快。出人意料的是,近期的两项老年人研究数据未找到这种可能性的证据。例如,研究 2 对糖尿病和非糖尿病患者随访了 4 年之久,虽然执行功能的表现(不是处理速度和记忆)随时间的推移而逐渐下降,但两组受试者的下降水平是平行的:没有组别-时间的相互作用。在另一项研究中也有注意到类似的模式,即随访一组"老寿星"(85 岁患和未患糖尿病的老人)5 年多的时间。在需要快速反应的测试中,虽然糖尿病受试者比非糖尿病对照受试者的得分更低,但没有证据表明糖尿病受试者的表现有特异性的下降。这些结果表明,糖尿病相关的认知功能障碍发展的病理生理过程,至今仍不太清楚,它可能不是持续的,这种方式与退化过程不同。它不像阿尔茨海默病那样不可避免地导致痴呆发生,而是可能在特定时间里发生了认知功能障碍,也许是某个机会的特定窗口期或关键时期。

综述的数据与几个大型纵向研究结果的差异表明,糖尿病大大增加了痴呆发生的风险,虽然这仍存在争议。对这个主题的全面讨论超出了本章的范围,但一篇优秀的系统综述(包含 14 篇高品质的流行病学研究结果)指出,糖尿病增加患者痴呆的风险。对于阿尔茨海默病,糖尿病增加风险的范围是 50%～100%,而糖尿病增加血管性痴呆的风险是从 100%～150%。多种激素、代谢和血管异常与糖尿病和痴呆都相关,包括缺血性脑血管疾病,高血糖症相关的神经毒性(葡萄糖毒性),胰岛素和淀粉样蛋白代谢改变,氧化应激增加,以及 C 反应蛋白、白介素 6 和肿瘤坏死因子-α 等炎症因子释放增加,但是目前,T2D 和痴呆之间统计关联的因果途径仍然不明。

我们专注于研究 T2D 老年人,却忽视了儿童和青少年患 T2D 的风险也在增加,这主要是因为西方国家肥胖的流行。到目前为止,只有一个研究系统评估了一小群患 T2D 的病态肥胖的青少年,并与无糖尿病或胰岛素抵抗的同龄肥胖青少年进行了比较。尽管只是相对较短的时间内被诊断为糖尿病(平均 23.4 个月),但在多个神经认知域,糖尿病患者比非糖尿同龄者表现更差。其效应值大概是先前已报告的 1 型或 2 型糖尿病的成人患者的 2 倍，范围是 d =1.3（IQ 值）至 d =0.7（语言记忆、神经运动速度、执行功能）。脑部结构异常也存在，全脑和额叶白质体积减小，以及多个脑区灰质和白质微结构的显著改变。虽然糖尿病受试者没有血管异常的临床证据，单作者推测，这些脑部结构和功能的变化可能是亚临床血管改变，葡萄糖和脂质代谢改变和胰岛素异常的结果。这项工作可以明确的是，在青少年中，这些糖尿病相关的神经认知异常可能在相对较短的时间内出现，而他们的大脑仍处于正常发育的状态。

电生理特性

感觉诱发电位、事件相关电位和静息脑电图的记录显示 T2D 老年人神经迟缓，这与 T1D 患者的报道相似。糖尿病诊断后不久便会出现诱发电位潜伏期延长，这在患有外周神经病变的患者更为明显。随着时间的推移，这种现象也相当稳定。尽管在 4 年的时间里 HbA1C 值显著增加（6.7%～7.5%），视觉诱发电位潜伏期没有随着时间的推移而恶化加剧。事件相关电位潜伏期——当受试者正在关注传入的刺激和识别不常发生的目标时进行的测试——在 T2D 年轻人和老人中均有 4%～11% 的延迟。患有糖尿病似乎足以引起这些变化，因为无论是代谢控制程度，还是糖尿病病程的持续时间都与潜伏期测试无关。

静息状态下的 EEG 记录显示 T2D 患者神经迟缓，这与之前 T1D 儿童和成人的报道相似。在使用这种方法的为数不多的报告中，有一个报告指出 α 波活动减少和 θ 波（表示慢波活动增多）活动增加，特别是在中央和顶叶电极。δ 波也稍有增加，但如此小的样本量（13 名糖尿病患者和 8 名对照对象）限制了这些研究结果的敏感性和普遍性。

脑血管结果

脑血流量减少是 T2D 老年人患者确定的现象。一个使用 SPELT 技术的早期研究显示，在所研究的两个半球中的所有脑区 CBF 都减少 15%。这种影响的大小与疾病严重程度相关，而疾病的严重程度依据治疗类型来定义。例如，那些用胰岛素治疗的严重的糖尿病类型，与那些只需饮食改变来治疗的较轻的糖尿病类型相比，大脑额叶的脑血流量显著降低。

使用连续动脉自旋标记 MRI 技术的近期研究也指出，与健康对照组相比，糖尿病患者（平均年龄 60 岁）的脑血流量显著减少。虽然对于所有的受试者来说，顶枕区的脑血流量比额区或颞区更高，但糖尿病组的 CBF 值明显低于对照组。在糖尿病患者中存在大脑皮质和皮质下萎缩的证据，表现为灰质和白质体积减小及脑脊液（CSF）容积增大。CBF 减少与脑体积相关，两者都与慢性高血糖症（视网膜病、高血压和升高的 HbA1C 值）的标记物相关。这些结果，与前面 T1D 患者的报道类似，为大脑皮质和皮质下萎缩、脑灌注和慢性高血糖的生物标志物之间强力的相互作用，提供了最好的证据。

然而，人们对脑血流量和认知测试表现之间的关系仍缺乏理解。在为数不多的研究中，有一项研究测量了糖尿病成人患者和非糖尿病成人患者的 CBF 和认知功能，在这两组受试者中，CBF 总量与任务中更好的表现相关，这些任务要求快速的信息处理能力、注意力和执行能力。糖尿病组的认知功能测试表现比对照组更差，他们的大脑体积更小，CBF 绝对值更低。然而，当 CBF 绝对值用脑体积校正后，校正的 CBF 值在两组中相似。这些意外的发现表明，至少在静息状态下，糖尿病患者相对较差的认知功能与校正的 CBF 总量值没有明显的相关性。目前仍有待确定是否其他血管机制（例如，对于血管的变化，脑血管反应性异常）参与糖尿病相关的神经认知功能障碍。

脑结构异常

脑萎缩和脑白质病变在 2 型糖尿病老年人患者的研究报道中经常出现，但细节的变化差异取决于患者群体状态和所使用的神经成像技术。

从社区招募的糖尿病成人患者和非糖尿病成人患者的大样本研究结果表明，T2D 与较小的灰质容积（减少 22ml），更大的皮质下萎缩（侧脑室体积增加 7ml）和更大的白质病变体积（增加 57%）有关。用磁共振（MR）图像的自动评估可确定结构的变化，并且（意外地）发现女性比男性更显著，这与较高的 HbA1C 值和老龄有关，与高血压、糖尿病病程或高血脂无关。一项针对相同群体的早期的 MRI 数据的定性分析也表明这群人较差的认知功能，尤其是在信息处理速度和抽象推理的测试上更为显著，这与皮质萎缩的程度和白质病变有关。此外，皮质萎缩的程度与微血管和大血管并发症的存在呈正相关，与降脂药物的使用呈负相关。

当使用相同的神经影像学和神经认知评估参数来比较在年龄（平均61 岁）、性别、智商评估上相匹配的 2 型和 1 型糖尿病受试者时，2 型糖尿病的患者被发现有更大的皮质萎缩和更深的脑白质病变，效应值范围是 0.5～0.66。这一点引起人们的注意是因为，作为一个群体，2 型糖尿病受试者代谢控制更好，糖尿病病程较短（7 年 vs34 年），且临床上显著的微血管病变率较低（激光治疗视网膜病变：8%vs38%）。因为他们有更高的大血管疾病发生率和更多的动脉粥样硬化危险因素（如高胆固醇血症、高三酰甘油血症、高血压、高 BMI），所以，很有可能 T2D 患者脑异常的病理生理过程在性质上与 1 型糖尿病患者不同。这项研究强烈提示动脉粥样硬化的危险因素与 T2D 患者的大脑异常有关，但其他一些针对患有前驱糖尿病的高龄者的研究表明，糖耐量受损和（或）胰岛素调节也有助于 2 型糖尿病患者大脑异常的发展。

海马体萎缩在 T2D 患者中也很明显，而且这些变化可能在病程相对早期出现。45～70 岁且无临床大血管并发症的糖尿病成人患者，与年龄匹配的健康对照组相比，其海马体积明显较小（5.4 cm^3 vs. 6.2 cm^3；d =1.4），但额叶/颞叶脑体积却相似。即时记忆表现也受损，这些表现得分与海马体积相关（r=0.25）。最好的海马体积萎缩预测因子是 HbA1C，这解释了多元建模中 33%的方差，高血压和血脂异常对此结果均无影响。

因为只有海马体在这项研究中表现为体积减小，作者认为该结构尚未在其他近期的神经成像研究中进行特定评估，特别易受到糖尿病相关的代谢和血管变化的损害。这种可能性与证明海马体对代谢事件（如低血糖）的敏感性的其他数据相一致，并且这种可能性也被海马体积与代谢控制之间的强关联性所加强，对年纪相对较轻且没有白质高信号和其他脑异常的糖尿病老年人患者进行研究得出了这种强关联性。由于针对糖耐量受损的非糖尿病老人的早期研究指出了类似的结果模型，因此 2型糖尿病成人 CNS 的变化可能是代谢和微血管变化的结果——与胰岛素抵抗、葡萄糖失调和葡萄糖进入大脑结构的高效运输有关，这种解释是合理的。

在鹿特丹研究和檀香山-亚洲老龄化研究中也发现了糖尿病老年人患者显著的海马萎缩。不仅在后者的研究中，糖尿病患者的海马体萎缩风险比非糖尿病患者增加 2 倍，而且一个辅助尸检的研究证实了糖尿病和载脂蛋白 Eε4（ApoEε4）等位基因的存在有协同作用，而 ApoEε4 等位基因是公认的阿尔茨海默病的遗传危险因素。同时具有糖尿病和阿尔茨海默病的受试者与单独只有一种疾病的受试者相比，他们在海马体有更多的神经炎斑，在海马体和皮质有更多的神经原纤维缠结，脑淀粉样血管病的风险显著提高。认知评估还指出，T2D 的诊断增加了患阿尔茨海默病或血管性痴呆的危险，特别是那些携带 ApoEε4 等位基因的人。

T2D 患者的皮质萎缩随着时间的推移而进展在近期才被研究，现在很清楚的是，尽管可察觉的脑萎缩增加在 4 年的时间内才会明显，但这种影响的幅度非常小。在基线水平，糖尿病患者与人口学上相似的非糖尿病受试者相比，其大脑总体积更小（1.36%），CSF 量更大（0.98%），但在其他两项测试数据中水平相当：侧脑室体积和白质高信号。4 年后，55个糖尿病受试者只在一种脑萎缩检测结果上表现出了相对较高的增加（0.11%），即侧脑室体积。随着时间的推移，预测糖尿病患者变化最强的因素是年龄和高血压病史，不是 HbA1C，也不是任何与大脑体积变化相关联的其他代谢变量。这些神经影像学研究结果与从这些受试者身上收集的认知数据相似，这在前面已经讨论。这些结果加在一起，并没有为这一假设——糖尿病加快大脑退化速率与在阿尔茨海默病中看到的情况相类似——提供支持。至于在随访更长时间之后、评估时年龄更大（平均年龄为 65 岁）、代谢控制更差（平均 HbA1C 为 7.0%）或有更多的血管并发症时，这些受试者是否会出现更大的变化，这还有待确定。

神经化学异常

用质子磁共振波谱评估的 T2D 成人患者表明，一些脑代谢产物的改变，与年龄较大的青少年和 1 型糖尿病成人患者中所报道的稍有不同。肌醇（mI）浓度的变化是最突出的，尤其是在额叶白质区域，在代谢控制良好（HbA1C=7.1%）的相对健康的患者中肌醇增加的范围是 16%（左半球）～26%（右半球）。尽管与 HBAIC 值无关，肌醇值与脑血管危险因素量表的评分有关，这表明该额叶胶质增生继发于脑血管的变化。对其他的神经代谢因子也进行了测定，包括 N-乙酰基-天门冬氨酸（NAA）、谷氨酸、谷氨酰胺、胆碱，但这些值在糖尿病和非糖尿受试者之间没有差异，这与 1 型糖尿病成人患者的研究所报道的结果相反。

其他研究代谢控制较差的（HbA1C 为 8.0%）胰岛素治疗的 2 型糖尿病患者的调查者，在白质和灰质也发现肌醇浓度升高，以及灰质的胆碱（CHO）值增加。此外，那些大脑代谢物和 HbA1C 值无关，但与并发症有很大的关系。与那些没有周围神经病变的受试者相比，有周围神经病变的患者有更高的胆碱值及更高的白质肌醇浓度。另外，神经病变、白质异常和糖尿病病程之间有很大的相关性，这与以下的观点相一致，即脑代谢产物的变化反映了胶质增生，反过来，胶质增生继发于渗透性改变和（或）胰岛粥样多肽的脑沉积。谷氨酸/谷氨酰胺水平在本研究中没有测量，NAA 测量值与非糖尿病对照者相似。合并考虑，这些研究和那些对 T1D 患者进行的研究表明，大脑的神经代谢改变可以在这两种疾病中发生明显变化，但 T1D 成人发生的变化最大。需要更多的研究使用 MRS 技术来直接比较两种类型的糖尿病患者，并仔细确定生物医学并发症的性质和程度。

生物医学风险因素

现象学上，T2D 老年人（和青少年）患者的神经认知特征类似于 T1D 成人（和儿童）患者。两个群体都有神经和运动减慢的证据——这是一个普遍存在的发现，并且两者在注意力和执行功能上都有相近幅度的减慢（d 为 0.3～0.4）。一个主要的特点是 T2D 患者通常（但不总是）在学习和记忆上表现更差，而相关的记忆障碍在 T1D 患者中很少报道。像 T1D 患者一样，T2D 成年人患者也有神经迟缓，脑灌注不足，更多的皮质萎缩和脑白质束微观结构异常，以及相似的但不完全相同的脑神经代谢改变。

潜藏于 2 型糖尿病相关神经并发症的发展背后的生物危险因素，我们仍然知之甚少，尽管不少研究因素已经被提出。我们知道，慢性高血糖和糖尿病的长病程都与认知功能障碍有很强的相关性，血管危险因素

（如高血压、高胆固醇和肥胖）和微血管、大血管并发症的存在也是一样。胰岛素失调在 T2D 患者中常见，也可能通过多种机制对神经认知进程产生影响。一些近期的文章也认为，低血糖可能对 T2D 患者的认知有不利的影响，并且这可能是后期发展为痴呆的关键危险因子。表 5-3 总结了一些与 T2D 相关的脑功能障碍最合理的潜在路径。不幸的是，除非研究人员对接受全面神经认知和生物医学/代谢评估的糖尿病患者和非糖尿病成人患者进行大样本的研究，否则这些候选预测变量的贡献将仍然是未知的。

表 5-3　2 型糖尿病 CNS 损害的潜在路径

血糖水平改变
- 低血糖反应
- 蛋白糖化
- 神经细胞内钙离子稳态改变
- 血管升压素增加

血管疾病
- 微血管疾病
- 大血管疾病
- 内皮功能紊乱
- 氧化应激
- 血-脑屏障通透性改变

胰岛素抵抗
- CNS 血糖利用率改变
- CNS 胰岛素信号缺失
- β-淀粉样沉积
- Tau 蛋白磷酸化

广义上来说，如果代谢控制不佳，是神经认知并发症的发生发展的主要危险因素，人们则期望通过努力改进代谢控制来提高相应的认知情况。对这一观点的支持来自单一的大规模随机临床试验，旨在检验这一假设。用二甲双胍治疗的 T2D 老人患者随机在治疗方案中加入 2 种药物中的一种，他们要么接受噻唑烷二酮胰岛素增敏剂——罗格列酮治疗，要么接受磺酰脲类降糖药——格列本脲治疗，并且随访 6 个月。在随机分配之前及研究完成之后，都对患者进行了认知测试，患者也随着时间的推移进行了空腹血糖值的测量。无论使用哪种药物，在一个具有挑战性的工作记忆测试中的表现显著改善与 FPG 的改善有关，而且，FPG 的改善幅度与工作记忆测试中的错误数量之间存在线性关系。这项研究首次为糖尿病相关的认知功能障碍可能是可逆的这一观点提供了有力的证据。

临床实践建议

糖尿病相关的认知功能障碍在大多数情况下是轻微的，很少能满足临床上显著损害的标准。然而，无论是哪种类型的糖尿病成人（和儿童）患者，其心理效率降低是常见的，这种情况足以使患者精气神减弱，破坏其在课堂、工作场所和家庭中的最佳表现。虽然没有前瞻性研究证明心理效率开始发生变化的确切时间，初步证据表明，这些变化在病程早期开始，并会随着时间的推移而加重。也就是说，糖尿病患者可能会在诊断后不久就出现轻微的功能变化，但是那些长期代谢控制较差及有并发症的患者可能会出现持续的神经认知下降。如果患者报告说，他/她在学校、工作及日常活动能力方面（包括糖尿病自我管理行为）正在经历功能下降，或者如果患者询问糖尿病对功能的影响，建议使用下面的方法来筛选和评估。

1. **与患者进行开放式的讨论以记录患者的认知损伤和现有的功能水平，尤其要关注对优势功能缺陷的感知**　临床医生应要求患者以现象学的方式描述自己的经历，并提供他们所观察到的具体实例，如他们所犯错误的类型或心理效率发生的各种变化。尽可能获得来自于患者环境的个体认知功能下降的证据。患者还应该描述这些事件发生的频率及它们如何影响日常活动。收集患者并发的情感状态（郁闷、焦虑、压力），事件发生时（如低血糖症或最近血糖下降）代谢状态，以及代谢控制的整体水平这方面的信息，也非常重要。

2. **确定导致认知能力下降的其他潜在的生物医学病因来源**　常见病症包括高血压、高胆固醇血症、肥胖症和睡眠质量差。

3. **告知患者认知功能障碍的可能原因**　急性低血糖是公认的导致

短暂的认知功能障碍的原因，患者应知道它是如何引起心理效率短暂降低的。情绪也可以干扰认知功能。患者应了解认知功能障碍和长期代谢控制不佳的关系——尤其是当它与临床上显著的微血管并发症相关时。提高代谢控制和改善认知功能之间的连接可能会促使患者更积极地改善高血糖。应对患者提出忠告，即他们也许能够减少认知问题的严重性或阻止其变得更加严重。

4. **如果患者报告有日常活动和（或）执行疾病管理的任务有显著的困难时，应参考临床神经心理学家的评估/服务** 神经心理学家可以系统地记录认知优势和劣势，确定受损程度，并与医疗护理团队合作，以确定除糖尿病之外可能会破坏认知能力的其他因素。因为这种评估的费用较高，我们应该有对患者熟悉的其他人证实的一些证据，来说明此人有认知的缓慢变化。

5. **推荐认知矫正服务应当谨慎** 没有研究调查认知康复是否能有效地扭转糖尿病相关的认知功能障碍，但其他情况的研究表明，当运用这些方法治疗证据充分的认知功能障碍的患者时，其效果一般。只有在完成全面的神经心理学评估之后才能进行转诊。在另一方面，建议将临床努力集中在改善血糖控制上。

6. **一旦确定认知能力的下降，建议专业人员对其进行持续监测** 除了监测神经认知功能以外，如果认知能力继续下降，应该排除其他生物医学的解释。

7. **患者可能需要帮助来适应他们新的"正常的"认知水平** 如果烦躁不安或焦虑伴随认知障碍，可以使用精神药物治疗。

参 考 文 献

Abbatecola AM, Lattanzio F, Spazzafumo L, Molinari AM, Cioffi M, Canonico R, DiCioccio L, Paolisso G: Adiposity predicts cognitive decline in older persons with diabetes: a 2-year follow-up. *PLoS ONE* 5:e10333, 2010

Ajilore O, Haroon E, Kumaran S, Darwin C, Binesh N, Mintz J, Miller J, Thomas MA, Kumar A: Measurement of brain metabolites in patients with type 2 diabetes and major depression using proton magnetic resonance spectroscopy. *Neuropsychopharmacology* 32:1224–1231, 2007

Akisaki T, Sakurai T, Takata T, Umegaki H, Araki A, Mizuno S, Tanaka S, Ohashi Y, Iguchi A, Yokono K, Ito H: Cognitive dysfunction associates with white matter hyperintensities and subcortical atrophy on magnetic resonance imaging of the elderly diabetes mellitus Japanese Elderly Diabetes Intervention Trial (J-EDIT). *Diabetes/Metabolism Research and Reviews* 22:376–384, 2006

Allen KV, Frier BM, Strachan MWJ: The relationship between type 2 diabetes and cognitive dysfunction: longitudinal studies and their methodological limitations. *European Journal of Pharmacology* 490:169–175, 2004

Araki Y, Nomura M, Tanaka H, Yamamoto H, Yamamoto T, Tsukaguchi I, Nakamura H: MRI of the brain in diabetes mellitus. *Neuroradiology* 36:101–103, 1994

Arvanitakis Z, Wilson RS, Li Y, Aggarwal NT, Bennett DA: Diabetes and function in different cognitive systems in older individuals without dementia. *Diabetes Care* 29:560–565, 2006

Asimakopoulou KG, Hampson SE, Morrish NJ: Neuropsychological functioning in older people with type 2 diabetes: the effect of controlling for confounding factors. *Diabetic Medicine* 19:311–316, 2002

Auer RN: Hypoglycemic brain damage. *Metabolic Brain Disease* 19:169–175, 2004

Auer RN, Hugh J, Cosgrove E, Curry B: Neuropathologic findings in three cases of profound hypoglycemia. *Clinical Neuropathology* 8:63–68, 1989

Auer RN, Wieloch T, Olsson Y, Siesjo BK: The distribution of hypoglycemic brain damage. *Acta Neuropathologica* 64:177–191, 1984

Awad N, Gagnon M, Messier C: The relationship between impaired glucose tolerance, type 2 diabetes, and cognitive function. *Journal of Clinical and Experimental Neuropsychology* 26:1044–1080, 2004

Biessels GJ, Deary IJ, Ryan CM: Cognition and diabetes: a lifespan perspective. *Lancet: Neurology* 7:184–190, 2008

Biessels G-J, Staekenborg S, Brunner E, Scheltens P: Risk of dementia in diabetes mellitus: a systematic review. *Lancet: Neurology* 5:64–74, 2006

Brands AMA, Biessels GJ, Kappelle LJ, de Haan EHF, de Valk HW, Algra A, Kessels RPC, Utrecht Diabetic Encephalopathy Study Group: Cognitive functioning and brain MRI in patients with type 1 and type 2 diabetes mellitus: a comparative study. *Dementia and Geriatric Cognitive Disorders* 23:343–350, 2007

Brands AMA, Kessels RPC, Biessels GJ, Hoogma RPLM, Henselmans JML, van der Beek Boter JW, Kappelle LJ, de Haan EHF: Cognitive performance, psychological well-being, and brain magnetic resonance imaging in older patients with type 1 diabetes. *Diabetes* 55:1800–1806, 2006

Brands AMA, Biessels G-J, de Haan EHF, Kappelle LJ, Kessels RPC: The effects of type 1 diabetes on cognitive performance: a meta-analysis. *Diabetes Care* 28:726–735, 2005

Brismar T, Hyllienmark L, Ekberg K, Johansson B-L: Loss of temporal lobe beta power in young adults with type 1 diabetes mellitus. *Neuroreport* 13:2469–2473, 2002

Bruehl H, Sweat V, Hassenstab J, Polyakov V, Convit A: Cognitive impairment in nondiabetic middle-aged and older adults is associated with insulin resistance. *Journal of Clinical and Experimental Neuropsychology* 32:487–493, 2010

Cardoso S, Correia S, Santos RX, Carvalho C, Santos MS, Oliveira CR, Perry G, Smith MA, Zhu X, Moreira PI: Insulin is a two-edged knife on the brain. *Journal of Alzheimer's Disease* 18:483–507, 2009

Cavalieri M, Ropele S, Petrovic K, Pluta-Fuerst A, Homayoon N, Enzinger C, Grazer A, Katschnig P, Schwingenschuh P, Berghold A, Schmidt R: Metabolic syndrome, brain magnetic resonance imaging, and cognition. *Diabetes Care* 33:2489–2495, 2010

Chalmers J, Risk MTA, Kean DM, Grant R, Ashworth B, Campbell IW: Severe amnesia after hypoglycemia. *Diabetes Care* 14:922–925, 1991

Cicerone KD, Dahlberg C, Malec JF, Langenbahn DM, Felicetti T, Kneipp S, Ellmo W, Kalmar K, Giacino JT, Harley JP, Laatsch L, Morse PA, Catanese J: Evidence-based cognitive rehabilitation: updated review of the literature from 1998 through 2002. *Archives of Physical Medicine and Rehabilitation* 86:1681–1692, 2005

Cole AR, Astell A, Green C, Sutherland C: Molecular connexions between dementia and diabetes. *Neuroscience and Biobehavioral Review* 31:1046–1063, 2007

Convit A: Links between cognitive impairment in insulin resistance: an explanatory model. *Neurobiology of Aging* 26(Suppl. 1):S31–S35, 2005

Convit A, Wolf OT, Tarshish C, de Leon MJ: Reduced glucose tolerance is associated with poor memory performance and hippocampal atrophy among normal elderly. *Pro Nat Acad Sci* 100:2019–2022, 2003

Cooper LS, Wong TY, Klein R, Sharrett AR, Bryan N, Hubbard LD, Couper DJ, Heiss G, Sorlie PD: Retinal microvascular abnormalities and MRI-defined subclinical cerebral infarction: the Atherosclerosis Risk in Communities Study. *Stroke* 37:82–86, 2006

Craft S, Watson GS: Insulin and neurodegenerative disease: shared and specific mechanisms. *Lancet: Neurology* 3:169–178, 2004

Cukierman T, Gerstein HC, Williamson JD: Cognitive decline and dementia in diabetes: systematic overview of prospective observational studies. *Diabetologia* 48:2460–2469, 2005

Cukierman-Yaffe T, Gerstein HC, Anderson C, Zhao F, Sleight P, Hilbrich L, Jackson SHD, Yusuf S, Teo K, ONTARGET/TRANSCEND Investigators: Glucose intolerance and diabetes as risk factors for cognitive impairment in people at high cardiovascular risk: results from the ONTARGET/TRANSCEND Research Programme. *Diabet Res Clin Prac* 83:387–393, 2009

de Bresser J, Tiehuis AM, van den Berg E, Reijmer YD, Jongen C, Kappelle LJ, Mali WP, Viergever MA, Biessels GJ: Progression of cerebral atrophy and white matter hyperintensities in patients with type 2 diabetes. *Diabetes Care* 33:1309–1314, 2010

de la Torre JC: Alzheimer's disease is a vasocognopathy: a new term to describe its nature. *Neurological Research* 26:517–524, 2004

Deary I, Crawford J, Hepburn DA, Langan SJ, Blackmore LM, Frier BM: Severe hypoglycemia and intelligence in adult patients with insulin-treated diabetes. *Diabetes* 42:341–344, 1993

Dejgaard A, Gade A, Larsson H, Balle V, Parving A, Parving H: Evidence for diabetic encephalopathy. *Diabet Med* 8:162–167, 1991

den Heijer T, Vermeer SE, van Dijk EJ, Prins ND, Koudstaal PJ, Hofman A, Breteler MMB: Type 2 diabetes and atrophy of medial temporal lobe structures on brain MRI. *Diabetologia* 46:1604–1610, 2003

Dey J, Misra A, Desai NG, Mahapatra AK, Padma MV: Cerebral function in a relatively young subset of NIDDM patients. *Diabetologia* 38:251, 1995

Diabetes Control and Complications Trial / Epidemiology of Diabetes Interventions and Complications Study Research Group, Jacobson AM, Musen G, Ryan CM, Silvers N, Cleary P, Waberski B, Burwood A, Weinger K, Bayless M, Dahms W, Harth J: Long-term effects of diabetes and its treatment on cognitive function. *N Engl J Med* 356:1842–1852, 2007

Dik MG, Jonker C, Comijs HC, Deeg DJH, Kok A, Yaffe K, Penninx BW: Contribution of metabolic syndrome to components of cognition in older individuals. *Diabetes* 30:2655–2660, 2007

Elderkin-Thompson V, Kumar A, Bilker W, Dunkin JJ, Mintz J, Moberg PJ, Mesholam RI, Gur RE: Neuropsychological deficits among patients with late-onset minor and major depression. *Archives of Clinical Neuropsychology* 18:529–549, 2003

Elias M, Elias P, Sullivan L, Wolf P, Dagostino R: Obesity, diabetes and cognitive deficit: the Framingham Heart Study. *Neurobiology of Aging* 26:11–16, 2005

Ferguson SC, Blanc A, Perros P, McCrimmon RJ, Best JJK, Wardlaw JM, Deary IJ, Frier BM: Cognitive ability and brain structure in type 1 diabetes: relation to microangiopathy and preceding severe hypoglycemia. *Diabetes* 52:149–156, 2003

Flory JD, Manuck SB, Ferrell RE, Ryan CM, Muldoon MF: Memory performance and the apolipoprotein E polymorphism in a community sample of middle-aged adults. *American Journal of Medical Genetics (Neuropsychiatric Genetics)* 96:707–711, 2000

Frier BM: How hypoglycaemia can affect the life of a person with diabetes. *Diabetes/Metabolism Research and Reviews* 24:87–92, 2008

Fujioka M, Okuchi K, Hiramatsu K, Sakaki T, Sakaguchi S, Ishii Y: Specific changes in human brain after hypoglycemic injury. *Stroke* 28:584–587, 1997

Fülesdi B, Limburg M, Bereczki D, Michels RPJ, Neuwirth G, Legemate D, Valikoics A, Csiba L: Impairment of cerebrovascular reactivity in long-term type 1 diabetes. *Diabetes* 46:1840–1845, 1997

Gaudieri PA, Chen R, Greer TF, Holmes CS: Cognitive function in children with type 1 diabetes: a meta-analysis. *Diabetes Care* 31:1892–1897, 2008

Geissler A, Fründ R, Schölmerich J, Feuerbach S, Zietz B: Alterations of cerebral metabolism in patients with diabetes mellitus studied by proton magnetic resonance spectroscopy. *Experimental and Clinical Endocrinology and Diabetes* 111:421–427, 2003

Gold AE, Deary IJ, Frier BM: Recurrent severe hypoglycaemia and cognitive function in type 1 diabetes. *Diabet Med* 10:503–508, 1993

Gold SM, Dziobek I, Sweat V, Tirsi A, Rogers K, Bruehl H, Tsui W, Richardson S, Javier E, Convit A: Hippocampal damage and memory impairments as possible early brain complications of type 2 diabetes. *Diabetologia* 50:711–719, 2007

Gunstad J, Lhotsky A, Wendell CR, Ferrucci L, Zonderman AB: Longitudinal examination of obesity and cognitive function: results from the Baltimore Longitudinal Study of Aging. *Neuroepidemiology* 34:222–229, 2010

Haan MN: Therapy insight: type 2 diabetes mellitus and the risk of late-onset Alzheimer's disease. *Nature Clinical Practice: Neurology* 2:159–166, 2006

Hallschmid M, Schultes B: Central nervous insulin resistance: a promising target in the treatment of metabolic and cognitive disorders? *Diabetologia* 52:2264–2269, 2009

Hassing LB, Hofer SM, Nilsson SE, Berg S, Pedersen NL, McClearn G, Johansson B: Comorbid type 2 diabetes mellitus and hypertension exacerbates cognitive decline: evidence from a longitudinal study. *Age and Ageing* 33:355–361, 2004

Hissa MN, D'Almeida JA, Cremasco F, de Bruin VM: Event related P300 potentials in NIDDM patients without cognitive impairment and its relationship with previous hypoglycemic episodes. *Neuroendocrinology Letters* 23:226–230, 2002

Hyllienmark L, Maltez J, Dandenell A, Ludviggson J, Brismar T: EEG abnormalities with and without relation to severe hypoglycaemia in adolescents with type 1 diabetes. *Diabetologia* 48:412–419, 2005

Jacobson AM, Ryan CM, Cleary PA, Waberski BH, Weinger K, Musen G, Dahms W; Diabetes Control and Complications Trial / EDIC Research Group: Biomedical risk factors for decreased cognitive functioning in type 1 diabetes: an 18 year follow-up of the Diabetes Control and Complications Trial (DCCT) cohort. *Diabetologia* 54:245–255, 2011

Jiménez-Bonilla JF, Quirce R, Hernández A, Vallina NK, Guede C, Banzo I, Amado JA, Carril JM: Assessment of cerebral perfusion and cerebrovascular reserve in insulin-dependent diabetic patients without central neurological symptoms by means of 99mTc-HMPAO SPET with acetazolamide. *European Journal of Nuclear Medicine* 28:1647–1655, 2001

Jongen C, Biessels GJ: Structural brain imaging in diabetes: a methodological perspective. *European Journal of Pharmacology* 585:208–218, 2008

Jongen C, van der Grond J, Kappelle LJ, Biessels GJ, Viergever MA, Pluim JPW; Utrecht Diabetic Encephalopathy Study Group: Automated measurement of brain and white matter lesion volume in type 2 diabetes mellitus. *Diabetologia* 50:1509–1516, 2007

Kent S: Is diabetes a form of accelerated aging? *Geriatrics* 31:140–154, 1976

Keymeulen B, Jacobs A, de Metz K, de Sadeleer C, Bossuyt A, Somers G: Regional cerebral hypoperfusion in long-term type 1 (insulin-dependent) diabetic patients: relation to hypoglycaemic events. *Nuclear Medicine Communications* 16:10–16, 1995

Kim J, Basak JM, Holtzman DM: The role of apolipoprotein E in Alzheimer's disease. *Neuron* 63:287–303, 2009

Kloppenborg PR, van den Berg E, Kappelle LJ, Biessels GJ: Diabetes and other vascular risk factors for dementia: what factor matters most? A systematic review. *European Journal of Pharmacology* 585:97–108, 2008

Kodl CT, Franc DT, Rao JP, Anderson FS, Thomas W, Mueller BA, Lim KO, Seaquist ER: Diffusion tensor imaging identifies deficits in white matter microstructure in subjects with type 1 diabetes that correlate with reduced neurocognitive function. *Diabetes* 57:3083–3089, 2008

Korf ESC, White LR, Scheltens P, Launer LJ: Brain aging in very old men with type 2 diabetes. *Diabetes Care* 29:2268–2274, 2006

Kramer L, Fasching P, Madl C, Schneider B, Damjancic P, Waldhäusl W, Irsigler K, Grimm G: Previous episodes of hypoglycemic coma are not associated with permanent cognitive brain dysfunction in IDDM patients on intensive insulin treatment. *Diabetes* 47:1909–1914, 1998

Kreis R, Ross BD: Cerebral metabolic disturbances in patients with subacute and chronic diabetes mellitus: detection with proton MR spectroscopy. *Radiology* 184:123–130, 1992

Kumar A, Haroon E, Darwin C, Pham D, Ajilore O, Rodriguez G, Mintz J: Gray matter prefrontal changes in type 2 diabetes detected using MRI. *Journal of Magnetic Resonance Imaging* 27:14–19, 2008

Kumar A, Anstey KJ, Cherbuin N, Wen M, Sachdev PS: Association of type 2 diabetes with depression, brain atrophy, and reduced fine motor speed in a 60- to 64-year-old community sample. *American Journal of Geriatric Psychiatry* 16:989–998, 2008

Kumari M, Brunner E, Fuhrer R: Minireview: mechanisms by which the metabolic syndrome and diabetes impair memory. *Journal of Gerontology: Biological Sciences* 55:B228–B232, 2000

Kumari M, Marmot M: Diabetes and cognitive function in a middle-aged cohort: findings from the Whitehall II study. *Neurology* 65:1597–1603, 2005

Kurita A, Katayama K, Mochio S: Neurophysiological evidence for altered higher brain functions in NIDDM. *Diabetes Care* 19:361–364, 1996

Last D, Alsop DC, Abduljalil AM, Marquis RP, de Bazelaire C, Hu K, Cavallerano J, Novak V: Global and regional effects of type 2 diabetes on brain tissue volumes and cerebral vasoreactivity. *Diabetes Care* 30:1193–1199, 2007

Lesage SR, Mosley TH, Wong TY, Szklo M, Knopman DS, Catellier DJ, Cole SR, Klein R, Coresh J, Coker LH, Sharrett AR: Retinal microvascular abnormalities and cognitive decline: the ARIC 14-year follow-up. *Neurology* 73:862–868, 2009

Longstreth WT, Marino-Larson EK, Klein R, Wong TY, Sharrett AR, Lefkowitz D, Manolio T: Associations between findings on cranial magnetic resonance imaging and retinal photography in the elderly: the Cardiovascular Health Study. *American Journal of Epidemiology* 165:78–84, 2006

Lyoo IK, Yoon SJ, Musen G, Simonson DC, Weinger K, Ryan CM, Kim JE, Renshaw PF, Jacobson AM: Altered prefrontal glutamate-glutamine-γ-aminobutyric acid levels and relation to low cognitive performance and depressive symptoms in type 1 diabetes mellitus. *Archives of General Psychiatry* 66:879–887, 2009

MacLullich AMJ, Seckl JR: Diabetes and cognitive decline: are steroids the missing link? *Cell Metabolism* 7:286–287, 2008

Mäkimattila S, Malmberg-Cêder K, Häkkinen A-M, Vuori K, Salonen O, Summanen P, Yki-Järvinen H, Kaste M, Heikkinen S, Lundbom N, Roine RO: Brain metabolic alterations in patients with type 1 diabetes-hyperglycemia-induced injury. *Journal of Cerebral Blood Flow and Metabolism* 24:1393–1399, 2004

Manschot SM, Biessels GJ, de Valk HW, Algra A, Rutten GEHM, van der Grond J, Kappelle LJ, Utrecht Diabetic Encephalopathy Study Group: Metabolic and vascular determinants of impaired cognitive performance and abnormalities on brain magnetic resonance imaging in patients with type 2 diabetes. *Diabetologia* 50:2388–2397, 2007

Manschot SM, Brands AMA, van der Grond J, Kessels RPC, Algra A, Kappelle LJ, Biessels GJ, Utrecht Diabetic Encephalopathy Study Group: Brain magnetic resonance imaging correlates of impaired cognition in patients with type 2 diabetes. *Diabetes* 55:1106–1113, 2006

McNay EC: Insulin and ghrelin: peripheral hormones modulating memory and hippocampal function. *Current Opinion in Pharmacology* 7:628–632, 2007

Messier C, Gagnon M: Cognitive decline associated with dementia and type 2 diabetes: the interplay of risk factors. *Diabetologia* 52:2471–2474, 2009

Mooradian AD, Perryman K, Fitten J, Kavonian GD, Morley JE: Cortical function in elderly non-insulin dependent diabetic patients: behavioral and electrophysiologic studies. *Archives of Internal Medicine* 148:2369–2372, 1988

Moreo G, Mariani E, Pizzamiglio G, Colucci GB: Visual evoked potentials in NIDDM: a longitudinal study. *Diabetologia* 38:573–576, 1995

Musen G, Lyoo IK, Sparks CR, Weinger K, Hwang J, Ryan CM, Jimerson DC, Hennen J, Renshaw PF, Jacobson AM: Effects of type 1 diabetes on gray matter density as measured by voxel-based morphometry. *Diabetes* 55:326–333, 2006

Nagamachi S, Nishikawa T, Ono S, Ageta M, Matsuo T, Jinnouchi S, Hoshi H, Ohnishi T, Futami S, Watanabe K: Regional cerebral blood flow in diabetic patients: evaluation by N-isopropyl-123I-IMP with SPECT. *Nuclear Medicine Communications* 15:455–460, 1994

Nakamura Y, Takahashi M, Kitaguti M, Imaoka H, Kono N, Tarui S: Abnormal brainstem evoked potentials in diabetes mellitus: evoked potential testings and magnetic resonance imaging. *Electromyography and Clinical Neurophysiology* 31:243–249, 1991

Northam EA, Rankins D, Lin A, Wellard RM, Pell GS, Finch SJ, Werther GA, Cameron FJ: Central nervous system function in youth with type 1 diabetes 12 years after disease onset. *Diabetes Care* 32:445–450, 2009

Northam EA, Rankins D, Cameron FJ: Therapy insight: the impact of type 1 diabetes on brain development and function. *Nature Clinical Practice: Neurology* 2:78–86, 2006

Northam EA, Anderson PJ, Jacobs R, Hughes M, Warne GL, Werther GA: Neuropsychological profiles of children with type 1 diabetes 6 years after disease onset. *Diabetes Care* 24:1541–1546, 2001

Northam EA, Anderson PJ, Werther GA, Warne GL, Adler RG, Andrewes D: Neuropsychological complications of IDDM in children 2 years after disease onset. *Diabetes Care* 21:379–384, 1998

Obisesan TO, Obisesan OA, Martins S, Alamgir L, Bond V, Maxwell C, Gillum RF: High blood pressure, hypertension, and high pulse pressure are associated with poorer cognitive function in persons aged 60 and older: the Third National Health and Nutrition Examination Survey. *Journal of the American Geriatric Society* 56:501–509, 2008

Patiño-Fernández AM, Delamater AM, Applegate EB, Brady E, Eidson M, Nemery R, Gonzalez-Mendoza L, Richton S: Neurocognitive functioning in preschool-age children with type 1 diabetes mellitus. *Pediatric Diabetes* 11:424–430, 2010

Peila R, Rodriguez BL, Launer LJ: Type 2 diabetes, APOE gene, and the risk for dementia and related pathologies: the Honolulu-Asia Study. *Diabetes* 51:1256–1262, 2002

Perlmuter LC, Hakami MK, Hodgson-Harrington C, Ginsberg J, Katz J, Singer DE, Nathan DM: Decreased cognitive function in aging non-insulin-dependent diabetic patients. *American Journal of Medicine* 77:1043–1048, 1984

Perros P, Deary IJ, Sellar RJ, Best JJK, Frier BM: Brain abnormalities demonstrated by magnetic resonance imaging in adult IDDM patients with and without a history of recurrent severe hypoglycemia. *Diabetes Care* 20:1013–1018, 1997

Petrak F, Herpertz S: Treatment of depression in diabetes: an update. *Current Opinion in Psychiatry* 22:211–217, 2009

Pozzessere G, Rizzo PA, Valle E, Mollica MA, Meccia A, Morano S, Di Mario U, Andreani D, Morocutti C: Early detection of neurological involvement in IDDM and NIDDM: multimodal evoked potentials versus metabolic control. *Diabetes Care* 11:473–480, 1988

Qiu C, Cotch MF, Sigurdsson S, Klein R, Jonasson F, Klein BEK, Garcia M, Jonsson PV, Harris TB, Eiriksdottir G, Kjartansson O, van Buchem MA, Gudnason V, Launer LJ: Microvascular lesions in the brain and retina: the Age, Gene/Environment Susceptibility–Reykjavik Study. *Annals of Neurology* 65:569–576, 2009

Quirce R, Carril JM, Jiménez-Bonilla JF, Amado JA, Gutiérrez-Mendiguchía C, Banzo I, Blanco I, Uriarte I, Montero A: Semi-quantitative assessment of cerebral blood flow with 99mTc-HMPAO SPET in type 1 diabetic patients with no clinical history of cerebrovascular disease. *European Journal of Nuclear Medicine* 24:1507–1513, 1997

Reijmer YD, van den Berg E, Ruis C, Jaap Kappelle L, Biessels GJ: Cognitive dysfunction in patients with type 2 diabetes. *Diab Metab Res Re* 27:195–202, 2010

Reitz C, Tang M-X, Manly J, Mayeux R, Luchsinger JA: Hypertension and the risk of mild cognitive impairment. *Archives of Neurology* 64:1734–1740, 2007

Reske-Nielsen E, Lundbaek K, Rafaelsen OJ: Pathological changes in the central and peripheral nervous system of young long-term diabetics. *Diabetologia* 1:232–241, 1965

Reske-Nielsen E, Lundbaek K: Diabetic encephalopathy: diffuse and focal lesions of the brain in long-term diabetes. *Acta Neurologica Scandinavica* 39:273–290, 1963

Rohling ML, Faust ME, Beverly B, Demakis G: Effectiveness of cognitive rehabilitation following acquired brain injury: a meta-analytic re-examination of Cicerone et al.'s (2000, 2005) systematic reviews. *Neuropsychology* 23:20–39, 2009

Romero JR, Beiser A, Seshadri S, Benjamin FJ, Polak JF, Vasan RS, Au R, DeCarli C, Wolf PA: Carotid artery atherosclerosis, MRI indices of brain ischemia, aging, and cognitive impairment: the Framingham Study. *Stroke* 40:1590–1596, 2009

Ruis C, Biessels GJ, Gorter KJ, van den Donk M, Kappelle IJ, Rutten GEHM: Cognition in the early stage of type 2 diabetes. *Diabetes Care* 32:1261–1265, 2009

Ryan CM: Searching for the origin of brain dysfunction in diabetic children: going back to the beginning. *Pediatric Diabetes* 9:527–530, 2008

Ryan CM: Diabetes and brain damage: more (or less) than meets the eye? *Diabetologia* 49:2229–2233, 2006a

Ryan CM, Freed MI, Rood JA, Cobitz AR, Waterhouse BR, Strachan MWJ: Improving metabolic control leads to better working memory in adults with type 2 diabetes. *Diabetes Care* 29:345–351, 2006b

Ryan CM: Diabetes, aging, and cognitive decline. *Neurobiology of Aging* 26(Suppl. 1):S21–S25, 2005

Ryan CM, Geckle MO, Orchard TJ: Cognitive efficiency declines over time in adults with type 1 diabetes: effects of micro- and macrovascular complications. *Diabetologia* 46:940–948, 2003

Ryan CM, Geckle MO: Circumscribed cognitive dysfunction in middle-aged adults with type 2 diabetes. *Diabetes Care* 23:1486–1493, 2000

Sabri O, Hellwig D, Schreckenberger M, Schneider R, Kaiser H-J, Wagenknecht G, Mull M, Buell U: Influence of diabetes mellitus on regional cerebral glucose metabolism and regional cerebral blood flow. *Nuclear Medicine Communications* 21:19–29, 2000

Sabri O, Ringelstein E-B, Hellwig D, Schneider R, Schreckenberger M, Kaiser H-J, Mull M, Buell U: Neuropsychological impairment correlates with hypoperfusion and hypometabolism but not with severity of white matter lesions on MRI in patients with cerebral microangiopathy. *Stroke* 30:556–566, 1999

Saczynski JS, Jónsdóttir MK, Garcia MF, Jonsson PV, Peila R, Eiriksdottir G, Olafsdottir E, Harris TB, Gudnason V, Launer LJ: Cognitive impairment: an increasingly important complication of type 2 diabetes: the Age, Gene/Environment Susceptibility-Reykjavik Study. *American Journal of Epidemiology* 168:1132–1139, 2008

Schott JM, Price SL, Frost C, Whitwell JL, Rossor MN, Fox NC: Measuring atrophy in Alzheimer disease: a serial MRI study over 6 and 12 months. *Neurology* 65:119–124, 2005

Seidl R, Birnbacher R, Hauser E, Gernert G, Freilinger M, Schober E: Brainstem auditory evoked potentials and visually evoked potentials in young patients with IDDM. *Diabetes Care* 19:1220–1224, 1996

Shaw J: Epidemiology of childhood type 2 diabetes and obesity. *Pediatric Diabetes* 8:7–15, 2007

Stocco A, Lebiere C, Anderson JR: Conditional routing of information to the cortex: a model of the basal ganglia's role in cognitive coordination. *Psychological Review* 117:541–574, 2010

Strachan MWJ, Reynolds RM, Frier BM, Mitchell RJ, Price JF: The relationship between type 2 diabetes and dementia. *British Medical Bulletin* 88:131–146, 2008

Strachan MWJ, Deary IJ, Ewing FME, Frier BM: Is type II diabetes associated with an increased risk of cognitive dysfunction? A critical review of published studies. *Diabetes Care* 20:438–445, 1997

Tiehuis AM, Mali WPTM, van Raamt AF, Visseren FLJ, Biessels GJ, van Zandvoort MJE, the SMART Study Group: Cognitive dysfunction and its clinical and radiological determinants in patients with symptomatic arterial disease and diabetes. *Journal of the Neurological Sciences* 283:170–174, 2009

Tiehuis AM, Vincken KL, van den Berg E, Hendrikse J, Manschot SM, Mali WPTM, Kappelle LJ, Biessels GJ: Cerebral perfusion in relation to cognitive function and type 2 diabetes. *Diabetologia* 51:1321–1326, 2008

van den Berg E, Reijmer YD, de Bresser J, Kessels RPC, Kappelle LJ, Biessels GJ, Utrecht Diabetic Encephalopathy Study Group: A 4 year follow-up study of cognitive functioning in patients with type 2 diabetes mellitus. *Diabetologia* 53:58–65, 2010

van den Berg E, Kloppenborg RP, Kessels RPC, Kappelle LJ, Biessels GJ: Type 2 diabetes mellitus, hypertension, dyslipidemia and obesity: a systematic comparison of their impact on cognition. *Biochimica et Biophysica Acta* 1792:470–481, 2009

van den Berg E, De Craen AJM, Biessels GJ, Gussekloo J, Westendorp RGJ: The impact of diabetes mellitus on cognitive decline in the oldest old: a prospective population-based study. *Diabetologia* 49:2015–2023, 2006

van Harten B, Oosterman J, Muslimovic D, van Loon B-J, Scheltens P, Weinstein HC: Cognitive impairments and MRI correlates in the elderly patients with type 2 diabetes mellitus. *Age and Ageing* 36:164–170, 2007

van Harten B, de Leeuw F-E, Weinstein HC, Scheltens P, Biessels GJ: Brain imaging in patients with diabetes: a systematic review. *Diabetes Care* 29:2539–2548, 2006

van Harten B, Oosterman J, Muslimovic D, van Loon B-J, Scheltens P, Weinstein HC: Cognitive impairments and MRI correlates in the elderly patients with type 2 diabetes mellitus. *Age and Ageing* 36:164–170, 2007

van Harten B, de Leeuw F-E, Weinstein HC, Scheltens P, Biessels GJ: Brain imaging in patients with diabetes: a systematic review. *Diabetes Care* 29:2539–2548, 2006

Várkonyi TT, Pető T, Dégi R, Keresztes K, Lengyel C, Janáky M, Kempler P, Lonovics J: Impairment of visual evoked potentials: an early central manifestation of diabetic neuropathy? *Diabetes Care* 25:1161–1162, 2002

Vázquez LA, Amado JA, Carcía-Unzueta MT, Quirce R, Jiménez-Bonilla JF, Pazos F, Pesquera C, Carril JM: Decreased plasma endothelin-1 levels in asymptomatic type 1 diabetic patients with regional cerebral hypoperfusion assessed by Spect. *Journal of Diabetes and Its Complications* 13:325–331, 1999

Verhaeghen P, Salthouse TA: Meta-analysis of age-cognition relations in adulthood: estimates of linear and nonlinear age effects and structural models. *Psychological Bulletin* 122:231–249, 1997

Virtaniemi J, Laakso M, Kärjä J, Nuutinen J, Karjalainen S: Auditory brainstem latencies in type 1 (insulin-dependent) diabetic patients. *American Journal of Otolaryngology* 14:413–418, 1993

Waldstein SR: The relation of hypertension to cognitive function. *Current Directions in Psychological Science* 12:9–12, 2003

Warren RE, Frier BM: Hypoglycaemia and cognitive function. *Diabetes, Obesity and Metabolism* 7:493–503, 2005

Watari K, Letamendi A, Elderkin-Thompson V, Haroon E, Miller J, Darwin C, Kumar A: Cognitive function in adults with type 2 diabetes and major depression. *Archives of Clinical Neuropsychology* 21:787–796, 2006

Waters F, Bucks RS: Neuropsychological effects of sleep loss: implications for neuropsychologists. *Journal of the International Neuropsychological Society* 17:571–586, 2011

Wessels AM, Scheltens P, Barkhof F, Heine RJ: Hyperglycaemia as a determinant of cognitive decline in patients with type 1 diabetes. *European Journal of Pharmacology* 585:88–96, 2008

Wessels AM, Simsek S, Remijnse PL, Veltman DJ, Biessels GJ, Barkhof F, Scheltens P, Snoek FJ, Heine RJ, Rombouts SARB: Voxel-based morphometry demonstrates reduced gray matter density on brain MRI in patients with diabetic retinopathy. *Diabetologia* 49:2474–2480, 2006

Whitmer RA, Karter AJ, Yaffe K, Quesenberry CP, Selby JV: Hypoglycemic episodes and risk of dementia in older patients with type 2 diabetes mellitus. *JAMA* 301:1565–1572, 2009

Whitmer RA: Type 2 diabetes and risk of cognitive impairment and dementia. *Current Neurology and Neuroscience Reports* 7:373–380, 2007

Winblad B, Palmer K, Kivipelto M, Jelic V, Fratiglioni L, Wahlund L-O, Nordberg A, Bäckman L, Albert M, Almkvist O, Arai H, Basun H, Blennow K, De Leon M, DeCarli C, Erkinjuntti T, Giacobini E, Graff C, Hardy J, Jack C, Jorm A, Ritchie K, van Duijn C, Visser P, Petersen RC: Mild cognitive impairment—beyond controversies, towards a consensus: report of the International Working Group on Mild Cognitive Impairment. *Journal of Internal Medicine* 256:240–246, 2004

Wong TY, Mosley TH, Klein R, Klein BEK, Sharrett AR, Couper DJ, Hubbard L, for the Atherosclerosis Risk in Communities (ARIC) Study Investigators: Retinal microvascular changes and MRI signs of cerebral atrophy in healthy, middle-aged people. *Neurology* 61:806–811, 2003

Wong TY, Klein R, Sharrett AR, Nieto FJ, Boland LL, Couper DJ, Mosley TH, Klein BEK, Hubbard LD, Szklo M: Retinal microvascular abnormalities and cognitive impairment in middle-aged persons: the Atherosclerosis Risk in Communities Study. *Stroke* 33:1487–1492, 2002

Wong TY, Klein R, Klein BEK, Tielsch JM, Hubbard L, Nieto FJ: Retinal microvascular abnormalities and their relationship with hypertension, cardiovascular disease, and mortality. *Survey of Ophthalmology* 46:59–80, 2001

Yau PL, Javier DC, Ryan CM, Tsui WH, Ardekani BA, Ten S, Convit A: Preliminary evidence for brain complications in obese adolescents with type 2 diabetes mellitus. *Diabetologia* 53:2298–2306, 2010

Zammitt NN, Frier BM: Hypoglycemia in type 2 diabetes: Pathophysiology, frequency, and effects of different treatment modalities. *Diabetes Care* 28:2948–2961, 2005

Ziegler D, Langen K-J, Herzog H, Kuwert T, Mühlen H, Feinendegen LE, Gries AF: Cerebral glucose metabolism in type 1 diabetic patients. *Diabetic Medicine* 11:205–209, 1994

第二篇
患者自我管理

第六章

问卷评估糖尿病知识、自我管理技能和自我管理行为

Garry Welch，PhD，Sofija E. Zagarins，PhD

糖尿病是一种治疗成本很高并且常见的慢性疾病，每个患者的生存质量存在明显的差别。尽管每年花费高额的临床治疗费用（2007 年花费1740 亿美元），只有 7%的患者 HbA1C、血压、血脂达标，初级保健医生在帮助这些患者达标时面临着相当大的挑战。评估糖尿病知识、技能及自我护理行为可能给临床医生提供一种更加个性化的糖尿病治疗和教育方式，但是要做到这一点，临床医生需要一种在忙碌的临床工作中易于管理和评分，对变化比较敏感的评估方法，而且产生的结果可直接用于临床护理。

在这篇文章中已经确定了大量可能的评估方式，如果适当地进行修改，它们就可以应用在常规护理中。有证据表明，许多可用的措施可为临床医生提供有用的信息。然而，仍有大量的工作有待完成，以创建一个标准、清晰、可应用于大量临床事件和患者群体的实践措施。两大新兴的计算机评估工具（如 AADE7TM 和 DSCP，后文中将要阐述）在可用度和早期的研究结果方面具有一定的价值，如果能够充分利用信息技术，它们将极有可能被整合到糖尿病临床信息系统和医疗关怀中。

虽然此前描述的患者评估策略有帮助众多患者的可能性，特别是医学高危人群和很少来医院就诊的患者容易获益。健康素养低、认知和眼界的限制、文化和激励障碍、患者和医疗工作者的偏好等都是在制订评估策略中需要考虑的重要因素。

系统化与标准化评估方法的必要性

此文讨论患者在初级保健机构的自我管理评估时，值得注意的是，以病人为中心的医疗之家（PCMH）和责任医疗组织（ACO）模式的出现。PCMH/ACO 方法强调初级护理提供者的核心作用，他们协调了患者护理的方方面面（如初级者、专家、医院、家庭保健、临终关怀），无缝地共享所有护理提供者和护理中心的数据和信息，并且关注预防，综合护理和以病人为中心的护理。为了实现这些目标，PCMH/ACO 模型将促进基层医疗的日常工作，促进以人群为基础的糖尿病自我管理教育的应用，系统地且有针对性地扩展 DSME 评估的使用。用可扩展的且实用的问卷来评估糖尿病知识、自我护理技能和自我护理行为是非常有必要的，这些问卷可通过各种评估渠道获得，并且适应每个医疗机构和病患的需要。这些评估可以通过安全的网站、病人门户网站、交互式语音留言服务、固定电话、手机应用程序、平板电脑或者医疗服务社区、养老院进行访问。以电子模式代替传统的纸笔模式，这样的患者评估最终可能通过临床团队中适当的工作人员无缝地融入电子病历系统，患者或（签协议的）监护人或社区健康工作者可通过个人控制健康记录（PCHRs）来得到这些评估。

虽然已经发明了大量的患者自我报告的方法来评估糖尿病知识、自我护理技能和自我护理行为，值得注意的是，这些方法主要被用作糖尿病研究。在不考虑治疗背景的情况下，尽管早有预期，但这些方法在美国的临床实践中并没有被普遍使用。研究问卷的设计是为了满足特定的研究目标，它们往往是冗长的且需要考虑文化水平、理解水平及文化契合水平才能完成的。研究还通常要测试行为理论或评估与行为、教育或临床的干预有关的机制和结果。相比之下，实用的及相关的评估——适合那些在初级保健机构工作的忙碌的糖尿病护理人员——用以确定可以受益于干预措施的患者，告知他们干预措施的设计，或者帮助评估一些关键的结果。

为了在临床护理中发挥作用，糖尿病知识，自我管理技能和自我管理行为的评估需要广泛应用于需要自我管理的患者，并适合于各种年龄、文化及社会经济地位（SES）的人，他们需要有合理的可靠性和有效性，尤其是对变化的反应度。除了用于研究，许多现有的评估知识、技能和行为的患者自我报告都有可能成为简单的临床工具，它可以提高初级护理者对糖尿病治疗计划的裁减（并且很可能成功）。

临床评估工具的使用

大部分的糖尿病治疗计划是在患者每日的日常生活中进行的，而与医疗团队面对面时间只是占很少的一部分。因此，从门诊中获得的每个患者糖尿病知识、自我管理能力和日常自我管理行为的档案可以帮助护理人员减少针对 DSME 的努力，以便能更准确地满足患者的偏好、需求和自我管理的屏障蓝图。因为所获得的信息可能对患者具有重要意义，因此有效的利用这些评估，可以进一步提高临床护理水平，促进患者参与护理计划。当评估结合有效的沟通时，患者的资料档案可以促进合作目标的设定，确定自我管理的特殊障碍，鼓励直接解决问题的培训，并且支持治疗及随访的计划与实施。

在罗列目前可用的评估工具以前，需要评估患者临床护理中存在的现实障碍。如果这样的评估被广泛地接受，那么就需要陈述这些结构性和逻辑性的问题。这些障碍包括：护理人员缺乏执行知识、技能和行为评估的资格认证和监管规则（例如，这些评估通常不是由认可的组织或权威人士执行或推荐的）；缺乏对临床管理人员和护理者执行评估的财务激励；缺乏对这些相关概念、评估和临床应用的专业培训；并且存在临床综合评估程序的实际障碍（例如，需要额外的支持人员，整合现有的临床数据库和电子医疗记录，标准化的解释和评估数据的实际应用，以及临床工作人员的个人目标与年度业绩指标的对接）。

初级保健机构实施糖尿病知识、技能及行为常规评估的进一步障碍是缺乏实用的评估工具、支持材料和培训计划，以帮助临床医生解释和使用这些评估的结果。虽然针对这个讨论的书面措施知识库已经存在于互联网中（例如，少数民族人口老龄化研究的资源中心，生命仪器数据库的质量问卷【QOLID】，Robert Wood Johnson 的糖尿病倡议，Michigan 和 Vanderbilt 糖尿病研究培训中心，糖尿病健康意识研究中心），但它们可能很难访问或不经常更新。一些潜在的有用的问题只有通过系统的文献检索才能找到，其次是非正式的专业网络（例如，糖尿病组间交换行为的研究【BRIDGE】，行为医学糖尿病特别兴趣小组协会，美国糖尿病医学与心理学协会）。

尽管有关于在美国繁忙的医疗机构中进行患者评估的可行性的警告，但对于那些想要改善特定患者（例如，那些血液代谢控制较差的患者或那些不定期就诊的患者）的临床护理的"采用者"，仍有可用的实际策略。另外，这些评估可以纳入所有糖尿病患者的年度糖尿病检查程序中。后者的策略是用于注重糖尿病生活质量的大型的跨国监测糖尿病的个人需求（MIND）程序。MIND 提供一种免费、标准、简洁的 CD-ROM，而这个 CD-ROM 可以被纳入年度临床审查访问和用于提升以病人为中心的护理。

知识、技能和自我管理行为的评估

许多糖尿病知识、技能和自我管理行为的评估是有效的，下面将针对这一部分进行讨论。这次讨论不是基于一个系统的数据库搜索，所以它不是对所有可用的工具的详细陈述，而是集中陈述一系列已经应用于临床机构的常见的或有希望出版的评估。

以下问卷调查目前提供纸笔版本，可用于个人访谈或团体机构。互联网和交互式语音识别系统目前正在开发一些问卷调查来简化数据收集、评分，以及问题解读，并能够把评估整合到常规临床过程中。

糖尿病知识

许多美国个人糖尿病教育服务或专科诊所使用未发表的和非正式的糖尿病知识问卷。尽管这些问卷很少受到经验审查或者发表在同行评议期刊中，但有几个已出版的知识评估测试是可用的，已用于以下临床研究。

1. 糖尿病知识测试（DKT） 由 23 个知识问题组成，测试患者一般的糖尿病知识。虽然最开始的 14 个项目只适合那些不使用胰岛素，但所有的 23 个项目都可以用于使用胰岛素的糖尿病患者。该 DKT 以正确答案的百分比计分，分数越高表示患者拥有更多的糖尿病知识。DKT 的内容是以专家意见为根据，并且被使用于美国社区 1 型和 2 型糖尿病患者。实证分析结果包括良好的可靠性，与 HbA1C 正相关，适当的难度水平（例如，患者每一项正确得分的百分比不高也不低），能够区分不同组的治疗强度和糖尿病教育程度，糖尿病教育计划实施后有响应性的改变。这些发现表明，DKT 可能在临床上是有用的，并且可能适合各种临床环境和患者群体。

2. 糖尿病审计（ADKnowl）　最近更新是在 2009 年，有 138 项糖尿病相关知识的测试，已被用于识别两种糖尿病患者的性质和程度及健康专业知识的缺乏。内容的有效性是以临床共识和一系列糖尿病专家正在进行的评议过程为根据。胰岛素调整技能培训的临床试验和新确诊的 2 型糖尿病患者的生活方式教育项目（以视频的方式）可以支持 ADKnowl 对变化的反应度。虽然 ADKnowl 内容冗长，特殊项目和组成部分可以恰当地用在临床环境中。这些项目包括糖尿病治疗和检测；病假管理；胰岛素使用；低血糖管理；体育锻炼；饮食和食品；饮酒；并发症减少；戒烟；足部护理和血糖水平。

3. 糖尿病知识量表（DKN A，B，C）　由 3 个相等的 15 个项目的调查问卷（A，B，C）组成，应用于一些临床环境中的 1 型和 2 型糖尿病患者，这些环境需要快速、可靠、反复地评估糖尿病知识。DKN 问卷由澳大利亚的研究人员根据一个专家意见小组和文献综述发展而来，已被用于糖尿病教育研究。创建 3 个平行的形式来允许重复测量，并消除由于在重复的场合使用相同的形式造成的最小的回忆偏差。DKN 项目覆盖了基础生理和胰岛素作用，低血糖症，食物种类和替代食物，病假管理及一般的糖尿病护理。DKN 分数范围为 0～100 分，分数越高表明其具有更多的糖尿病知识。DKN 量表具有很高的可靠性，在强化的教育项目实施前后，它对变化有反应度。尽管最初的项目和特定的地方性用词需要不断更新，研究表明 DKN 量表在临床上仍是有用的。

4. 糖尿病和心血管疾病测试（DCDT）　这 14 个项目的问卷是用来评估糖尿病患者发生心血管疾病的风险意识。项目包括对"好"与"坏"胆固醇的识别评估；临床目标包括空腹血糖、血压、低密度脂蛋白（LDL）、高密度脂蛋白（HDL）；自我监测血糖的知识（SMBG），营养和体育活动。这些评估表明我们意识到血糖、血压、血脂是糖尿病并发症进展的关键控制因素。DCDT 已被用于一些研究，包括糖尿病自我管理的问题解决能力评估，在密集且高强度的教育干预后，其知识分数显著提高。因此，这个简洁的量表可用于临床医生对于糖尿病患者的心血管疾病风险评估。

5. 其他知识问卷调查　其他有临床应用前景、更具体的糖尿病问卷调查已经出版，例如，成人糖类测试是一个由 43 个项目组成的问卷，评估病人 6 大领域的糖类知识计算：识别，单一食物中糖类的计算，食物标签，血糖目标，低血糖的预防和管理及餐食中糖类的计算。AdultCarbQuiz 表现出了鼓舞人心的判别和规范关联效度。例如，患者在AdultCarbQuiz 上的得分与患者从注册营养师那获得的糖类计算知识显著相关。

大多数糖尿病知识评估是根据其表面效度而使用，反映当地的临床共识。一般来说，糖尿病知识测试带来了挑战，因为问题包括了评估工具可能与实践或个人教育工作者提供的特定教育内容不匹配，或问题随着 DSME 实践或证据基础的变化而变得过时。实施评估首先应确定在任何给定的环境中该评估都具备了良好的问卷内容匹配。如果在评估过程中患者不能得到辅助，那么也需要考虑患者的文化、语言偏好、视觉和认知功能障碍。目前，糖尿病知识问卷并没有与临床结果的变化相链接。

糖尿病的自我管理技能

1. 解决问题　如果治疗糖尿病的方案是有效的，就要求患者进行高度的日常参与和积极的决策。特别是，患者必须学习各种各样的自我护理技能来有效地执行糖尿病治疗计划。具体的技能可能包括有效解决问题以克服自我管理障碍，日常压力的管理，计划和处理自我适应，以及接受来自他人的社会支持。特别是解决问题的技能是有效的糖尿病自我管理的关键，但这些技能很难教授，而让患者获得这些技能也是一个挑战。解决问题被定义为：运用一系列的思维操作来弄清楚什么时候该做，什么时候达到一个不太明显的目标。它主要作为多层面 DSME 干预的一部分来教授，但也作为一个独立的策略来应用。它通常侧重于一系列问题评估，例如，障碍识别、解决方案的产生、计划制订、计划实施、成果评价，以及障碍的重新审查。一个近期的综述发现了目前关于解决问题干预研究的一系列方法学弱点。然而，有几种方法可用来评估解决问题的技能，包括糖尿病问题解决清单、糖尿病问题解决量表。这些量表已经表现出了内在信度、结构效度和反应度，这些证据表明他们可能会成为临床实践中有用的工具。

2. 自我效能 较强的糖尿病自我效能感知是有效的糖尿病自我管理的又一重要特性,可以通过临床医生的影响和 DSME 来加强。自我效能感是源于 Bandura 的社会认知理论(SCT),为自我认知和特定的行为之间提供联系。Bandura 把自我效能描述为一种认知过程,涉及执行需要产生一定结果的特定行为的自我能力判定。个体对他们完成任务的能力的信心决定了他们将参与的行为,他们会坚持多久,他们将花费多少精力来达到他们的目标。从实践和理论的角度来看,有四个重要的信息来源可提高患者某一特定行为的自我效能:成就表现(掌握)、替代学习(同行建模)、言语劝说、情绪和生理反应的自我评价。这些可以进行系统评估,并且用来精心构建糖尿病患者的教育和行为改变策略。最近一项综述表明糖尿病自我效能措施方法的增多(如多于 10 种),并且很多其他研究已经被报道,包括那些早期量表的修订。Frei 等指出了这些量表在研究方式和方法上显著的弱点。此外,关于评估方法的目的和它们与 SCT 的关系缺乏一个整体的清晰度。它们在项目内容、测试特点、长度、全球多维关注点,可靠性、有效性及反应度的证据方面存在很大的不同。尽管存在这些问题,一些有用的自我效能量表可以帮助识别在检查中对特定自我管理任务信心较差的患者并且追踪患者进展的情况。

糖尿病自我管理行为

自我管理行为的评估是糖尿病研究文献中一致关注的焦点。通常情况下 SMBG、饮食、运动、药物依从性是自我管理调查问卷中糖尿病自我活动评估的关键点。其他评估可能涉及心血管风险评估(如服用阿司匹林和戒烟)和(或)足、眼及肾脏的筛查。公开发表的有效的评估糖尿病患者自我管理行为的方法包括以下几种。

1. 糖尿病自我管理活动的总结(SDSCA) SDSCA 是一份简短的有关糖尿病自我管理行为的自我报告式调查问卷,它评估了一般饮食、特定的饮食、运动、血糖测试、足病管理和吸烟。针对患者感知自我管理行为的频率或时间百分比的问题,我们进行了几周的随访。正如所预期的那样,SDSCA 分量表与一系列标准方法的相关性和可靠性都非常充分,7 个回顾性研究的变化敏感性分数表明 SDSCA 是糖尿病患者自我管理简单而可靠并且有效的自我报告式调查问卷，对临床实践是有用的。

2. 自我管理库——修订版（SCI-R）　　和 SDSCA 一样，SCI-R 是应用于繁忙的临床实践和科学研究的自我管理行为的评估。这是糖尿病患者对自我管理行为的感知依从性的衡量方法，并由护理工作者实施。实证研究表明，它是充分可靠的，并且根据它与糖尿病相关的心理痛苦、自尊、自我效能感、抑郁、焦虑和血糖控制（HbA1C）的相关性来证明其有效性。依据一系列糖尿病教育干预的使用，它也显示了其对变化的良好反应度。因此，SCI-R 是一个简短、可靠且有效的方法，用以评估患者自我管理行为依从性的自我感知能力。

基于技术的知识、技能和行为评估

一些使用 CD-ROM、互联网、电话进行自我管理行为和障碍评估的工具已经被开发和出版。尽管有些评估工具仍然处于早期的发展阶段，也没有有效的结果数据，但其他一些工具与 HBA1C 显著改善有关。

目前有两种评估方式可向卫生保健提供者宣传，并且会在后文中进行更详细的讨论。这两种评估都被融入更广泛的糖尿病自我管理教育保健系统中，但依据患者的目标、技能和障碍，它们也经常被临床医生和其他保健提供者当作独立的工具来使用。

美国糖尿病协会教育者的 AADE7™ 自我管理行为工具

国家糖尿病教育成果系统（NDEOS）是由 AADE 开发的，用以提高糖尿病教育和结果追踪效果。该系统及其组件包括原始的糖尿病自我管理评估报告工具（D-SMART），现已被纳入 AADE7™ 自我管理行为工具的开发，它提供了标准化的糖尿病自我管理培训的概念框架。

该 AADE7™ 框架为患者的糖尿病教育和管理提供了一个结构化的模式，并为七大定向的糖尿病管理行为提供了重要信息（如体育锻炼、健康饮食、药物治疗、血糖监测、问题解决、风险降低的活动以及心理适应）。该 AADE7™ 系统的测量工具，包括原来的 D-SMART，是一个比 SDSCA 和 SCI-R 调查问卷更加综合、全面的工具，它不仅评估行为改变意图，而且还评估自我管理的障碍。它可用来指导临床计划的发展，并关注对患者重要的领域，因此它有可能增强患者对治疗的参与性和行为改变的积极性。它被用于更广泛的临床环境，可重复进行患者测量以评估随时间变化的行为。糖尿病教育工具（D-ET）也包括在 AADE7^{TM} 自我管理行为工具中，它是一种补充性的教育者-完备化工具，可用来记录患者的知识、技能、自信和障碍。

虽然 AADE7^{TM} 自我管理行为工具仍处于评估的早期阶段，使用 D-SMART 的一些初级研究已经完成。D-SMART 已经在功能上被整合入一个近期对计算机和电话系统的研究中，通过五项糖尿病自我管理项目来验证其可行性和患者的可接受性。一个涉及糖尿病患者的评估过程正在实施，即患者可以在家里通过电话或电脑完成问题。实现 D-SMART 评估的自动化技术的发展，可以加强其临床应用潜能，因为调查问卷由于专业时间、空间和资源限制等原因很难完成这些评估。D-SMART 研究结果表明，76%的患者认为这些问题是容易理解的，而只有 12%需要协助来完成问题。总之，D-SMART 可以通过一次尝试很容易地在家里完成，患者对问题的措辞、答案的选择及易用性方面普遍是满意的。

对 D-SMART 和 D-ET 进行了二次分析，AADE7TM 成果系统在 8 种不同的糖尿病自我管理项目中被整合入以互联网、触摸屏和电话为基础的系统内。这次的研究包含了 954 例糖尿病患者，有 527 例患者确定了其糖尿病教育者所推荐的目标，包括健康的饮食（94%）、积极的运动（59%）及血糖监测（49%）。

基于计算机和电话的 D-SMART 版本在临床实践中似乎是可行的评价方法。这些发现表明，D-SMART 依据专家小组谨慎的研发展现了良好的表面效度，能够被糖尿病患者接受且可行，具有自动化模式获取的优势，这也许能够克服 SDSCA 和 SCI-R 纸笔评估工具所面临的障碍。此外，它对 AADE7^{TM} 的自我管理行为工具的整合及其与临床现场登记表的联系表明，随着时间的推移，D-SMART 在各种临床环境中持续测量糖尿病管理和成果方面具有相当大的潜力。

糖尿病自我管理档案（DSCP）

DSCP 是糖尿病综合管理项目（CDMP）的一部分，是一个互动、基于互联网、以 ADA 的实践指南为基础的糖尿病管理工具。CDMP 侧重于临床管理、生活方式的改变和心理健康，并为长期护理管理人员提供了一组临床和行为的警告，用以指导治疗意见、建立医学管理和糖尿病教育计划。

DSCP——之前在 CD-ROM 版本中叫做 Accu-Chek 访谈——是一个用互联网对患者进行评估的工具，旨在支持护理工作者与患者之间的沟通，并协助患者与护理工作者进行合作，以改善患者的血糖控制和生活质量。DSCP 可识别当前的自我管理行为和心理问题，这些问题可损害糖尿病患者的自我管理并提高血糖水平，它也可在 HbA1C、血压、血脂控制方面给予视觉反馈。该系统的目标是以一个系统、简洁、用户友好的方式来获取患者自我管理的关键信息。这种方法使得糖尿病教育者花费更少的时间来评估 DSME 需求，从而有更多的时间与患者和谐交往，并且依据患者的需求和兴趣提供糖尿病教育和技能培训。

DSCP 评估饮食、锻炼、药物治疗及体育活动对血糖控制的影响，高度突出了糖尿病患者的行为选择。此外，DSCP 可以评估开始用胰岛素治疗的态度和障碍（如果只单独口服药物治疗），并且记录妨碍最佳自我管理的问题，包括抑郁症、糖尿病心理痛苦、低血糖症、低社会支持、暴食、酗酒和对胰岛素治疗的消极态度。当患者完成了 DSCP 的评估，就确定患者目前自我管理问题的报告就会被打印出来。这份报告可使患者和医师之间的谈话重点集中在潜在的行为改变领域和制订改变策略上面。

一项对原来的罗氏血糖仪访谈系统（现在的 DSCP 网络工具的前身）的分析发现，在前面完成了卫生保健专业人员的门诊咨询的患者能够更多地参与这个评估系统。这些患者在咨询问题的时候会问两倍多的问题（$P<0.01$），并且超过一半完成访谈评估的患者报告说他们的咨询有积极的获益。

在前后分析 59 例 2 型糖尿病患者中，所有的患者均完成 DSCP 的评估，并且完成了一项 4 期、6 个月的糖尿病教育干预。DSCP 包含的四个自我管理的话题中，大多数患者将用餐计划定为第一要务（76.3%）；低社会支持（49.2%）、抑郁（42.4%）及情绪困扰（42.9%）被选定为主要的生活挑战。当 DSCP 被应用于 DSME 时，HbA1C 在超过 6 个月时间里显著改善（均值标准差：$-1\%\pm1.3\%$，$P<0.01$）。总体而言，这些早期的研究结果表明，DSCP 有相当大的潜力来把糖尿病管理的重点放在可改变的糖尿病具体问题上和影响血糖控制的生活习惯上。

总结

　　美国的卫生保健系统目前通过鼓励其服务收费系统、计费代码和还款时间表来运作，专注于急性医疗问题、特殊条款、晚期的临终护理或复杂的医疗情况。通常在管理慢性病相关的医疗并发症时需要这些努力，而这些并发症本来是可以避免的。我们对医疗保健系统中医疗管理的预防方面关注较少，包括提供全面、以病人为中心的慢性病患者的自我管理支持，如糖尿病等。支持地方初级保健诊所，以综合医院为基础的糖尿病项目通常会面临一个持续的斗争以产生足够多的利润来满足项目开销，并且倾向于削减预算、调整强调项目有效性的人员。有意义的全面系统改革的成果旨在提高糖尿病和其他慢性疾病患者的自我管理支持，这些支持包括提高患者的访问、护理的满意度、护理质量的提高及临床疗效的提高，并降低医疗总费用。

　　如同在本章中讨论的那样，评估糖尿病知识、技能和自我管理行为，可为临床医生在繁忙的临床工作中提供更多个性化的糖尿病管理和教育手段。在 1994 年糖尿病问卷调查实施之后，尽管在数量、类型、质量措施方面评估糖尿病知识、技能和自我管理行为具有了显著的扩大，然而有趣的是，我们注意到很少或者没有后续措施运用到临床实践中来。尽管缺乏采用，但医疗 PCMH/ACO 模式的出现带来了巨大的希望，旨在产生一个更加全面综合、以病人为中心的糖尿病护理模式，包括更加有效的患者自我管理教育和支持，并促进患者 DSME 及其评估更加广泛地应用。国家糖尿病研究和护理社区的支持等措施，如紧急 PCMH/ACO 模型及其糖尿病试点示范项目，和国家质量保证委员会（NCQA）认证项目目前正在美国实施，这些措施可能会增加本章所讨论的以科研为基础的患者评估的使用。

　　目前存在的各种糖尿病研究措施都可能应用于临床实践中。然而，还需要更多的研究来确定适合初级护理实践的能力。具体来说，他们必须能够广泛使用，由患者自行管理，适合各种年龄、文化、SES 及文学团体，并有合理的可靠度和效度，特别是对变化的反应度。

　　目前可获得的糖尿病知识、技能和自我管理行为措施缺乏连贯性和标准化，这阻碍了研究见解和有效的临床实践方面系统的进步。在主要的心理测量学、理论和实践问题上缺乏国际的共识，包括对"一流的评估"的共识。

临床护理的建议

总之，目前有以下几个有关糖尿病知识、技能和自我管理行为的评估建议被用于临床实践中。

1. 在知识这一问题上，应该使用正式的工具进行评估。简短的知识评估措施可以获取患者知识水平的定性评估，更长的措施可以获取相对详细而全面的知识评估。这些工具可以对具体的知识差距和教育工作进行详细评估的指导。

2. 当自我管理行为和结果都不太理想时，应该使用自我管理技能评估。评估解决问题的技能、健康知识和自我效能这些因素的工具可能会优于临床医生给予的非系统性评估。

3. 评估患者自我管理行为的关键是识别自我管理的差距，当临床医生没有时间来执行一个全面、详细的行为评估措施时，这些评估工具就应该被使用。

4. 获取和存储患者自我管理评估的电子系统是可用的，当随着时间推移需要增加自我管理的追踪时，它可以减少护理工作者的负担。

参 考 文 献

American Association of Diabetes Educators (AADE): AADE7™ Self-Care Behaviors. *Diabetes Educ* 34:445–449, 2008

American Association of Diabetes Educators: AADE position statement: cultural sensitivity and diabetes education: recommendations for diabetes educators. *Diabetes Educ* 33:41–44, 2007a

American Association of Diabetes Educators: AADE position statement: individualization of diabetes self management education. *Diabetes Educ* 33:45–49, 2007b

American Diabetes Association: Executive summary: standards of medical care in diabetes—2011. *Diabetes Care* 34 (Suppl. 1):S4–S10, 2011

Anderson RM, Funnell MM: *The Art of Empowerment: Stories and Strategies for Diabetes Educators.* Alexandria, VA, American Diabetes Association, 2000

Barnard KD, Cradock S, Parkin T, Skinner TC: Effectiveness of a computerised assessment tool to prompt individuals with diabetes to be more active in consultations. *Pract Int Diab* 24:36–41, 2007

Beeney LJ, Dunn SM, Welch GW: Measurement of diabetes knowledge: the development of the DKN scales. In *Handbook of Psychology and Diabetes: A Guide to Psychological Measurement in Diabetes Research and Practice.* Bradley C, Ed. London, Harwood Academic Publishers, 1994, p. 159–190

Bojadzievski T, Gabbay RA: Patient-centered medical home and diabetes. *Diabetes Care* 34:1047–1053, 2011

Boren SA: A review of health literacy and diabetes: opportunities for technology. *J Diabetes Sci Technol* 3:202–209, 2009

Bradley C: *Handbook of Psychology and Diabetes: A Guide to Psychological Measurement in Diabetes Research and Practice.* 1st ed. Chur, Switzerland, Harwood Academic Publishers, 1994

Charron-Prochownik D, Zgibor JC, Peyrot M, Peeples M, McWilliams J, Koshinsky J, et al.: The diabetes self-management assessment report tool (D-SMART): process evaluation and patient satisfaction. *Diabetes Educ* 33:833–838, 2007

Dose Adjustment For Normal Eating (DAFNE) Study Group: Training in flexible, intensive insulin management to enable dietary freedom in people with type 1 diabetes: dose adjustment for normal eating (DAFNE) randomised controlled trial. *BMJ* 325:746, 2002

Dyson PA, Beatty S, Matthews DR: An assessment of lifestyle video education for people newly diagnosed with type 2 diabetes. *J Hum Nutr Diet* 23:353–359, 2010

Fisher KL: Assessing psychosocial variables: a tool for diabetes educators. *Diabetes Educ* 32:51–58, 2006

Fitzgerald JT, Funnell MM, Hess GE, Barr PA, Anderson RM, Hiss RG, Davis WK: The reliability and validity of a brief diabetes knowledge test. *Diabetes Care* 21:706–710, 1998

Fonda SJ, Paulsen CA, Perkins J, Kedziora RJ, Rodbard D, Bursell SE: Usability test of an internet-based informatics tool for diabetes care providers: the comprehensive diabetes management program. *Diabetes Technol Ther* 10:16–24, 2008

Frei A, Svarin A, Steurer-Stey C, Puhan MA: Self-efficacy instruments for patients with chronic diseases suffer from methodological limitations: a systematic review. *Health Qual Life Outcomes* 7:86, 2009

Glasgow RE, Ory MG, Klesges LM, Cifuentes M, Fernald DH, Green LA: Practical and relevant self-report measures of patient health behaviors for primary care research. *Ann Fam Med* 3:73–81, 2005

Glasgow RE, Toobert DJ, Barrera M Jr, Strycker LA: Assessment of problem-solving: a key to successful diabetes self-management. *J Behav Med* 27:477–490, 2004

Glasgow RE, Boles SM, McKay HG, Feil EG, Barrera M Jr: The D-Net diabetes self-management program: long-term implementation, outcomes, and generalization results. *Prev Med* 36:410–419, 2003

Glasgow RE, Toobert DJ, Hampson SE, Strycker LA: Implementation, generalization and long-term results of the "choosing well" diabetes self-management intervention. *Patient Educ Couns* 48:115–122, 2002

Hill-Briggs F, Lazo M, Peyrot M, Doswell A, Chang YT, Hill MN, et al.: Effect of problem-solving-based diabetes self-management training on diabetes control in a low income patient sample. *J Gen Intern Med* 26:972–978, 2011

Hill-Briggs F, Lazo M, Renosky R, Ewing C: Usability of a diabetes and cardiovascular education module in an African American, diabetic sample with physical, visual, and cognitive impairment. *Rehab Psychol* 53:1–8, 2008a

Hill-Briggs F, Smith AS: Evaluation of diabetes and cardiovascular disease print patient education materials for use with low-health literate populations. *Diabetes Care* 31:667–671, 2008b

Hill-Briggs F, Gemmell L, Kulkarni B, Klick B, Brancati FL: Associations of patient health-related problem solving with disease control, emergency department visits, and hospitalizations in HIV and diabetes clinic samples. *J Gen Intern Med* 22:649–654, 2007

Hurley AC, Shea CA: Self-efficacy: strategy for enhancing diabetes self-care. *Diabetes Educ* 18:146–150, 1992

Jackson CL, Bolen S, Brancati FL, Batts-Turner ML, Gary TL: A systematic review of interactive computer-assisted technology in diabetes care: interactive information technology in diabetes care. *J Gen Intern Med* 21:105–110, 2006

Khamis A, Hoashi S, Duffy SG, Forde R, Vizzard N, Keenan P, et al.: Diabetes knowledge deficits in adolescents and young adults with type 1 diabetes mellitus. *Endocrine Abstracts* 7:P71, 2004

Martin C, Daly A, McWhorter LS, Shwide-Slavin C, Kushion W, American Association of Diabetes Educators: The scope of practice, standards of practice, and standards of professional performance for diabetes educators. *Diabetes Educ* 31:487–488, 490, 492 passim, 2005

Mulcahy K, Maryniuk M, Peeples M, Peyrot M, Tomky D, Weaver T, Yarborough P: Diabetes self-management education core outcomes measures. *Diabetes Educ* 29:768–770, 773–784, 787–788 passim, 2003

Peeples M, Mulcahy K, Tomky D, Weaver T, National Diabetes Education Outcomes System (NDEOS): The conceptual framework of the National Diabetes Education Outcomes System (NDEOS). *Diabetes Educ* 27:547–562, 2001

Piette JD, Weinberger M, Kraemer FB, McPhee SJ: Impact of automated calls with nurse follow-up on diabetes treatment outcomes in a Department of Veterans Affairs health care system: a randomized controlled trial. *Diabetes Care* 24:202–208, 2001

Quackenbush PA: Physiologic and psychosocial stage-based differences for dietary fat consumption in women with type 2 diabetes. Texas Medical Center Dissertations (via ProQuest), 2005

Quinn CC, Gruber-Baldini AL, Shardell M, Weed K, Clough SS, Peeples M, et al.: Mobile diabetes intervention study: testing a personalized treatment/behavioral communication intervention for blood glucose control. *Contemp Clin Trials* 30:334–346, 2009

Quinn CC, Clough SS, Minor JM, Lender D, Okafor MC, Gruber-Baldini A: WellDoc mobile diabetes management randomized controlled trial: change in clinical and behavioral outcomes and patient and physician satisfaction. *Diabetes Technol Ther* 10:160–168, 2008

Rosal MC, Ockene IS, Restrepo A, White MJ, Borg A, Olendzki B, et al.: Randomized trial of a literacy-sensitive, culturally tailored diabetes self-management intervention for low-income Latinos: Latinos en Control. *Diabetes Care* 34:838–844, 2011

Sarkar U, Fisher L, Schillinger D: Is self-efficacy associated with diabetes self-management across race/ethnicity and health literacy? *Diabetes Care* 29:823–829, 2005

Schumann KP, Sutherland JA, Majid HM, Hill-Briggs F: Evidence-based behavioral treatments for diabetes: problem-solving therapy. *Diabetes Spectrum* 24:64–69, 2011

Snoek FJ, Kersch NY, Eldrup E, Harman-Boehm I, Hermanns N, Kokoszka A, et al.: Monitoring of Individual Needs in Diabetes (MIND): baseline data from the Cross-National Diabetes Attitudes, Wishes, and Needs (DAWN) MIND study. *Diabetes Care* 34:601–603, 2011

Stetson B, Boren S, Leventhal H, Schlundt D, Glasgow R, Fisher EB, et al.: Embracing the evidence on problem solving in diabetes self management education and support. *Self Care* 1:83–99, 2010

Van der Ven NCW, Ader H, Weinger K, Van der Ploeg HM, Yi J, Pouwer F, Snoek FJ: The confidence in diabetes self-care scale: psychometric properties or a new measure of diabetes-specific self-efficacy in Dutch and US patients with type 1 diabetes. *Diabetes Care* 26:713–718, 2003

Watts SA, Anselmo JM, Ker E: Validating the AdultCarbQuiz: a test of carbohydrate counting knowledge for adults with diabetes. *Diabetes Spectrum* 24:154–160, 2011

Weinger K, Butler HA, Welch GW, La Greca AM: Measuring diabetes self-care: a psychometric analysis of the Self-Care Inventory-Revised with adults. *Diabetes Care* 28:1346–1352, 2005

Welch G, Allen NA, Zagarins SE, Stamp KD, Bursell SE, Kedziora RJ: Comprehensive diabetes management program for poorly controlled Hispanic type 2 patients at a community health center. *Diabetes Educ* 37:680–688, 2011

Welch G, Shayne R, Zagarins S, Garb J: A web-based self-management assessment tool that improves HbA1c. *J Diab Nursing* 13:319, 2009

Welch G, Shayne R: Interactive behavioral technologies and diabetes self-management support: recent research findings from clinical trials. *Curr Diab Rep* 6:130–136, 2006

Welch GW, Guthrie DW: Supporting lifestyle change with a computerized psychosocial assessment tool. *Diabetes Spectrum* 15:203–207, 2002

Zgibor JC, Peyrot M, Ruppert K, Noullet W, Siminerio LM, Peeples M, et al.: Using the American Association of Diabetes Educators Outcomes System to identify patient behavior change goals and diabetes educator responses. *Diabetes Educ* 33:839–842, 2007

第七章
医疗方案的依从性

Suzanne Bennett Johnson，PhD

依从性的定义

30 多年以前，Haynes 定义医疗方案的顺应性为"一个人的行为（服药、饮食的控制或生活方式的改变）与医嘱相符合的程度"。由于顺应性意味着患者被动地接受医生的建议，所以尽管这个术语（顺应性）已经过时，但这个定义至今仍是有用的。现在更多的使用术语"依从性"，在接受医生的建议时，这个术语表示承认患者的积极作用。患者在知情的情况下有目的的拒绝医学建议（故意的或者有意的或者有目的的不依从）可导致医学建议依从性的失败，或者尽管患者按着医学建议努力（疏忽、意外、非有目的的不依从）但仍可导致依从性失败。疏忽引起的依从性失败可能是患者没有理解医学建议和（或）缺乏正确的执行医疗方案的技能（如不正确地抽取胰岛素、胰岛素注射技术差），忘记或者在患者的能力范围内不能克服执行任务的困难。大约 25 年前，Glasgow 等提出，由于糖尿病是患者管理的疾病，"糖尿病自我管理行为"是患者能够控制的更好的治疗糖尿病的方法。"自我管理"目前是糖尿病自我管理教育中被接受的国际标准术语。

不依从的概率

糖尿病一个治疗复杂且花费高的疾病，患者通常很难依从日常的服药、血糖测定、饮食和锻炼的建议。美国 2007 年糖尿病患者的医疗花费超过 1160 亿，目前美国出生人口的 1/3 预期可能会发生糖尿病，他们的花费会逐步增加。糖尿病治疗依从性差的患者花费会更高。

流行病学研究一般不能区分有意的还是疏忽引起的依从性差。然而，大量的文献显示对医疗方案较差的理解和回忆及缺乏正确执行医疗方案的必要技能是问题的重要组成部分。大量的研究显示患者经常不能理解或者准确地回忆医生的建议，不能正确地服用药物或进行血糖监测，不能理解"健康饮食"的意思或缺乏正确计算糖类的技能。儿童和老年人倾向于表现为技术缺陷。儿童在进行复杂的疾病管理时经常缺乏认知的成熟性和灵活性。老年患者可能存在视力问题或者对糖尿病自我管理的认知缺陷。

其他的许多因素也与糖尿病治疗依从性差相关：较高的医疗花费，治疗复杂性增加，患者抑郁程度增加，青少年可能与不太理想的自我管理有关。其他的引起依从性差的因素包括社会经济地位低、健康知识缺乏、家庭矛盾或者缺少家庭支持、儿童治疗过度、过度关注低血糖。

依从性和血糖控制

尽管假设较好的糖尿病治疗依从性可导致较好的血糖控制，但是经验性的证据显示这种相关性在 1 型糖尿病患者中最明显，血糖监测的频率与低水平的 HbA1C 值相关。2 型糖尿病的人群中，一些研究显示血糖测定次数增加与较好的血糖控制有关，其他一些研究显示没有临床意义。多数的 2 型糖尿病患者使用口服降糖药物，一些研究显示血糖监测可能对胰岛素治疗的患者的剂量调整适应更为重要。

Gramer 在系统性回顾中试图评估糖尿病药物依从性和血糖控制之间的关系，但是没有充足的证据证明依从性和血糖控制之间有关。在最近的 Cochrane 关于干预改善 2 型糖尿病患者依从性的综述中，这个研究的设计和测量的问题再次突显。

尽管有足够多的方法可以检测依从性和血糖，但是两者之间的关系仍很难明确，糖尿病治疗的依从性和血糖控制之间的关系很复杂并且取决于多种因素，而不仅仅是患者本身。最重要的是，患者依从性的影响完全取决于处方治疗的有效性。不适当的治疗建议——或者对血糖控制没有作用的建议——即使患者有较好的依从性，这对患者健康的作用很小或者没有作用。即使是最好的治疗也并不总是如我们想象的一样强大。

或许更令人担忧的事实是很多医生没有给予患者适当的治疗建议。

医生的依从性

我们引用 Haynes 依从性的定义来开始这一章,这个定义已经使用了 30 多年:"一个人的行为（服药、饮食或者生活方式的改变）与医嘱相符合的程度"。当讨论依从性时,有一种强烈的趋势认为那只是患者的行为。然而,"医嘱"同样重要;医生给患者的建议对健康结局、患者的能力和遵从"医嘱"的意愿一样关键。尽管 ADA 每年都发表标准的治疗流程,但是有足够的证据显示很多提供者不遵守这些建议。提高医生对 ADA 治疗标准的依从性与增强患者对医嘱的依从性一样重要。

患者依从性的评估

糖尿病患者自我管理有很多方面,包括药物服用、血糖监测、饮食的注意、日常锻炼。许多患者在糖尿病治疗的依从性上存在很大的差异;有一些患者认真的服用所有药物,但是很少监测血糖或饮食不注意。其他的一些人严格地禁甜食但是不锻炼。患者自我管理的差异对依从性的评估存在很大的挑战。

可以下载数据的血糖仪能为血糖监测提供客观的方法,1 型糖尿病患者自我管理与血糖控制密切相关,然而,对服用药物的 2 型糖尿病患者自身管理的依从性没有 1 型糖尿病那么重要。对于胰岛素泵治疗的患者,可以把数据下载下来评估用药的依从性,但是这仅限于少数使用胰岛素泵治疗的患者。在大量的研究中,药物事件管理系统（如药物事件管理系统盒子）成功的用于评估口服药物的依从性,但是 2 型糖尿病患者没有广泛地使用这个系统来评估口服药物的依从性。

糖尿病治疗依从性的自我报告的方法已经发展了较好的心理测量学功能,包括自我管理记录和糖尿病治疗方案依从性问卷调查。通常与其他的评估方法相比,自我报告的方法对依从性的评估更好,能更全面地反映糖尿病的治疗。然而,自我报告只能关注个体行为而不能提供总体的依从性。

　　有些人认为使用 24 小时回忆随访可以作为依从性评估的金标准，因为这种方法能评估有关糖尿病治疗的总体情况；这种方法也能与下载的数据或者直接的观察进行客观的比较，这种方法对依从性的评估通常比自我报告的数据要低。典型的随访就是受训访谈人员进行电话随访，通常集中于工作日和周末进行。这种方法很花费时间，需要对大量的数据进行管理和分析。迄今为止，这种方法在科研中仍占有重要地位，在临床工作中也没有发现更简单的方法。

　　依从性方案的选择取决于依从性评估的方法（如服药和血糖监测），是关注一个方面还是关注患者糖尿病的整体治疗，也取决于心理测量策略的质量及实际问题。不推荐使用 HbA1C 水平作为依从性评估的指标。尽管 HbA1C 水平是糖尿病患者血糖控制的重要指标，但是它不能反映患者每日是否进行了糖尿病管理。高质量的依从性评估需要使用目的明确的测量工具。高质量的糖尿病特异性的依从性评估数据的缺乏——现存的文献严重地妨碍了我们对糖尿病患者依从性和血糖控制之间关系的理解。

提高患者依从性的方法

　　通过再次取药可以反应药物的依从性，显示出了价格敏感性。一些研究显示提高药物的依从性可以减少或者消除患者的个人负担费用或者共担费用。有几个研究也报道当患者依从性提高时医疗花费会下降，相应地降低了患者糖尿病药物的个人负担费用或共担费用。从健康体系的前景来讲，降低患者的药物和血糖监测的花费是最有效的提高患者依从性的方法。

　　其他类型的干预药物依从性的方法的系统性综述对 1 型和 2 型糖尿病分别进行了阐述。鉴于这两类人群的年龄和用药建议本质上是不同的，因此这不难理解。此外，多数 1 型和 2 型糖尿病患者的文献都来自"黑盒子"方法，只反映依从性干预对 HbA1C 的影响，而不反映患者依从性行为的改变。

　　1 型糖尿病患者依从性的干预措施的系统性综述显示，教育本身不太可能影响依从性或血糖控制。关注心理（而不是教育）干预的综述表明行为和多元干预措施的患者依从性可以产生实质性的变化。然而，这些干预措施对血糖控制的影响要温和得多，关注家庭过程的多元干预比单个依从性行为的干预更有效。

在 2 型糖尿病患者中，系统性综述再次支持教育对依从性或血糖控制没有实质性影响。然而，有充分的证据表明，通过简单的提醒（如日历记录）减少剂量频率可以提高药物的依从性。心理干预和自我管理的培训对血糖控制有积极的作用，至少在短期内是有效的。2 型糖尿病患者增加锻炼的干预对血糖控制和心血管健康都有积极的作用；这些发现并没有出现在 1 型糖尿病患者身上。此外，运动作为生活方式干预的一部分能预防高危人群发展为 2 型糖尿病。鉴于 2 型糖尿病在非裔美国人、拉丁美洲和美国原住居民中发病率高，文化干预计划越来越受到关注；护士案例管理者和社区卫生工作者在这方面似乎特别有前途。

提高医务人员的依从性

说教的指令本身似乎不是有效的方法来提高医务人员对实践指南的依从性，如监测糖化血红蛋白、尿蛋白和血脂、足和眼睛的检查。然而，医务工作者的依从性行为可以通过组织的干预进一步加强，通过电脑追踪系统、标准化病人护理流程表、医疗记录审计和反馈来促进目标行为。这些干预措施对患者血糖控制影响的证据尚不明确。

尽管适当的医生监督是方案执行的重要的第一步，但这似乎不足以确保患者血糖控制的改善。患者必须有建设性的方法来保证日常有意义的糖尿病自我管理行为。为此，人们开始关注增加医患协作的方法，鼓励共同制订治疗目标和管理策略。研究报道，医患在治疗目标上协作性差，但当患者和医生的目标一致时，患者的糖尿病自我管理也能得到改善。增强医患互动的干预方法的系统性综述发现，几乎没有证据证明咨询医生的沟通方式能成功地提高医患互动；然而，旨在允许患者提问、参与医生治疗和糖尿病管理目标的干预是更有效的方法。结构化测试程序（STeP）是一个例子，2 型糖尿病患者和住院医生参与协作程序，在就诊前连续 3 天，记录和描绘患者的 7 点血糖测试结果，住院医生按公式改变患者的治疗方案。这种方法既能提高医生对治疗建议的修改，也能改善血糖控制。

临床护理的建议

医疗方案依从性是一个复杂的现象，囊括的内容很广，包括患者、患者的家庭、卫生保健系统、较大的社区。Fisher 等描述了一个这样的生态模型，为那些对设计有效的依从性干预方案的人提供了一个有用的结构。模型包括患者个人评估、医患协作目标设定、患者技能提高、随访和支持，增加患者的日常生活资源，临床治疗的连续性。

从健康保健系统前景来看，证据表明减少患者药物和血糖监测的成本可以提高患者的依从性。健康保健的提供者还必须保证他们的"医疗建议"符合 ADA 的标准。组织系统（如电脑追踪系统、审计、对医生的反馈）能让医生提供适当有效的医嘱。

患者对治疗计划认知和执行技能需要仔细评估。无意识的不依从极为常见，可以通过直接观察患者行为消除。知识和技能评分经常存在鉴别困难或误解，在诊所随访期间不能轻易显现（如认知、听力、视力或老人手的灵巧问题、儿童手灵巧度或误解）。这些评估为正确的反馈或治疗方案的修改提供依据。

对所有执行日常糖尿病护理工作的主要人员进行知识和技能的评估。如果是儿童糖尿病患者，这点是特别重要的，因为其他家庭成员也参与孩子的糖尿病管理。确定每一步方案由谁负责应该是评估的一部分，因为相当多的证据表明提高家长的参与度可以提高孩子的血糖控制。

每年对患者的糖尿病知识和技能进行评估，环境变化时评估频率要更多。生活在家庭和社区的患者，也因此接受许多不同来源的"医嘱"，其中一些可能与医生的建议冲突。孩子随着年龄的增长，糖尿病治疗会发生转变。成年患者可能产生认知、视力或手灵巧度问题，从而干扰他们正确执行治疗方案的能力。若不进行重复的知识和技能评估，那么无意的不依从会很容易重新出现。

成功地解决无意的不依从不能确保患者将成功地遵守治疗方案：糖尿病知识和技能是血糖控制必要的——但不充分的条件。因此，患者依从性评估应该作为常规治疗的一部分。有很多可靠和有效的评估策略；选择哪一种应该取决于它是否是特定糖尿病管理行为的重点（如下载数据评估血糖测定、MEMS 评估口服药物治疗、24 小时的回忆随访评估饮食行为），或取决于糖尿病管理要求的广泛的行为（如糖尿病护理、糖尿病方案依从性问卷、24 小时回忆随访）。HbA1C 不能用于依从性的评估，尽管它仍然是评估血糖控制的金标准。依从性行为和糖尿病知识和技能一样是可以随着时间而改变的。儿童成长和发育、患者生活环境的变化，依从性行为可能需要相应的改变。因此，依从性的重复评估——每年或环境改变时则需要更频繁——成为标准治疗的一部分。

良好的依从性评估将帮助医生确定哪些行为对患者来说是有问题的，应该有针对性的干预。有足够的证据表明，糖尿病自我管理可以改善。药物服用、降低用药成本、简化医疗方案、提示患者按时用药（如在日历上标注药物）可以提高依从性。对于更复杂的糖尿病管理行为，已经证明，行为的和多元的干预对 1 型和 2 型糖尿病患者来说是成功的方法。因为大多数研究，在相同调查中不包括足够的依从性和血糖控制的数据，目前尚不清楚依从性行为是否与改善血糖控制有密切的关系。尽管服用药物是必需的，但是数据表明，频繁的血糖监测与 1 型糖尿病患者良好的血糖控制相关，锻炼与 2 型糖尿病患者良好的血糖控制相关。随着对糖尿病患者依从性的干预研究质量的提高，临床医生可以提供更好的指导，为患者寻找最佳的治疗方案。专门针对少数民族人群的干预措施（2 型糖尿病的负担最重）尤其必要。

总结

1. 必须使用清楚的交流方式提供医嘱。健康护理体系要允许患者进行提问，强调治疗目标和糖尿病管理计划是促进医患合作最有效的方法。

2. 要对所有在糖尿病日常护理起主要作用的人员的知识和技能进行评估。

3. 要每年对患者的糖尿病知识和技能进行评估，如果患者出现不能解释的血糖控制不佳、出现并发症或有糖尿病治疗方案的重大改变，则需要增加评估频率。

4. 依从性的评估应该包括对管理的感知障碍和糖尿病知识、技能。

参 考 文 献

Alto WA, Meyer D, Schneid J, Bryson P, Kindig J: Assuring the accuracy of home glucose monitoring. *J Am Board Fam Pract* 15:1–6, 2002

Anderson B, Ho J, Brackett J, Finkelstein D, Laffel L: Parental involvement in diabetes management tasks: relationships to blood glucose monitoring adherence and metabolic control in young adolescents with insulin-dependent diabetes mellitus. *J Pediatr* 130:257–265, 1997

Athanasakis K, Skroumpelos AG, Tsiantou V, Milona K, Kyriopoulos J: Abolishing coinsurance for oral antihyperglycemic agents: effects on social insurance budgets. *American Journal of Managed Care* 17:130–135, 2011

Balkrishnan R, Rajagopalan R, Camacho F, Huston S, Murray F, Anderson R: Predictors of medication adherence and associated health care costs in an older population with type 2 diabetes mellitus: a longitudinal cohort study. *Clinical Therapeutics* 25:2958–2971, 2003

Berger J: Economic and clinical impact of innovative pharmacy benefit designs in the management of diabetes pharmacotherapy. *American Journal of Managed Care* 13 (Suppl. 2):S55–S58, 2007

Bouldin MJ, Low AK, Blackston JW, Duddleston DN, Holman HE, Hicks GS, Brown CA: Quality of care in diabetes: understanding the guidelines. *Am J Med Sci* 324:196–206, 2002

Breitscheidel L, Stamenitis S, Dippel FW, Schoffski O: Economic impact of compliance to treatment with antidiabetes medication in type 2 diabetes mellitus: a review paper. *Journal of Medical Economics* 13:8–15, 2010

Centers for Disease Control and Prevention: Strategies for reducing morbidity and mortality from diabetes through health-care system interventions and diabetes self-management education in community settings: a report on recommendations of the Task Force on Community Preventive Strategies. *Morbidity and Mortality Weekly Report* 50 (RR–16):1–15, 2001

Cooke JB: A practical guide to low vision management of patients with diabetes. *Clin Exp Optom* 84:155–161, 2001

Coon P, Zulkowski K: Adherence to American Diabetes Association standards of care by rural health care providers. *Diabetes Care* 25:2224–2229, 2002

Cramer J: A systematic review of adherence with medications for diabetes. *Diabetes Care* 27:1218–1224, 2004

Davis WA, Bruce DG, Davis TM: Is self-monitoring of blood glucose appropriate for all type 2 patients? The Fremantle Diabetes Study. *Diabetes Care* 29:1764–1770, 2006

Deakin T, McShane CE, Cade JE, Williams RD: Group based training for self-management strategies in people with type 2 diabetes mellitus. *Cochrane Database Syst Rev* CD003417, 2005

Faas A, Schellevis F, van Eijk J: The efficacy of self-monitoring of blood glucose in NIDDM subjects: a criteria-based review. *Diabetes Care* 20:1482–1486, 1997

Fisher EB, Brownson CA, O'Toole ML, Shetty G, Anwuri VV, Glasgow RE: Ecological approaches to self-management: the case of diabetes. *Am J Public Health* 95:1523–1535, 2005

Follansbee DS: Assuming responsibility for diabetes management: what age? what price? *Diabetes Educ* 15:347–353, 1989

Fonagy P, Moran GS, Lindsay MK, Kurtz AB, Brown R: Psychological adjustment and diabetic control. *Arch Dis Child* 62:1009–1013, 1987

Fontbonne A, Billault B, Acosta M, Percheron C, Varenne P, Besse A, Eschwege I, Monnier L, Slama G, Passa P: Is glucose self-monitoring beneficial to non-insulin-treated patients? Results of a randomized comparative trial. *Diabete Metab* 15:255–260, 1989

Fu AZ Qui Y, Radican L: Impact of fear of insulin or fear of injection on treatment outcomes of patients with diabetes. *Current Medical Research Opinion* 25:1413–1420, 2009

Funnell MM, Brown TL, Childs BP, Haas LB, Hosey GM, Jensen B, Maryniuk M, Peyrot M, Piette JD, Reader D, Siminerio LM, Weinger K, Weiss M: National Standards for Diabetes Self-Management Education. *Diabetes Care* 34 (Suppl. 1):S89–S96, 2011

Gary TL, Genkinger JM, Guallar E, Peyrot M, Brancati FL: Meta-analysis of randomized educational and behavioral interventions in type 2 diabetes. *Diabetes Educ* 29:488–501, 2003

Glasgow R, Wilson W, McCaul D: Regimen adherence: a problematic construct for diabetes research. *Diabetes Care* 8:300–301, 1985

Goldman DP, Joyce GF, Zheng Y: Prescription drug cost sharing: association with medication and medical utilization and spending and health. *JAMA* 298:61–69, 2007

Grey M, Boland EA, Yu C, Sullivan-Bolyai S, Tamborlane WV: Personal and family factors associated with quality of life in adolescents with diabetes. *Diabetes Care* 21:909–914, 1998

Gu Q, Zeng F, Patel BV, Tripoli LC: Part D coverage gap and adherence to diabetes medications. *American Journal of Managed Care* 16:911–918, 2010

Haller MJ, Stalvey MS, Silverstein JH: Predictors of control of diabetes: monitoring may be be the key. *J Pediatr* 144:660–661, 2004

Harkavy J, Johnson SB, Silverstein J, Spillar R, McCallum M, Rosenbloom A: Who learns what at diabetes camp. *Journal of Pediatric Psychology* 8:143–153, 1983

Haynes R: Introduction. In *Compliance in Health Care*. Haynes R, Taylor D, Sackett D, Eds. Baltimore, MD, Johns Hopkins Press, 1979, p. 2–3

Heisler M, Piette JD, Spencer M, Kieffer E, Vijan S: The relationship between knowledge of recent HbA1c values and diabetes care understanding and self-management. *Diabetes Care* 28:816–822, 2005

Heisler M, Vijan S, Anderson RM, Ubel PA, Bernstein SJ, Hofer TP: When do patients and their physicians agree on diabetes treatment goals and strategies, and what difference does it make? *Journal of General Internal Medicine* 18:893–902, 2003

Helgeson VS, Honcharuk E, Becker D, Escobar O, Siminerio L: A focus on blood glucose monitoring: relation to glycemic control and determinants of frequency. *Pediatr Diabetes* 12:25–30, 2011

Herman M: The economics of diabetes prevention. *Medical Clinics of North America* 95:373–384, 2011

Holmes CS, Chen R, Streisand R, Marschall DE, Souter S, Swift EE, Peterson CC: Predictors of youth diabetes care behaviors and metabolic control: a structural equation modeling approach. *J Pediatr Psychol* 31:770–784, 2006

Hood KK, Rohan JM, Peterson CM, Drotar D: Interventions with adherence-promoting components in pediatric type 1 diabetes. *Diabetes Care* 33:1658–1664, 2010

Hood KK, Peterson CM, Rohan JM, Drotar D: Association between adherence and glycemic control in pediatric type 1 diabetes: a meta-analysis. *Pediatrics* 124:e171–1179, 2009

Ismail K, Winkley K, Rabe-Hesketh S: Systematic review and meta-analysis of randomised controlled trials of psychological interventions to improve glycaemic control in patients with type 2 diabetes. *Lancet* 363:1589–1597, 2004

Johnson SB: Measuring adherence to medical regimens. Invited address, NIH Conference on Non-Adherence in Adolescents with Chronic Illness, Bethesda MD, September 2008

Johnson SB: Health behavior and health status: concepts, methods and applications. *Journal of Pediatric Psychology* 19:129–141, 1994

Johnson SB: Methodological issues in diabetes research: measuring adherence. *Diabetes Care* 15:1658–1672, 1992

Johnson SB, Pollak RT, Silverstein J, Rosenbloom A, Spillar RP, McCallum M, Harkavy J: Cognitive and behavioral knowledge about insulin-dependent diabetes among children and parents. *Pediatrics* 69:708–713, 1982

Kahana S, Drotar D, Frazier T: Meta-analysis of psychological interventions to promote adherence to treatment in pediatric chronic health conditions. *Journal of Pediatric Psychology* 33:590–611, 2008

Kavookjian J, Elswick BM, Whetsel T: Interventions for being active among individuals with diabetes: a systematic review of the literature. *Diabetes Educ* 33:962–988, 2007

Kirkman MS, Williams SR, Caffrey HH, Marrero DG: Impact of a program to improve adherence to diabetes guidelines by primary care physicians. *Diabetes Care* 25:1946–1951, 2002

Krane NK, Anderson D, Lazarus CJ, Termini M, Bowdish B, Chauvin S, Fonseca V: Physician practice behavior and practice guidelines: using unannounced standardized patients to gather data. *J Gen Intern Med* 24:53–56, 2008

Lawler FH, Viviani N: Patient and physician perspectives regarding treatment of diabetes: compliance with practice guidelines. *J Fam Pract* 44:369–373, 1997

Lerman I: Adherence to treatment: the key to avoiding the long-term complications of diabetes. *Archives of Medical Research* 36:300–306, 2005

Levine BS, Anderson BJ, Butler DA, Antisdel JE, Brackett J, Laffel LM: Predictors of glycemic control and short-term adverse outcomes in youth with type 1 diabetes. *J Pediatr* 139:197–203, 2001

Lin D, Hale S, Kirby E: Improving diabetes management. *Canadian Family Physician* 53:73–77, 2007

Lindenmeyer A, Hearnshaw H, Vermeire E, Van Royen P, Wens J, Biot Y: Interventions to improve adherence to medication in people with type 2 diabetes mellitus: a review of the literature on the role of pharmacists. *Journal of Clinical Pharmacy and Therapeutics* 31:409–419, 2006

Maciejewski ML, Farley JF, Parker J, Wansink D: Copayment reductions generate greater medication adherence in targeted populations. *Health Affairs* 29:2002–2008, 2010

Magione CM, Gerzoff RB, Williamson DF, Steers WN, Kerr EA, Brown AF, Waitzfelder BE, Marrero DG, Dudley A, Kim C, Herman W, Thompson TJ, Safford MM, Selby JV: The association between quality of care and the intensity of diabetes disease management programs. *Annals of Internal Medicine* 145:107–116, 2006

Mahoney JJ: Reducing patient drug acquisition costs can lower diabetes health claims. *American Journal of Managed Care* 11 (Suppl. 5):S170–S176, 2005

Messier C: Impact of impaired glucose tolerance and type 2 diabetes on cognitive aging. *Neurobiol Aging* 26 (Suppl. 1):26–30, 2005

Misono AS, Cutrona SL, Choudhry NK, Fischer MA, Stedman MR, Liberman JN, Brennan TA, Jain SH, Shrank WH: Healthcare information technology interventions to improve cardiovascular and diabetes medication adherence. *American Journal of Managed Care* 16 (Suppl. 12 HIT):SP82–SP92, 2010

Moore H, Summerbell C, Hooper L, Cruickshank K, Vyas A, Johnstone P, Ashton V, Kopelman P: Dietary advice for treatment of type 2 diabetes mellitus in adults. *Cochrane Database Syst Rev* CD004097, 2004

Moreland EC, Tovar A, Zuehlke JB, Butler DA, Milaszewski K, Laffel LM: The impact of physiological, therapeutic and psychosocial variables on glycemic control in youth with type 1 diabetes mellitus. *J Pediatr Endocrinol Metab* 17:1533–1544, 2004

Newman KD, Weaver MT: Insulin measurement and preparation among diabetic patients at a county hospital. *Nurse Practitioner* 19:44–45, 48, 1994

Norris SL, Lau J, Smith SJ, Schmid CH, Engelgau MM: Self-management education for adults with type 2 diabetes: a meta-analysis of the effect on glycemic control. *Diabetes Care* 25:1159–1171, 2002a

Norris SL, Nichos PJ, Caspersen CJ, Glasglow RE, Engelgau MM, Jack L, Isham G, Snyder SR. Carnade-Kulis VG, Garfield S, Briss P, McCulloch D: The effectiveness of disease and case management for people with diabetes: a systematic review. *American Journal of Preventive Medicine* 22 (Suppl. 4):15–38, 2002b

Norris SL, Engelgau MM, Naryan KMV: Effectiveness of self-management training in type 2 diabetes: a systematic review of randomized controlled trials. *Diabetes Care* 24:561–587, 2001

Odegard PS, Cappocia K: Medication taking and diabetes: a systematic review of the literature. *Diabetes Educ* 33:1014–1029, 2007

Page P, Verstraete DG, Robb JR, Etzwiler DD: Patient recall of self-care recommendations in diabetes. *Diabetes Care* 4:96–98, 1981

Patton SR: Adherence to diet in youth with type 1 diabetes. *Journal of the American Dietetic Association* 111:550–553, 2011

Peek ME, Cargill A, Huang ES: Diabetes health disparities: a systematic review of health care interventions. *Med Care Res Rev* 64 (Suppl. 5):S101–S156, 2007

Peeters B, Van Tongelen I, Boussery K, Mehys E, Remon JP, Willems S: Factors associated with medication adherence to oral hypoglycaemic agents in different ethnic groups suffering from type 2 diabetes: a systematic literature review and suggestions for further research. *Diabet Med* 28:262–275, 2011

Perwien A, Johnson SB, Dymtrow D, Silverstein J: Blood glucose monitoring skills in children with type 1 diabetes. *Clinical Pediatrics* 39:351–357, 2000

Polonsky WH, Fisher L, Schikman CH, Hinnen DA, Parkin CG, Jelsovsky Z, Axel-Schweitzer M, Petersen, B, Wagner RS: A structured self-monitoring of blood glucose approach to type 2 diabetes encourages more frequent, intensive, and effective physician interventions: results from the STeP Study. *Diabetes Technology and Therapeutics* 13:797–802, 2011a

Polonsky WH, Fisher J, Schikman CH, Hinnen DA, Parkin CG, Jelsovsky Z, Petersen B, Schweitzer M, Wagner RS: Structured self-monitoring of blood glucose significantly reduces A1C levels in poorly controlled noninsulin-treated diabetes: results from the Structured Testing Program study. *Diabetes Care* 34:262–267, 2011b

Quittner AL, Modi AC, Lermanek KL, Ievers-Landis CE, Rapoff MA: Evidence-based assessment of adherence to medical treatments in pediatric psychology. *Journal of Pediatric Psychology* 33:916–936, 2008

Reijmer YD, van den Berg E, Ruis C, Kappelle LJ, Biessels GJ: Cognitive dysfunction in patients with type 2 diabetes. *Diabetes Metab Res Rev* 26:507–519, 2010

Renders CM, Valk GD, Griffin S, Wagner EH, Eijk Van JT, Assendelft WJ: Interventions to improve the management of diabetes mellitus in primary care, outpatient and community settings: a systematic review. *Diabetes Care* 24:1821–1833, 2001

Roblin DW, Platt R, Goodman MJ, et al.: Effect of increased cost sharing on oral hypoglycemic use in five managed care organizations: how much is too much? *Medical Care* 43:951–959, 2005

Roumen C, Blaak EE, Corpeleijn E: Lifestyle intervention for prevention of diabetes: determinants of success for future implementation. *Nutrition Reviews* 67:132–146, 2009

Rubin RR: Adherence to pharmacologic therapy in patients with type 2 diabetes mellitus. *Am J Med* 118 (Suppl. 5A):S27–S34, 2005

Savage E, Farrell D, McManus V, Grey M: The science of intervention development for type 1 diabetes in children: systemic review. *Journal of Advanced Nursing* 66:2604–2619, 2010

Silverstein J, Klingensmith G, Copeland K, Plotnick L, Kaufman F, Laffel L, Deeb L, Grey M, Anderson B, Holzmeister LA, Clark N: Care of children and adolescents with type 1 diabetes: a statement of the American Diabetes Association. *Diabetes Care* 28:186–212, 2005

Stewart SM, Lee PW, Waller D, Hughes CW, Low LC, Kennard BD, Cheng A, Huen KF: A follow-up study of adherence and glycemic control among Hong Kong youths with diabetes. *Journal of Pediatric Psychology* 28:67–79, 2003

Thomas DE, Elliott EJ, Naughton GA: Exercise for type 2 diabetes mellitus. *Cochrane Database Syst Rev* CD002968, 2006

Thompson CJ, Cummings F, Chalmers J, Newton RW: Abnormal insulin treatment behaviour: a major cause of ketoacidosis in the young adult. *Diabet Med* 12:429–432, 1995

van Dam HA, van der Horst F, van den Borne B, Ryckman R, Crebolder H: Provider-patient interaction in diabetes care: effects on patient self-care and outcomes: a systematic review. *Patient Education and Counseling* 51:17–28, 2003

Vermeire E, Wens J, Van Royen P, Biot Y, Hearnshaw H, Lindenmeyer A: Interventions for improving adherence to treatment recommendations in people with type 2 diabetes mellitus. *Cochrane Database Syst Rev* CD003638, 2009

Wens J, Vermeire E, Hearnshaw H, Lindenmeyer A, Biot Y, Van Royen: Educational interventions aiming at improving adherence to treatment recommendations in type 2 diabetes: a sub-analysis of a systematic review of randomised controlled trials. *Diabet Res Clin Pract* 79:377–388, 2008

Winkley K, Landau S, Eisler I, Ismail K: Psychological interventions to improve glycaemic control in patients with type 1 diabetes: systematic review and meta-analysis of randomised controlled trials. *BMJ* 333:65, 2006

World Health Organization. *Report on Medication Adherence*. Geneva, WHO, 2003

Wysocki T: Behavioral assessment and intervention in pediatric diabetes. *Behavior Modification* 30:72–92, 2006

Ziegler YD, Heidtmann B, Hilgard D, Hofer S, Rosenbauer J, Holl R: Frequency of SMBG correlates with HbA1c and acute complications in children and adolescents with type 1 diabetes. *Pediatr Diabetes* 12:11–17, 2011

Zoorob RJ, Mainous AG: Practice patterns of rural family physicians based on the American Diabetes Association standards of care. *J Community Health* 21:175–182, 1996

第八章
生活方式改变：营养学

Judith Wylie-Rosett，EdD，RD

Linda M. Delahanty，MSRD

医学营养学治疗

营养学的定义是提供维持生命的必需物质（以食物的形式）。社会心理和营养学评估交织在一起，营养学评估需要考虑社会心理因素，同时要考虑营养学干预对社会心理结局的影响，包括身体和心理的健康。美国糖尿病协会（ADA）的营养学共识指出"为糖尿病医学营养治疗（MNT）提供有证据支持的推荐和干预"。糖尿病治疗营养学部分的目标是预防或至少减慢糖尿病并发症的发生率。营养与饮食学会（原美国营养学协会）定义 MNT 为"营养学治疗的发展和规定是基于对患者的病史、社会心理史、身体检查及饮食情况的详细评估"。MNT 社会心理学评估包括患者个体经济状况、种族、文化背景、健康知识、居住环境、教育水平、执业、精神状况的评估及为维持健康获取充分的食物来源。尽管 MNT的长期目标是为了减少糖尿病相关的死亡率，但是短期目标集中在完成超重或者肥胖患者的体重目标（通常减少 7%～10%），以及完成根据 ADA 推荐的代谢指标的控制（血糖、血压和血脂）。膳食评估方法包括 24 小时回顾、食物记录和各种冗长的问卷调查。膳食评估方法的比较在www.p3gobservatory.org/repository/nutritionComparisonChart.Htm 上可以获取。

社会生态学观点

这一章关注糖尿病 MNT 的行为策略和处理环境问题的基本原理和策略。MNT 的讨论是处理如何进行动机访谈，以及有助发展协同目标而设定的改进方法。应用动机访谈，包括开放式结局的问题、反映式聆听、肯定和总结，这些有助于患者陈述他们改变生活方式所关心的内容。对于那些有改变意愿的人，动机访谈提供了一个训练的机会，包括帮助患者设定目标和制订改变计划。考虑动机后，紧接着要审查糖尿病 MNT 相关障碍的评估工具，以及审查与 ADA 营养学建议相关的证据。使用 2010 年美国饮食指南上推荐的社会生态学模型来讨论处理环境问题的理论依据和策略，将证据转换为操作计划（在饮食指南的官网上可找到）。这一章包括了以社会生态学角度考虑糖尿病特性的建议。

影响医学营养治疗的因素

　　动机的评估提供了一种合作目标的框架，这一目标依据动机访谈原则来提高 MNT 的参与动机。动机访谈和改进中使用的评估包括探寻行为改变中的犹豫不决；它观察个体目前的行为与他们的核心价值观或个人目标之间的差异。动机访谈，无论是以减少体重还是改善血糖为目标，既包括反应性聆听来明确目标和关心，也包括引诱患者用自己的语言表述改变原因。临床医生可以应用动机访谈与患者"在其间"和谐相处，而不是在生活方式推荐上进行争斗。学习如何使用动机访谈需要培训，不应当认为这是一门技术，应当用培训卫生职业人员的方式来教，"看一个，做一个，教一个"。然而，动机访谈可与简短的咨询课程合并，这些课程是由动机访谈培训者网站（MINT）开发的培训程序。动机访谈培训的信息可从 MINT 中获取，网址为 http://www.Motivationalinterview.net/training/trainers.html。尽管动机访谈能与多种行为原理结合使用，但是对于动机访谈的误解通常包括：认为它是行为改变的跨理论模型，哄骗人们做出改变的方法，认知行为治疗，或是以客户为中心的疗法。体重或血糖控制的客观回馈显示没有促进个人目标讨论的调整和目前行为与个人预期之间差异的判断。

　　在糖尿病营养学管理中评估社会心理因素作用的工具很少。一篇关于糖尿病和肥胖调查的论著列出了如下工具：①评估食谱改变障碍的工具（已经形成评估非裔美籍女性 2 型糖尿病患者的一个范例）；②评估关于糖类摄入和自我血糖监测的质量的工具（工具和量表内部一致性的心理评估）；③资深的体重管理调查，有评估体重管理障碍的患者版本和提供者版本；④评估与饮食影响相关的糖尿病特定的生活质量的工具（例如，与选择或准备食物，预防和治疗低血糖和高血糖有关的麻烦事）。

与糖尿病和肥胖患病率平行增加的社会和环境因素评估（例如，在食品超市和快餐店中过多获取高热量食物），已经关注与美国人热量摄入增加相关的改变。饮食因素与肥胖型糖尿病的增加密切相关，包含大包装食物，每份更多食物量和热量，含糖甜饮料的摄入增加，小吃，商业化餐饮（特别是快餐），以及能量密集型食物。

糖尿病相关的健康悬殊与经济悬殊相关。低收入区的居民更可能居住在离市场（能获取健康食物）更远的地方，食物花费占收入更高的比例，更多地暴露于能量密集、低营养价值的食物中。国家健康与营养检测调查（NHANES）对食物不安全性进行分析，发现食物不安全性与糖尿病风险增加相关，这似乎可用收入和教育水平来解释。NHANES数据分析显示美国家庭食物花费占家庭可支配收入的9.8%，但是当绝对收入水平减少时，可支配收入中食物消费份额却增加。几乎没人知道最近经济低迷对与营养相关的糖尿病的影响。所有食物的消费者价格指数（CPI）在2008年增加5.5%，2009年下降1.8%，2010年下降0.8%。预计2011年增加3.0%～4.0%。据估算，2009年有14.7%的美国家庭遭遇了一定程度的食品的不安全（没钱购买食物）。

一个多级社会生态学评估方法提供了一个框架来检测遗传（食欲和饱腹感的基因及其他生物学决定因素）与环境（社会、文化、心理、经济和其他环境决定因素）复杂的相互作用，从而调节摄食。以社区为基础的糖尿病干预应用了混合方法评估，它的目标是解决营养问题的结构变化。饮食摄入和生活质量的改变使用定量测量和定性的方法进行评估，如关注成组的和半结构化访谈。多种陈述糖尿病管理中的肥胖和营养障碍问题的评估工具可在疾病控制和预防中心的糖尿病预防和控制项目中获得，网址为http：//cdc，gov/diabete/projects/index.html，也可在Robert Wood Johnson糖尿病机构中获得，网址为http：//diabetesnpo.im.wustl.edu/resources/type/program Training.html。混合方法的方式可以评估食物摄入如何与社会心理、社区、经济环境相关，同时评估与营养状态有关的糖尿病相关的健康差异，以及营养学是如何与糖尿病治疗相互关联的。

已知的（和已证实的）治疗方法

ADA 阐述了 MNT 在其健康标准中有益的证据。正如制定 1 型和 2 型糖尿病成人患者的营养实践指南那样，营养与饮食学会成立了证据分析图书馆（EAL）（http：//adaevidencelibrary.com），陈述了由注册营养师提供的 MNT 干预所带来的预期健康和社会心理结局。MNT 的临床试验/结果研究显示，根据糖尿病病程，1 型糖尿病患者 HbA1C 下降 1%，2 型糖尿病患者下降 1%～2%。在多中心糖尿病控制和并发症研究（DCCT）的实验中，营养干预是 1 型糖尿病患者强化治疗的重要部分。参与者被随机分配到传统治疗组或强化治疗组。强化治疗，用每日多次注射（MDI）胰岛素（每日 3 次或更多次注射），或者持续皮下胰岛素泵入（CSII），自我检测血糖（SMBG），并使用多种营养策略（如菜单计划、依据糖类摄入和体力活动进行胰岛素调整的计算法则、管理低血糖的方案）来帮助维持接近正常的血糖水平以达到治疗目标。自我研究报告显示，在强化治疗组饮食行为与较好的 HbA1C 水平相关，包括坚持制订饮食计划，根据血糖调整食物和（或）胰岛素，并且根据餐量和餐食种类较小程度地调整胰岛素剂量，以及持续摄入夜宵。过度治疗低血糖和摄入饮食计划以外的小吃与高 HbA1C 水平相关。另外，在 DCCT 中，标准糖尿病治疗组与强化治疗组在糖尿病特定的生活质量上没有差别。尽管与饮食、自我血糖监测和胰岛素管理相关的自我管理需求增加，但是没有报道提示生活质量恶化。普通饮食剂量调整（DAFNE）随机临床试验，使用了 6 个月的延迟干预，显示训练 1 型糖尿病患者进行灵活的强化胰岛素管理，允许其自由地摄入食物，他们的 HbA1C 水平、整体生活质量、总体幸福感和治疗满意度都有提高，而严重低血糖症、体重及血脂仍旧保持不变。Look AHEAD（糖尿病健康行为）研究了 2 型糖尿病患者的减重干预，这是一项多中心的随机对照研究，旨在确定有计划的减重在 2 型糖尿病超重患者中能否减少心血管的患病率和死亡率。这项研究开始于 2001 年，持续到 2014 年得出结论。Look AHEAD 干预的证据基础是随机对照研究，包括糖尿病预防项目，这个项目在 16～26 周联合应用饮食使体重减少 7%～10%（如建立脂肪和能量摄入的目标以造成能量缺乏）、运动（如每周中等强度运动 150 分钟）和行为治疗。研究显示 7%～10%的体重下降导致 2 型糖尿病患者血糖控制改善，血压也有改善。证据也支持提供膳食替代，制订菜单来关注控制购物列表，应用低能量密度饮食。另外，一个六项随机对照研究的 Meta 分析显示液态食物替代比传统饮食结构多下降 3kg 的体重。观察资料显示，肥胖患者进食一份传统食物饮食时低估了 40%～50%的卡路里摄入，这与评估分量、元素组成、卡路里含量和记录食物消耗的问题相关。Look AHEAD 基础数据显示，规律的自我检测体重和进食早餐的体重控制策略及少食用快餐，与研究人群中的 BMI 减低相关，这些变量占 BMI 变量的 24%。一项 2 型糖尿病超重女性的随机对照研究中，West 等评估了动机访谈的效果来帮助制订干预目标。在这项研究中，动机访谈方法达到的长期（2 年）体重下降和短期（6 个月）血糖控制都比对照组更好。使用 Meta 分析和系统性综述来评估营养干预和社会心理变量的关系是受限的，因为试验样本小，不能包含生活质量或其他社会心理变量作为终点事件，以及设计和研究方法相关的问题。

在超重和肥胖的胰岛素抵抗的患者中，适当减重能改善胰岛素抵抗。因此，减重对于已经患有糖尿病或者有患病风险的人群是推荐的。糖尿病预防项目和 Look AHEAD 研究显示 14～16 周的核心周项目平均可减重 7%～9%，伴有代谢情况改善。与此同时，Look AHEAD 研究的第 1 年中，强化生活方式干预（ILI）减重治疗的 2 型糖尿病患者的配偶体重也减少 2.7%，而参与随机普通护理项目组（DSE，糖尿病支持和教育）的配偶减重 0.2%。ILI 患者前 6 个月每周访视 1 次，接下来的 6 个月里每月访视 1 次，以获得核心的行为技能，如自我监测、问题解决、目标设定和预防复发。尽管配偶并不需要参加小组访谈，但是我们教授 ILI 参与者加强社会支持的方式（例如，如何与家庭成员沟通渴望改变食谱，如何使朋友和家庭成员参与他们的常规锻炼）。DSE 参与者每年参加 3 次信息小组访谈，这些访谈提供了糖尿病、营养和体力活动的基本信息。配偶不需要或被预期参加访谈，征得社会支持的策略也未被讨论。

配偶的体重减轻与参与者减重及高脂肪食物摄入减少相关，建议利用社会网络来促进减重的传播，进而创造涟漪效应。在 2 型糖尿病的管理中，减重干预对身体功能和社会心理结局的作用包括评估健康相关的生活质量（HRQOL）。Look AHEAD 参与者中接受 ILI 的人与那些接受

DSE 的人相比，其形体不满、身体功能和膝部疼痛有显著的减轻。体重减轻介导了生活方式干预对膝部疼痛和身体功能的影响。HRQOL 措施也显著地提高了实施 1 年后的体重减轻。HRQOL 的改善部分由减重、健康改善和身体问题相关的抱怨减少所介导。另外，那些极低 HRQOL 的参与者在参加生活方式干预项目中取得了最大获益。经过 4 年随访，与普通支持组相比，减重干预组的行动丢失风险降低了 48%。减重和健康改善也是这一效果的显著媒介。体重减少 1%和健康改善 1%，都使移动丢失的风险分别减少 7.3%和 1.4%。这些结果强调年龄增加、肥胖的风险如何与 2 型糖尿病患病率相结合来减低身体功能和流动性，这会影响生活质量，也会影响营养和生活方式干预在维持健康的体重、健康、身体功能和健康相关的生活质量中的重要作用。

2 型糖尿病患者中，糖尿病特有的情感痛苦与低龄、女性、高 HbA1C 水平相关，他们很少能坚持饮食、运动和药物疗法，而能更好地坚持血糖监测，血糖监测通常与胰岛素治疗和更严重的糖尿病相关。另外，即使轻度的抑郁症状似乎对自我管理的依从性也有消极影响，包括饮食、锻炼和用药管理。Cochrane 数据的系统性综述表明，迫切需要设计良好的饮食建议研究来调查在 2 型糖尿病患者中进行不同间隔随访的一系列干预和 MNT 方法。

ADA 营养学相关管理建议

根据延伸管理设施中营养学管理的系统性综述，营养与饮食学会推荐，MNT 可平衡医学需求和患者需求并且维持生活质量。

1. **糖尿病患者应该接受个体化的 MNT**　这项治疗最好由熟悉糖尿病 MNT 内容（以证据为基础）的注册营养师提供。医疗保险和其他第三方支付包括糖尿病有益的基础保险（1 年）中的 MNT 保险 3 小时。管理的时间通常包括 1 小时的初级评估，以及 1 年内 4 次 30 分钟的随访干预。如果治疗医师决定改变医疗条件，或者 MNT 的治疗方案需要改变，管理阶段要求额外的时间，那么有必要在医疗上考虑增加额外的时间。第二年随访是 2 小时。更多信息可登录 http：//www.diabetesarchive.net/for-health-professionals-and-scientists/recognition/mnt-guide.jsp。国家糖尿病信息票据交换所为无法进行 MNT 或获取其他资源的糖尿病患者提供信息。详见 http：//diabetes.niddk.nih.gov/dm/pubs/financialhelp/。

2. **营养学咨询**　应当针对糖尿病患者的个人需求、改变意愿和做出改变的能力体察入微。

临床管理的社会心理学推荐

1. **发展患者/当事者 MNT 自我管理技能和支持计划**　为最大程度发挥作用，证据支持的 MNT 的条款需要关注社会心理因素。例如，沮丧或抑郁、糖尿病特有的心理痛苦、改变的意愿、竞争生活优先权和自我效能，这些可能对实施 MNT 推荐表现出障碍。因此，进行 MNT 的营养学家需要精通专注而移情的倾听、口头表达的敏感，并且使用体贴而深思的评价——这些技能是良好的临床管理的标志。考虑知识和技能基础、行为改变的过去经验（成功或失败的），和目前改变障碍的营养学评估进程，是决定如何将营养学优势转换成患者能遵从的计划的基础。例如，与由于生活环境（与糖尿病无关）而痛苦的患者相比，那些报告有糖尿病相关心理痛苦的患者，可能需要不同的干预措施，这些痛苦来自于无法预测高血糖发作的挫败或害怕并发症。

冬季访谈和认知行为策略的使用，如目标设定、问题解决、自我监测、预防复发，对于促进行为改变进程非常重要。另外，策略的使用可改善行为改变的自效性，对于 MNT 的成功实施非常重要。例如，制订营养学和行为目标的进程是根据他们显著降低 HbA1C 水平的潜力及参与者自我报告中至少有 80% 的自信达成目标。

2. **使用环境策略来改善健康食物选择和体育运动**　美国健康和人类服务组织的 2010 年饮食指南和美国农业组织把社会生态模型作为一个多层框架（图 8-1），把有证据的研究转换为推荐指南。2010 年指南的原则是：①确保有权使用营养食品和体育运动的机会；②通过环境战略促进个人行为改变；③分阶段制订长期生活的健康饮食、体育活动和体重管理行为。尽管这一"呼吁"承认美国人在个人或家庭水平可随意选择食物和体育活动，但也强调提供以社区为基于的机会来做出这种选择。多层框架为把社会心理学/行为问题整合入推荐指南提供了基础，包括从个人水平的糖尿病 MNT 实施到生活方式和糖尿病相关的社会和政策推荐。糖尿病管理健康进程训练需要传达相关技能，包括帮助糖尿病患者/参与者做出正式的营养学决定和使用心理咨询技术，如动机增强，来管理他们的糖尿病。

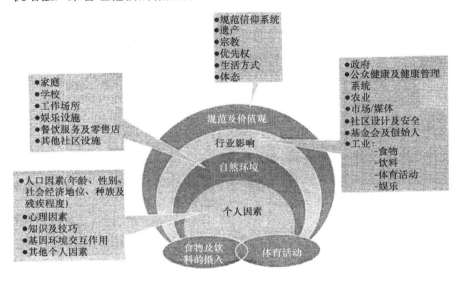

图 8-1　一个决定个人营养及身体活动的社会生态框架图

资料来源：（1）Centers ror Disease Control and Prevention. Division of Nutrition，Physical Activity，and Obesity. State Nutrition，Physical Activity and Obesity（NPAO）Program：Technical Assistance Manual. January 2008，Page 36. Accessed April 21，2010. http：//www.cdc. gov/obesity/downloads/TA_Manual_1_31_08. pdf.（2）Institute of Medicine. Preventing Childhood Obesity：Health in the Balance，Washington，DC：The National Academies Press；2005，Page 85.（3）Story M，Kaphingst KM，Robinson-O'Brien R，Glanz K. Creating healthy food and eating environments：Policy and environmental approaches. Annu Rev Public Health 2008；29：253-272. From USDA 2010.

3. 基于证据的政策和预防控制糖尿病合作的优化资源　政府和私人组织的协作及合伙企业需要陈述与糖尿病发病有关的食物摄入和肥胖趋势。潜在的合作者可能包括健康组织、社区花园和农民市场创业者、食品储藏室、学校、娱乐设施、医院、志愿卫生机构和企业。

　　机构需要制定政策或计划来支持健康体重。促进健康体重的学校和工作举措包括环境改变和咨询支持。糖尿病预防策略需要向民众讲述肥胖。尽管第三方保险包括明显糖尿病的 MNT，但是第三方保险和服务也需要对肥胖进行评估来陈述糖尿病差异，包括对于与体重或者种族/民族固有观念相关的内隐偏见。研究需要陈述在诊断糖尿病时推荐二甲双胍是如何与糖尿病 MNT 的态度和有益性相关的。

参 考 文 献

Academy of Nutrition and Dietetics (formerly American Dietetic Association): Medical nutrition therapy protocols: an introduction. *J Am Diet Assoc* 99:351, 1999a

Academy of Nutrition and Dietetics (formerly American Dietetic Association): Medicare Medical Nutrition Therapy Act of 1999: Effort to secure MNT coverage still popular with lawmakers (Public Policy News). *J Am Diet Assoc* 99:796, 1999b

Academy of Nutrition and Dietetics (formerly American Dietetic Association): Position of the American Dietetic Association: Medical nutrition therapy and pharmacotherapy. *J Am Diet Assoc* 99:227–230, 1999c

Albright A: What is public health practice telling us about diabetes? *Journal of the American Dietetic Association* 108 (Suppl. 1):S12–S18, 2008

American Diabetes Association: Standards of medical care in diabetes—2012. *Diabetes Care* 35 (Suppl. 1):S11–S63, 2012

Anderson EJ, Richardson M, Castle G, Cercone S, Delahanty L, Lyon R, Mueller D, Snetselaar L: Nutrition interventions for intensive therapy in the Diabetes Control and Complications Trial: the DCCT Research Group. *J Am Diet Assoc* 93:768–772, 1993

Appel LJ: Lifestyle modification as a means to prevent and treat high blood pressure. *J Am Soc Nephrol* 14 (Suppl. 2):S99–S102, 2003a

Appel LJ, Champagne CM, Harsha DW, Cooper LS, Obarzanek E, Elmer PJ, Stevens VJ, Vollmer WM, Lin PH, Svetkey LP, Stedman SW, Young DR: Effects of comprehensive lifestyle modification on blood pressure control: main results of the PREMIER clinical trial. *JAMA* 289:2083–2093, 2003b

Appel LJ, Espeland M, Whelton PK, Dolecek T, Kumanyika S, Applegate WB, Ettinger WH Jr, Kostis JB, Wilson AC, Lacy C, et al.: Trial of nonpharmacologic intervention in the elderly (TONE): design and rationale of a blood pressure control trial. *Annals of Epidemiology* 5:119–129, 1995

Bantle JP, Wylie-Rosett J, Albright AL, Apovian CM, Clark NG, Franz MJ, Hoogwerf BJ, Lichtenstein AH, Mayer-Davis E, Mooradian AD, Wheeler ML: Nutrition recommendations and interventions for diabetes: a position statement of the American Diabetes Association. *Diabetes Care* 31 (Suppl. 1):S61–78, 2008

Bell EA, Rolls BJ: Energy density of foods affects energy intake across multiple levels of fat content in lean and obese women. *American Journal of Clinical Nutrition* 73:1010–1018, 2001

Bleich S, Cutler D, Murray C, Adams A: Why is the developed world obese? *Annual Review of Public Health* 29:273–295, 2008

DAFNE Study Group: Training in flexible, intensive insulin management to enable dietary freedom in people with type 1 diabetes: Dose Adjustment for Normal Eating (DAFNE) randomised controlled trial. *BMJ* 325:746, 2002

Daly A, Michael P, Johnson EQ, Harrington CC, Patrick S, Bender T: Diabetes white paper: defining the delivery of nutrition services in Medicare medical nutrition therapy vs Medicare diabetes self-management training programs. *Journal of the American Dietetic Association* 109:528–539, 2009

Dattilo AM, Kris-Etherton PM: Effects of weight reduction on blood lipids and lipoproteins: a meta-analysis. *Am J Clin Nutr* 56:320–328, 1992

Delahanty L, Heinz, J: Tools and techniques to facilitate nutrition intervention. In *Nutrition in the Prevention and Treatment of Disease*. 2nd Ed. Coulston A, Boushey CJ, Eds. San Diego, CA, Academic Press, 2008a, p. 149–167

Delahanty LM, Nathan DM: Implications of the diabetes prevention program and Look AHEAD clinical trials for lifestyle interventions. *Journal of the American Dietetic Association* 108 (Suppl. 1):S66–S72, 2008b

Delahanty LM, Grant RW, Wittenberg E, Bosch JL, Wexler DJ, Cagliero E, Meigs JB: Association of diabetes-related emotional distress with diabetes treatment in primary care patients with type 2 diabetes. *Diabet Med* 24:48–54, 2007

Delahanty LM, Halford BN: The role of diet behaviors in achieving improved glycemic control in intensively treated patients in the Diabetes Control and Complications Trial. *Diabetes Care* 16:1453–1458, 1993a

Delahanty L, Simkins SW, Camelon K: Expanded role of the dietitian in the Diabetes Control and Complications Trial: implications for clinical practice: the DCCT Research Group. *J Am Diet Assoc* 93:758–764, 767, 1993b

Diabetes Control and Complications Trial Research Group: Influence of intensive diabetes treatment on quality-of-life outcomes in the diabetes control and complications trial. *Diabetes Care* 19:195–203, 1996

Duffey KJ, Popkin BM: Shifts in patterns and consumption of beverages between 1965 and 2002. *Obesity (Silver Spring)* 15:2739–2747, 2007

Ello-Martin JA, Roe LS, Ledikwe JH, Beach AM, Rolls BJ: Dietary energy density in the treatment of obesity: a year-long trial comparing 2 weight-loss diets. *American Journal of Clinical Nutrition* 85:1465–1477, 2007

Foy CG, Lewis CE, Hairston KG, Miller GD, Lang W, Jakicic JM, Rejeski WJ, Ribisl PM, Walkup MP, Wagenknecht LE: Intensive lifestyle intervention improves physical function among obese adults with knee pain: findings from the Look AHEAD trial. *Obesity (Silver Spring)* 19:83–93, 2011

Franz MJ, Boucher JL, Green-Pastors J, Powers MA: Evidence-based nutrition practice guidelines for diabetes and scope and standards of practice. *J Am Diet Assoc* 108:S52–S58, 2008

Galasso P, Amend A, Melkus GD, Nelson GT: Barriers to medical nutrition therapy in black women with type 2 diabetes mellitus. *Diabetes Educ* 31:719–725, 2005

Gonzalez JS, Fisher L, Polonsky WH: Depression in diabetes: have we been missing something important? *Diabetes Care* 34:236–239, 2011

Gorin AA, Wing RR, Fava JL, Jakicic JM, Jeffery R, West DS, Brelje K, Dilillo VG: Weight loss treatment influences untreated spouses and the home environment: evidence of a ripple effect. *Int J Obes* (Lond) 32:1678–1684, 2008

Guare JC, Wing RR, Grant A: Comparison of obese NIDDM and nondiabetic women: short- and long-term weight loss. *Obesity Research* 3:329–335, 1995

Hanni MD, Mendoza E, Snider J, Winkleby MA: A methodology for evaluating organizational change in community-based chronic disease interventions. *Preventing Chronic Disease* 4:A105, 2007

Heini AF, Weinsier RL: Divergent trends in obesity and fat intake patterns: the American paradox. *American Journal of Medicine* 102:259–264, 1997

Hersey J, Williams-Piehota P, Sparling PB, Alexander J, Hill MD, Isenberg KB, Rooks A, Dunet DO: Promising practices in promotion of healthy weight at small and medium-sized US worksites. *Prev Chronic Dis* 5:A122, 2008

Heymsfield SB, van Mierlo CA, van der Knaap HC, Heo M, Frier HI: Weight management using a meal replacement strategy: meta and pooling analysis from six studies. *Int J Obes Relat Metab Disord* 27:537–549, 2003

Horowitz CR, Colson KA, Hebert PL, Lancaster K: Barriers to buying healthy foods for people with diabetes: evidence of environmental disparities. *American Journal of Public Health* 94:1549–1554, 2004

Jeffery RW, Wing RR: Long-term effects of interventions for weight loss using food provision and monetary incentives. *Journal of Consulting and Clinical Psychology* 63:793–796, 1995

Kant AK, Graubard BI: Secular trends in the association of socio-economic position with self-reported dietary attributes and biomarkers in the US population: National Health and Nutrition Examination Survey (NHANES) 1971–1975 to NHANES 1999–2002. *Public Health Nutrition* 10:158–167, 2007a

Kant AK, Graubard BI, Kumanyika SK: Trends in black-white differentials in dietary intakes of U.S. adults, 1971–2002. *American Journal of Preventive Medicine* 32:264–272, 2007b

Kant AK, Graubard BI: Secular trends in patterns of self-reported food consumption of adult americans: NHANES 1971–1975 to NHANES 1999–2002. *American Journal of Clinical Nutrition* 84:1215–1223, 2006

Kant AK, Graubard BI: Energy density of diets reported by American adults: association with food group intake, nutrient intake, and body weight. *Int J Obes* (Lond) 29:950–956, 2005

Katz T: Shaping the marketplace for medical nutrition therapy: advocating for coverage. *Journal of the American Dietetic Association* 106:1027–1028, 2006

Knowler WC, Barrett-Connor E, Fowler SE, Hamman RF, Lachin JM, Walker EA, Nathan DM: Reduction in the incidence of type 2 diabetes with lifestyle intervention or metformin. *N Engl J Med* 346:393–403, 2002

Lenz A, Diamond FB Jr: Obesity: the hormonal milieu. *Current Opinion in Endocrinology, Diabetes, and Obesity* 15:9–20, 2008

Lichtman SW, Pisarska K, Berman ER, Pestone M, Dowling H, Offenbacher E, Weisel H, Heshka S, Matthews DE, Heymsfield SB: Discrepancy between self-reported and actual caloric intake and exercise in obese subjects. *N Engl J Med* 327:1893–1898, 1992

Look AHEAD Research Group, Wadden TA, West DS, Delahanty L, Jakicic J, Rejeski J, Williamson D, Berkowitz RI, Kelley DE, Tomchee C, Hill JO, Kumanyika S: The Look AHEAD study: a description of the lifestyle intervention and the evidence supporting it. *Obesity (Silver Spring)* 14:737–752, 2006

McCormack LA, Williams-Piehota PA, Bann CM, Burton J, Kamerow DB, Squire C, Fisher E, Brownson CA, Glasgow RE: Development and validation of an instrument to measure resources and support for chronic illness self-management: a model using diabetes. *Diabetes Educ* 34:707–718, 2008

Miller CK, Gutschall MD, Lawrence F: The development of self-efficacy and outcome expectation measures regarding glycaemic load and the nutritional management of type 2 diabetes. *Public Health Nutr* 10:628–634, 2007

Miller NH: Motivational interviewing as a prelude to coaching in healthcare settings. *Journal of Cardiovascular Nursing* 25:247–251, 2010

Miller WR, Rollnick S: Meeting in the middle: motivational interviewing and self-determination theory. *International Journal of Behavioral Nutrition and Physical Activity* 9:25, 2012

Miller WR, Rollnick S: Ten things that motivational interviewing is not. *Behavioural and Cognitive Psychotherapy* 37:129–140, 2009

Moore H, Summerbell C, Hooper L, Cruickshank K, Vyas A, Johnson M, Ashton V, Kopelman P: Dietary advice for treatment of type 2 diabetes mellitus in adults. *Cochrane Database Syst Rev* CD004097, 2004

Mossavar-Rahmani Y: Applying motivational enhancement to diverse populations. *Journal of the American Dietetic Association* 107:918–921, 2007

Niedert KC: Position of the American Dietetic Association: liberalization of the diet prescription improves quality of life for older adults in long-term care. *Journal of the American Dietetic Association* 105:1955–1965, 2005

Nielsen SJ, Popkin BM: Patterns and trends in food portion sizes, 1977–1998. *JAMA* 289:450–453, 2003

Norris SL, Zhang X, Avenell A, Gregg E, Brown TJ, Schmid CH, Lau J: Long-term non-pharmacologic weight loss interventions for adults with type 2 diabetes. *Cochrane Database Syst Rev* CD004095, 2005a

Norris SL, Zhang X, Avenell A, Gregg E, Schmid CH, Lau J: Long-term non-pharmacological weight loss interventions for adults with prediabetes. *Cochrane Database Syst Rev* CD005270, 2005b

Norris SL, Zhang X, Avenell A, Gregg E, Bowman B, Serdula M, Brown TJ, Schmid CH, Lau J: Long-term effectiveness of lifestyle and behavioral weight loss interventions in adults with type 2 diabetes: a meta-analysis. *American Journal of Medicine* 117:762–774, 2004

Pascale RW, Wing RW, Butler BA, Mullen M, Bononi P: Effects of a behavioral weight loss program stressing calorie restriction versus calorie plus fat restriction in obese individuals with NIDDM or a family history of diabetes. *Diabetes Care* 18:1241–1248, 1995

Pastors JG, Franz MJ, Warshaw H, Daly A, Arnold MS: How effective is medical nutrition therapy in diabetes care? *J Am Diet Assoc* 103:827–831, 2003

Pastors JG, Warshaw H, Daly A, Franz M, Kulkarni K: The evidence for the effectiveness of medical nutrition therapy in diabetes management. *Diabetes Care* 25:608–613, 2002

Polonsky WH, Fisher L, Earles J, Dudl RJ, Lees J, Mullan J, Jackson RA: Assessing psychosocial distress in diabetes: development of the diabetes distress scale. *Diabetes Care* 28:626–631, 2005

Polonsky WH, Anderson BJ, Lohrer PA, Welch G, Jacobson AM, Aponte JE, Schwartz CE: Assessment of diabetes-related distress. *Diabetes Care* 18:754–760, 1995

Raynor HA, Jeffery RW, Ruggiero AM, Clark JM, Delahanty LM: Weight loss strategies associated with BMI in overweight adults with type 2 diabetes at entry into the Look AHEAD (Action for Health in Diabetes) trial. *Diabetes Care* 31:1299–1304, 2008

Rejeski WJ, Ip EH, Bertoni AG, Bray GA, Evans G, Gregg EW, Zhang Q: Lifestyle change and mobility in obese adults with type 2 diabetes. *N Engl J Med* 366:1209–1217, 2012

Rolls BJ, Bell EA, Waugh BA: Increasing the volume of a food by incorporating air affects satiety in men. *American Journal of Clinical Nutrition* 72:361–368, 2000

Rowe S, Alexander N, Almeida NG, Black R, Burns R, Bush L, Crawford P, Keim N, Kris-Etherton P, Weaver C: Translating the Dietary Guidelines for Americans 2010 to bring about real behavior change. *Journal of the American Dietetic Association* 111:28–39, 2011

Ruelaz AR, Diefenbach P, Simon B, Lanto A, Arterburn D, Shekelle PG: Perceived barriers to weight management in primary care: perspectives of patients and providers. *J Gen Intern Med* 22:518–522, 2007

Schnepf R, Richardson J: Consumer and food price inflation. Congressional Research Service Report for Congress. R40545. April 14, 2011. Available at www.crs.gov.

Seligman HK, Laraia BA, Kushel MB: Food insecurity is associated with chronic disease among low-income NHANES participants. *J Nutr* 140:304–310, 2010

Seligman HK, Bindman AB, Vittinghoff E, Kanaya AM, Kushel MB: Food insecurity is associated with diabetes mellitus: results from the National Health Examination and Nutrition Examination Survey (NHANES) 1999–2002. *Journal of General Internal Medicine* 22:1018–1023, 2007

Spahn JM, Lyon JM, Altman JM, Blum-Kemelor DM, Essery EV, Fungwe TV, Macneil PC, McGrane MM, Obbagy JE, Wong YP: The systematic review methodology used to support the 2010 Dietary Guidelines Advisory Committee. *Journal of the American Dietetic Association* 111:520–523, 2011

U.S. Department of Agriculture, U.S. Department of Health and Human Services: *Dietary Guidelines for Americans, 2010.* 7th ed. Washington, DC, U.S. Government Printing Office, 2010

Wang YC, Bleich SN, Gortmaker SL: Increasing caloric contribution from sugar-sweetened beverages and 100% fruit juices among US children and adolescents, 1988–2004. *Pediatrics* 121:e1604–1614, 2008

West DS, DiLillo V, Bursac Z, Gore SA, Greene PG: Motivational interviewing improves weight loss in women with type 2 diabetes. *Diabetes Care* 30:1081–1087, 2007

Wildman RP, Muntner P, Reynolds K, McGinn AP, Rajpathak S, Wylie-Rosett J, Sowers MR: The obese without cardiometabolic risk factor clustering and the normal weight with cardiometabolic risk factor clustering: prevalence and correlates of 2 phenotypes among the US population (NHANES 1999–2004). *Arch Intern Med* 168:1617–1624, 2008

Williamson DA, Rejeski J, Lang W, Van Dorsten B, Fabricatore AN, Toledo K: Impact of a weight management program on health-related quality of life in overweight adults with type 2 diabetes. *Archives of Internal Medicine* 169:163–171, 2009

Wing RR, Jeffery RW: Food provision as a strategy to promote weight loss. *Obesity Research* 9 (Suppl. 4):S271–S275, 2001

Wing RR, Jeffery RW, Burton LR, Thorson C, Nissinoff KS, Baxter JE: Food provision vs structured meal plans in the behavioral treatment of obesity. *Int J Obes Relat Metab Disord* 20:56–62, 1996

Wing RR, Blair E, Marcus M, Epstein LH, Harvey J: Year-long weight loss treatment for obese patients with type II diabetes: does including an intermittent very-low-calorie diet improve outcome? *Am J Med* 97:354–362, 1994

Wing RR, Koeske R, Epstein LH, Nowalk MP, Gooding W, Becker D: Long-term effects of modest weight loss in type II diabetic patients. *Archives of Internal Medicine* 147:1749–1753, 1987

Wylie-Rosett J. The diabetes epidemic: what can we do? *Journal of the American Dietetic Association* 109:1160–1162, 2009

Wylie-Rosett J, Elmer P: Cardiovascular risk factor reduction: evaluating dietary intake in assessing nutrition education. *Journal of Patient Education and Counseling* 15:217–227, 1990

Zhang X, Norris SL, Chowdhury FM, Gregg EW, Zhang P: The effects of interventions on health-related quality of life among persons with diabetes: a systematic review. *Medical Care* 45:820–834, 2007

第九章

生活方式改变：运动

David G. Marrero，PhD
Paula M. Trief，PhD

运动的定义是"身体活动或运动，尤其是想要保持一个人……舒适和健康的时候"，这也反映出了运动在治疗糖尿病方面所扮演的角色。考虑到肥胖在 2 型糖尿病中的重要影响，第二种定义可能更加有用，那就是"运动指的是超出日常能量消耗的那部分增加的活动量"。在这种情况下，运动可以消耗卡路里，从而对减肥和体重的保持起到有效作用。

在 1953 年，Joslin 写到"在胰岛素之前运动被认为是有用的，但并没有认为其对糖尿病管理至关重要……我们应该重拾运动来帮助我们治疗所有的情况"。超过 40 年的研究表明 Joslin 的观察报告具有先驱性：规律的体育锻炼对 1 型和 2 型糖尿病患者都有很多好处。它之所以能够被人接受，是因为基于更深入的研究证明参与规律的体育锻炼对人体健康有直接的好处，尤其是对糖尿病患者。体育锻炼可以提高胰岛素的功效，控制血糖，减肥，还可以很好地减少体脂，降低血压、胆固醇和油脂，从而降低心血管疾病的风险。体育锻炼已经成为"生活方式改变"干预的一部分，从而避免或延缓一些糖尿病并发症的发展进程。此外，运动可以帮助维持减肥，这对预防 2 型糖尿病（T2D）患者风险因素的增长有很大贡献。

运动还可以帮助治疗抑郁，这是与糖尿病有关的一种共患病。Meta 分析表明运动可以减少社会人群的沮丧情绪。在 Look AHEAD 的试验中，参加强化生活方式干预的 2 型糖尿病患者在生活质量和抑郁方面有了改善，这是通过提升身体健康状况来介导的。

增加日常活动的行为干预未被充分利用

依据代谢效能中的心理获益和体重相关的改善，我们强烈建议启动包括体育锻炼在内的业余时间的活动。然而，现在许多资料表明糖尿病患者比正常人运动的少。一项对南卡罗莱纳州的居民调查发现，42%的成年糖尿病患者（包括1型和2型）很少运动，而无糖尿病的成人只有27%。同样的是，对美国墨西哥患有糖尿病的患者调研表明，只有61%的人在业余时间经常做运动，例如，修整花园（33.7%）或者走路（31.5%）。另一项针对不同种族之间体育锻炼差异的研究中，有32 440名美国成年人参与调研，这其中1850人患有糖尿病（包括1型和2型）。总的来说，只有25%的美国成年人每日进行适度的或强烈的体育锻炼，黑色人种（16%）要低于西班牙裔（23%）和白色人种（27%）。更多的细节分析发现显著的种族差异，几乎大部分是由于黑人女性低水平的体育锻炼。由于职业和家务不包括体育锻炼，所以研究需要复制并且扩展。不管怎样，这些研究结果强调一个事实，一般的美国成年人倾向于久坐，少数成人——有较高2型糖尿病风险——体育锻炼的比例都很低，把通过体育锻炼提高身体素质作为目标，对美国人民来说具有重大意义。

对于糖尿病患者来说，并发症的存在及其严重程度可能会影响体育锻炼。每种并发症都与特定的运动建议相关联，而且可能会限制患者的选择。如果患有增生性或严重的非增殖性视网膜疾病应尽量避免激烈的有氧运动，这有可能有视网膜脱落或者玻璃体积血的风险。当人们患有严重的精神性疾病，同时伴有疼痛和麻木，建议选择无负重的运动方式（如骑脚踏车、游泳）。自主神经病变将提高运动中受伤的风险，强烈建议要进行心脏评估。大多数对糖尿病患者运动的研究已经证实各式的运动对健康都有显著的益处，包括有氧锻炼、抗阻训练、机动性训练。鉴于健康的益处和增加风险的有限证据，大多数研究表明与其避免活动，不如确定一种将风险降到最小的同时又能增加体育锻炼的方式。把运动目标（应该被看作是一种自我管理行为）作为日常糖尿病管理的一部分进行系统的合并及监测，通常很难完成。

适应证

除非有特殊的禁忌，日常锻炼对所有人，特别是糖尿病患者有明显的作用。越来越多证据建议，应该开始以诊断为根据的日常体育锻炼。日常锻炼有助于降低死亡率和发病率，对血糖控制、减肥的维持及内心幸福感的提升有直接的影响。运动对体重管理有潜在的影响，对超重或肥胖的 2 型糖尿病患者尤其重要，因为这种情况可以增加胰岛素抵抗和心血管风险。糖尿病患者存在与运动相关的潜在风险，对于之前就存在糖尿病并发症的患者，运动也有一定的限制。这些包括低血糖的可能性，运动造成的高血糖及使特殊糖尿病并发症恶化的风险。尽管运动是为了降低血糖水平，但如果运动开始时血糖水平较高，它也有可能会导致血糖水平增高。

在运动计划开始之前，所有糖尿病患者都应该进行身体测试来确保可以进行安全的、个体化的运动计划。这个测试必须重点评估是否存在大血管和（或）微血管并发症，这种情况下将不会推荐某些形式的运动。这些并发症包括肌肉骨骼损伤或畸形，一些心血管疾病（CVD），以及禁用 Valsalva 动作的微血管的疾病。微血管疾病患者，尤其是视网膜疾病患者，应避免像举重这样的运动，因为在 Valsalva 过程中会增加微血管压力。在这种情况下，可能会用一些其他形式的替代运动（如走路）来提高体育锻炼的水平。另外，患有 2 型糖尿病的患者需要进行压力测试来评价他们的心血管系统和呼吸系统的完整性。压力测试的优势就是可以帮助建立目标心率界限值，以便患有自主神经疾病的患者能够安全地运动。另外，它可以识别运动引起的高血压，这将使患者进行最适合的运动，包括类型、强度及持续时间，以便使健康风险降到最低。是否对全部的糖尿病患者还是仅对那些有危险因素的患者进行运动心电图（ECG）压力测试，还存在一些分歧。然而，并发症的出现加强了人们对一种关系的关注，即运动强度和频率对心脏和呼吸功能的影响与需要使用压力测试进行筛选之间的关系。

干预的目标

运动处方应该根据患者自身的目标和患者在其所处的环境可以安全而现实地实施所给定的体育活动的这种能力评估来制订。可能的目标包括改善血糖控制，降低心血管的风险，减重和加强力量和耐力。一些人运动是为了保持身体健康，然而其他人可能有竞争性的运动员目标。不管目标如何，所有的糖尿病患者都需要进行体育锻炼，除非他们有禁忌参加体育活动的身体状况，正如上面所指出的那样。如果因为肌肉骨骼受伤或者畸形而不能进行承重运动，可以考虑降低身体负载的运动，如游泳和水中有氧运动。

已知的治疗方法

运动计划开始的第一步通常是来自患者医生的建议。向健康专家咨询是动机和支持的强有力来源。

在有职业认证的运动专家（运动生理学家，有认证的运动训练员或者心脏功能锻炼专家）的帮助下订制的个人运动计划将会使很多人受益。合格的运动工作者包括有以下资格证书的人员：美国运动医学学院的资格证书（ASCM）、美国运动协会的证书（ACE）、美国有氧健身协会的证书（AFFA）或者国际健康专业组织的认证（IFPA）。另外，针对所选择的不同种类的运动，应该使用在具体运动模式中训练的具有认证资格的指导者。当无法获得这些资源时，建议求助社区中心（如 YMCA），他们可以在合适的运动程序中提供一些指导。如果没有支持资源可用，建议实施日常的散步计划。如果要参与无人监管的运动计划，建议他/她关注基本的安全规程是非常重要的。这包括在运动的时长和强度方面要缓慢而平稳的提升，如果选择走路则需要选择合适的鞋，注意任何预示身体有潜在问题的感觉征兆，如剧痛、胸闷、呼吸困难或者意识混乱。如果有上述症状发生，除非可以进行医疗评估，否则需要暂停运动。这些建议不只针对糖尿病患者，它们代表了基本的指南，故临床医生在医疗管理访谈中也可以提出此类建议。

正式运动计划的发展

在正式的运动计划开始之前，应该进行运动评估以使患者获得个人合适的运动计划处方。糖尿病病史包括糖尿病的类型、患糖尿病的时间、糖尿病的并发症、控制血糖的治疗、自我监测血糖的频率、低血糖发生的频率，包括严重程度及其与运动的关系，目前糖尿病的控制情况。正如上文所提到的，运动可以根据其中一些因素来降低和提升血糖水平。如果患者血糖处在正常值低限时（例如，血糖为 80 mg/dl）开始运动，那么体育锻炼可能导致低的血糖水平，尤其是该患者是使用胰岛素来控制糖尿病的。因此，在运动开始之前，评估血糖和准备对抗低血糖的快速作用的糖类都非常重要。同样的是，1 型糖尿病患者在血糖水平较高时（例如，血糖＞250mg/dl）开始运动，可以通过刺激肝糖原储备的释放来升高血糖。因此，对于 1 型糖尿病患者来说，在运动之前进行血糖评估及定时的运动来确保血糖波动处于安全的范围：在 80～240mg/dl，这是非常重要的。不存在胰岛素严重缺陷时，例如，2 型糖尿病患者的早期病程阶段，轻微或中等强度的锻炼能够降低血糖。因此，假如 2 型糖尿病患者不存在脱水，并且尿液和（或）血酮呈阴性时，就没有必要将高血糖症作为唯一的推迟运动的标准。

如果运动计划的目标是为了帮助体重管理，那么目标的建立是为了完成热量的消耗。这就要求运动的续时间和强度要达到热量消耗的目标。

行为干预

许多研究已经确定了有效的生活方式干预。大规模的研究，像预防糖尿病项目和 Look AHEAD 已经使用多种干预措施，包括设定目标、自我监测、频繁联系，以及逐步的管理条款。这些干预措施可以在受过培训的辅导者那里得到一系列持续的课程指导。这些辅导者与患者协商减重目标，并且教他们特定的策略来实现减重，如追踪食物和减少脂肪克数的方法。有效的干预措施已经通过各种形式和模式被传播，包括出版物、互联网、电话，当然还有人与人之间相互传播。例如，体重监测者运用成熟的在线干预来帮助使用者追踪饮食摄取量并且进行食物选择，食物选择是根据能反应食物的成分和卡路里的分数系统进行的。尽管很多项目还没有进行长期效力和成本效益的评估，但现存的评估表明这些干预是有成本效益的。

干预中的社会心理因素

动机和社会心理问题的难题经常干扰运动方案的依从性和体育锻炼的水平。因此，一个明确的个人动机和支持性的资源的评估是选择一个可以坚持的运动方式的基本保证。这包括回顾个人的喜好，评估支持资源的有效性（也就是设施、培训人员、器材），以及评估常规地进行运动可能存在的障碍。在这一点上，询问患者过去在运动过程中的成功和挑战，并且让他们确定每日可以坚持运动的时间段，这是很有价值的。至关重要的因素是每个人需要选择有意义且有回报的，生活环境支持的，与社会经济及自身状态相符的运动形式。

如果要开始常规的运动，那么需要治疗沮丧、压抑和焦虑的情绪。就这一点而言，运动可以减少沮丧情绪症状是值得注意的。自我效能可以减少抑郁，是身体锻炼非常重要的决定性因素。一个现实的运动方案需要获得早期的成果，而且可以为了进一步的改变优化自我效能。这包括选择适合的运动模式、时长、频率及强度。一旦运动规划确定，为达到长期的运动目标可以逐步增加运动量。

参加社会支持系统也是有价值的，尤其是家庭，可以帮助人们开启及维持运动计划。因为家庭支持可以帮助人们将开启及维持常规运动计划的可能性发挥到最大，所以让家庭成员参与计划的决策制订是非常重要的。

管理环境

有多种多样的环境可以支持运动计划，而且合适环境的获取可能是影响日常身体锻炼的重要的因素。这取决于选择的运动形式。正式的运动设备是没有必要的。有一些可以在家里建立运动计划的选择。例如，Jette 等的研究表明，坐在椅子上的时候，可以利用家里平常的东西（如罐头）进行中等程度的耐力训练，从而完成有效的运动计划。大量的证据表明简单的走路有许多运动益处，尤其是对糖尿病患者。走路的好处是它在不需要花费金钱的环境里就可以完成，容易实现，而且可以根据天气情况随时调整计划。

成果的持续监测

日常运动计划包括多种形式的成果监测。这包括出勤记录和各种各样的绩效指标（例如，花费在运动上的时间增加；体重、血压和血糖水平的变化）。基本的组成部分包括使用一些自我监测的方式和在健康管理团队的帮助下，监测与体育锻炼次数和时间相关的生理变化。体育锻炼本身可以通过问卷表格、计步器或者加速计来进行测量。（评估体育锻炼的方法可以在以下网址获得 http://www.cde.gov/physical activity/ professionals /data/ explanation.heml）基于计步器的干预对增加体育锻炼是有效的，这在某种程度上是因为增加监测的意识本身就是一种有力的干预措施。

临床管理的建议

最近一项对运动和糖尿病的相关研究和立场声明的综述总结了关于运动、身体锻炼和糖尿病控制管理的现有建议。作者指出运动建议的不同取决于患者的健康目标。总之，他们建议以下几点。

1. 如果目标是改善血糖控制、减少心血管风险或维持体重，每周至少 150 分钟中等强度有氧运动和（或）每周 90 分钟高强度有氧运动。

2. 2 型糖尿病患者，经运动专家初步评估和定期评估，如果没有并发症禁忌，每周持续运动 3 次。

3. 30 岁以上合并其他危险因素和 40 岁以上所有糖尿病患者进行剧烈运动前需进行压力测试。

4. 在系统阐述运动方案或执行运动计划之前，应该进行心理评估，包括抑郁评估[应用 9 条目病人健康问卷（PHQ-9）标准抑郁自评工具]和受试者参加运动的自我效能的感觉评估（应用标准测量）。

　　5. 应该使用行为策略来帮助患者开启并维持运动计划，包括但是不局限于目标设定，还应该逐步实施但增加运动强度，为达到里程碑效果而整体巩固加强。

参 考 文 献

Aiello LP, Wong J, Cavallerano JD, Bursell SE, Aiello LM: Retinopathy. In *Handbook of Exercise in Diabetes*. 2nd ed. Ruderman N, Devlin JT, Schneider SH, Kriska A, Eds. Alexandria, VA, American Diabetes Association, 2002, p. 401-413

Ainsworth BE, et al.: 2011 compendium of physical activities: a second update of codes and MET values. *Med Sci Sports Exerc* 43:1575, 2011

Aljasem LI, Peyrot M, Wissow L, Rubin RR: The impact of barriers and self-efficacy on self-care behaviors in type 2 diabetes. *Diabetes Educ* 27:393-404, 2001

American Diabetes Association: Physical activity/exercise and diabetes (Position Statement). *Diabetes Care* 27 (Suppl. 1):S58-S62, 2004

Anderson RJ, Freedland KE, Clouse RE, Lustman PJ: The prevalence of comorbid depression in adults with diabetes: a meta analysis. *Diabetes Care* 24:1069-1078, 2001

Armit CM, Brown WJ, Marshall AL, Ritchie CB, Trost SG, Green A, Bauman AE: Randomized trial of three strategies to promote physical activity in general practice. *Prev Med* 48:156-163, 2009

Barrett-Connor EL, Wingard DL, Edelstein SL: Why is diabetes a stronger risk factor for fatal ischemic heart disease in women than in men? The Rancho Bernardo Study. *JAMA* 265:627-631, 1991

Basevi V, Di Mario S, Morciano C, Nonino F, Magrini N: Comment on: American Diabetes Association: Standards of Medical Care in Diabetes—2011. *Diabetes Care* 34 (Suppl. 1):S1-S61, 2011

Berlin JA, Colditz GA: A meta-analysis of physical activity in the prevention of coronary heart disease. *American Journal of Epidemiology* 132:612-628, 1990

Borghouts LB, Keizer HA: Exercise and insulin sensitivity: a review. *International Journal of Sports Medicine* 21:1-12, 2000

Boulé NG, Kenny GP, Haddad E, Wells GA, Sigal RJ: Meta-analysis of the effect of structured exercise training on cardiorespiratory fitness in type 2 diabetes mellitus. *Diabetologia* 46:1071-1081, 2003

Boulé NG, Haddad E, Kenny GP, Wells GA, Sigal RJ: Effects of exercise on glycemic control and body mass in type 2 diabetes mellitus: a meta-analysis of controlled clinical trials. *JAMA* 286:1218-1227, 2001

Bravata DM, Smith-Spangler C, Sundaram V, Gienger AL, et al.: Using pedometers to increase physical activity and improve health: a systematic review. *JAMA* 298:2296-2304, 2007

Carron AV, Hausenblas HA, Mack D: Social influence and exercise: a meta-analysis. *J Sport Exercise Psychology* 18:1-16, 1996

Caspersen CJ, Powell KE, Christenson GM: Physical activity, exercise, and physical fitness: definitions and distinctions for health-related research. *Public Health Rep* 100:126-131, 1985

Church TS, Cheng YJ, Earnest CP, Barlow CE, Gibbons LW, Priest EL, Blair SN: Exercise capacity and body composition as predictors of mortality among men with diabetes. *Diabetes Care* 27:83-88, 2004

Clark M, Hampson SE, Avery L, Simpson R: Effects of a tailored lifestyle self-management intervention in patients with type 2 diabetes. *Br J Health Psychol* 9:365-379, 2004

Colberg SR, Sigal RJ, Fernhall B, Regensteiner JG, Blissmer BJ, Rubin RR, Chasan-Taber L, Albright AL, Braun B: Exercise and type 2 diabetes: the American College of Sports Medicine and the American Diabetes Association: joint position statement. *Diabetes Care* 33:e147-e167, 2010

Craft LL, Perna FM: The benefits of exercise for the clinically depressed. *Prim Care Companion J Clin Psychiatry* 6:104-111, 2004

de Groot M, Anderson RJ, Freedland KE, Clouse RE, Lustman PJ: The association of depression and diabetes complications: a meta analysis. *Psychosomatic Medicine* 63:619-630, 2001

Delahanty LM, Conroy MB, Nathan DM: Psychological predictors of physical activity in the Diabetes Prevention Program. *J Am Diet Assoc* 106:698-705, 2006

Deshpande AD, Baker EA, Lovegreen SL, Brownson RC: Environmental correlates of physical activity among individuals with diabetes in the rural midwest. *Diabetes Care* 28:1012-1018, 2005

Diabetes Prevention Program (DPP) Research Group: The Diabetes Prevention Program (DPP): description of lifestyle intervention. *Diabetes Care* 25:2165-2171, 2002

Duncan P, Richards L, Wallace D, Stoker-Yates J, Pohl P, Luchies C, Ogle A, Studenski S: A randomized, controlled pilot study of a home-based exercise program for individuals with mild and moderate stroke. *Stroke* 29:2055-2060, 1998

Dutton GR, Tan F, Provost BC, Sorenson JL, Allen B, Smith D: Relationship between self-efficacy and physical activity among patients with type 2 diabetes. *J Behav Med* 32:270-277, 2009

Dutton GR, Provost BC, Tan F, Smith D: A tailored print-based physical activity intervention for patients with type 2 diabetes. *Preventive Medicine* 47:409-411, 2008

Eakin EG, Reeves MM, Lawler SP, Oldenburg B, et al.: The Logan Healthy Living Program: a cluster randomized trial of a telephone delivered physical activity and dietary behavior intervention for primary care patients with type 2 diabetes or hypertension from a socially disadvantaged community: rationale, design and recruitment. *Contemp Clin Trials* 29:439-454, 2008

Egede LE, Poston ME: Racial/ethnic differences in leisure-time physical activity levels among individuals with diabetes. *Diabetes Care* 27:2493-2494, 2004

Fisher NM, Kame VD Jr, Rouse L, Pendergast DR: Quantitative evaluation of a home exercise program on muscle and functional capacity of patients with osteoarthritis. *Am J Phys Med Rehabil* 73:413-420, 1994

Fowler-Brown A, Pignone M, Pletcher M, Tice JA, Sutton SF, Lohr KN: Exercise tolerance testing to screen for coronary heart disease: a systematic review for the technical support for the U.S. Preventive Services Task Force. *Ann Intern Med* 140:W9-W24, 2004

Ganda OP: Patients on various drug therapies. In *Handbook of Exercise in Diabetes*. 2nd ed. Ruderman N, Devlin JT, Schneider SH, Kriska A, Eds. Alexandria, VA, American Diabetes Association, 2002, p. 587-599

Glasgow RE, Nutting PA, King DK, Nelson CC, et al.: Randomized effectiveness trial of a computer-assisted intervention to improve diabetes care. *Diabetes Care* 28:33-39, 2005

Gleeson-Kreig J: Social support and physical activity in type 2 diabetes: a social-ecologic approach. *Diabetes Educ* 34:1037-1044, 2008

Gordon NF: The exercise prescription. In *Handbook of Exercise in Diabetes*. Ruderman N, Devlin JT, Schneider SH, Eds. Alexandria, VA, American Diabetes Association, 2001, p. 269-288

Grundy SM, Hansen B, Smith SC, Cleeman JI, Kahn RA, et al.: Clinical management of metabolic syndrome: report of the American Heart Association/National Heart, Lung, and Blood Institute/American Diabetes Association conference on scientific issues related to management. *Circulation* 109:551-556, 2004

Haskell WL, Lee IM, Pate RR, Powell KE, Blair SN, Franklin BA, et al.: Physical activity and public health: updated recommendation for adults from the American College of Sports Medicine and the American Heart Association. *Medicine and Science in Sports and Exercise* 39:1423-1434, 2007

Hayes C, Kriska A: Role of physical activity in diabetes management and prevention. *Journal of the American Dietetic Association* 108 (Suppl. 1):S19-S23, 2008

Hu FB, Sigal RJ, Rich-Edwards JW, Colditz GA, Solomon CG, Willet WC, Speizer FE, Manson JE: Walking compared with vigorous physical activity and risk of type 2 diabetes in women. *JAMA* 282:1433-1439, 1999

Jackson R, Asimakopoulou K, Scammell A: Assessment of the transtheoretical model as used by dietitians in promoting physical activity in people with type 2 diabetes. *J Hum Nutr Diet* 20:27-36, 2007

Jacobs-van der Bruggen MA, van Baal PH, Hoogenveen RT, Feenstra TL, et al.: Cost-effectiveness of lifestyle modification in diabetes patients. *Diabetes Care* 32:1453-1458, 2009

Jacobs-van der Bruggen MA, Bos G, Bemelmans WJ, Hoogenveen RT, Vijgen SM, Baan CA: Lifestyle interventions are cost-effective in people with different levels of diabetes risk: results from a modeling study. *Diabetes Care* 30:128-134, 2007

Jette AM, Rooks D, Lachman M, Lin TH, Levenson C, Helstein D, Giorgetti MM, Harris BA: Home-based resistance training predictors of participation and adherence. *Diabetes Care* 38:412-421, 1998

Joslin EP: *A Diabetic Manual for Doctor and Patient*. 9th ed. Philadelphia, Lea & Febiger, 1953

Keyserling TC, Samuel-Hodge CD, Ammerman AS, Ainsworth BE, et al.: A randomized trial of an intervention to improve self-care behaviors of African-American women with type 2 diabetes: impact on physical activity. *Diabetes Care* 25:1576–1583, 2002

Kirk A, Mutrie N, MacIntyre P, Fisher M: Effects of a 12-month physical activity counselling intervention on glycaemic control and on the status of cardiovascular risk factors in people with type 2 diabetes. *Diabetologia* 47:821–832, 2004a

Kirk AF, Mutrie N, Macintyre PD, Fisher MB: Promoting and maintaining physical activity in people with type 2 diabetes. *Am J Prev Med* 27:289–296, 2004b

Knowler WC, Barrett-Connor E, Fowler SE, Hamman RF, Lachin JM, Walker EA, Nathan DM, Diabetes Prevention Program Research Group: Reduction in the incidence of type 2 diabetes with lifestyle intervention or metformin. *N Engl J Med* 346:393–403, 2002

Kroenke K, Spitzer RL, Williams, JBW: The PHQ-9 validity of a brief depression severity measure. *Journal of General Internal Medicine* 16:606–613, 2001

Lee C, Bobko P: Self-efficacy beliefs: comparison of five measures. *Journal of Applied Psychology* 79:364–369, 1994

Liebreich T, Plotnikoff RC, Courneya KS, Boule N: Diabetes NetPLAY: a physical activity website and linked email counselling randomized intervention for individuals with type 2 diabetes. *Int J Behav Nutr Phys Act* 6:18, 2009

Look AHEAD Research Group, Wadden TA, West DS, Delahanty L, et al.: The Look AHEAD study: a description of the lifestyle intervention and the evidence supporting it. *Obesity (Silver Spring)* 14:737–752, 2006

Marrero DG: Initiation and maintenance of exercise in patients with diabetes. *Handbook of Exercise in Diabetes*. Ruderman N, Devlin JT, Schneider SH, Eds. Alexandria, VA, American Diabetes Association, 2001, p. 289–309

McGale N, McArdle S, Gaffney P: Exploring the effectiveness of an integrated exercise/CBT intervention for young men's mental health. *Br J Health Psychol* 16:457–471, 2011

Mier N, Medina AA, Ory MG: Mexican Americans with type 2 diabetes: perspectives on definitions, motivators, and programs of physical activity. *Prev Chronic Dis* 4:A24, 2007

Mulloolly CA, Hanson, CK: Physical activity/exercise. In *A Core Curriculum for Diabetes Education*. 5th ed. Franz M, Ed. Chicago, American Association of Diabetes Educators, 2003

Ogilvie D, Foster CE, Rothnie H, Cavill N, et al.: Interventions to promote walking: systematic review. *BMJ* 334:1204, 2007

Peyrot M, Rubin RR: Behavioral and psychosocial interventions in diabetes: a conceptual review. *Diabetes Care* 30:2433–2440, 2007

Ratner R, Goldberg R, Haffner S, Marcovina S, Orchard T, Fowler S, Temprosa M, Diabetes Prevention Program Research Group: Impact of intensive lifestyle and metformin therapy on cardiovascular disease risk factors in the diabetes prevention program. *Diabetes Care* 28:888–894, 2005

Sacco WP, Malone JI, Morrison AD, Friedman A, Wells K: Effect of a brief, regular telephone intervention by paraprofessionals for type 2 diabetes. *J Behav Med* 32:349–359, 2009

Scully D, Kremmer J, Meade MM, Dudgeon K: Physical exercise and psychological well being: a critical review. *British Journal of Sports Medicine* 32:111–120, 1998

Sigal RJ, Kenny GP, Wasserman DH, Castaneda-Sceppa C, White RD: Physical activity/exercise and type 2 diabetes: a consensus statement from the American Diabetes Association. *Diabetes Care* 29:1433–1438, 2006

Sigal RJ, Kenny GP, Wasserman DH, Castaneda-Sceppa C: Physical activity/exercise and type 2 diabetes. *Diabetes Care* 27:2518–2539, 2004

Sjosten N, Kivela SL: The effects of physical exercise on depressive symptoms among the aged: a systematic review. *Int J Geriatr Psychiatry* 21:410–418, 2006

Tudor-Locke C, Bell RC, Myers AM, Harris SB, et al.: Controlled outcome evaluation of the First Step Program: a daily physical activity intervention for individuals with type II diabetes. *Int J Obes Relat Metab Disord* 28:113–119, 2004

U.S. Preventive Services Task Force: Screening for coronary heart disease: recommendation statement. *Ann Intern Med* 140:569–572, 2004

Van Vrancken C, Bopp CM, Reis JP, DuBose KD, Kirtland KA, Ainsworth BE: The prevalence of leisure-time physical activity among diabetics in South Carolina. *Southern Medical Journal* 97:141–144, 2004

Waxman A: Why a global strategy on diet, physical activity and health? *World Review of Nutrition and Dietetics* 95,162–166, 2005

Wei M, Gibbons LW, Kampert JB, Nichaman MZ, Blair SN: Low cardiorespiratory fitness and physical inactivity as predictors of mortality in men with type 2 diabetes. *Ann Intern Med* 132:605–611, 2000

Williamson DA, Rejeski J, Lang W, Van Dorsten B, et al.: Impact of a weight management program on health-related quality of life in overweight adults with type 2 diabetes. *Arch Intern Med* 169:163–171, 2009

Wood FG: Leisure time activity of Mexican Americans with diabetes. *Journal of Advanced Nursing* 45:190–196, 2004

第三篇

治疗技术的应用

第十章
皮下胰岛素注射或胰岛素泵治疗

Jill Weissberg-Benchell，PhD，CDE

糖尿病控制和并发症试验研究小组（DCCT）和英国前瞻性糖尿病研究小组（UKPDS 1998）的数据强调实现严格的代谢控制在改善健康结果方面的重要性。推荐使用每日多次注射（MDI）或持续皮下胰岛素输注（CSII）的强化治疗方案来优化糖尿病控制。CSII 提供了一个比 MDI 更加精确的生理方法来进行胰岛素管理。尽管强化治疗技术得到不断改善，但确实还是增加了患者及其家庭的负担。日常护理任务的增加和糖尿病护理时间的增加使得患者需要在丰富的生活和糖尿病患者具体的医学需要方面达到一个平衡，这是一个所有人都关心的挑战。研究人员试图确定是否 CSII 不仅提高个人的医疗成果，也可提高个人的社会心理结果。这些研究结果的总结，将在这一章呈现。

血糖控制

大多数评估 CSII 效能的研究都关注其在血糖控制方面的影响。100 多个研究评估了 HbA1C，几乎所有研究都发现使用 CSII 患者的 HbA1C 比使用 MDI/CT（多个每日注射/传统治疗）的患者更低，同时有 4 个 Meta 分析也证实了这一发现。这些研究适用于学龄儿童、青少年和成年人。然而，关于学龄前儿童的数据还不太清楚。四个随机对照试验（相关的）已在学龄前儿童中开展。其中两个研究结果表明，在开始的 6 个月使用 CSII 可发现 HbA1C 的改善，而在一年后 HbA1C 回到基线水平。另外两个随机研究表明并没有发现 MDI 和 CSII 在 HbA1C 中的区别。

两项研究评估了使用 CSII 的青年人中次优控制的潜在因素，研究表明不及时进餐和很少进行血糖检查都是可能的原因。自 2003 年以来，已有 4 个 Meta 分析，10 个随机对照研究，5 个匹配控制研究，>25 个纵向前后研究来评估 CSII 中的血糖控制。总体而言，研究数据表明，使用 CSII 的糖尿病患者（除了学龄前儿童）的代谢控制比使用 MDI 治疗方案的患者更好。

胰岛素需求量

50 多项研究评估患者每日的胰岛素用量变化，2003 年后有 16 项研究已发表。几乎所有的研究表明，患者使用 CSII 方案时每日使用很少量的胰岛素，且这些研究结果不受研究对象的年龄（学龄前、学龄儿童、青少年或成年人）和糖尿病持续时间的限制。自 2003 年以来，3 个 Meta 分析，4 个随机试验研究，3 个匹配控制研究，9 个纵向前后研究已经评估了使用 CSII 方案的胰岛素用量。总的来说，数据表明与 MDI 疗法相比，使用 CSII 所需的每日胰岛素用量更少。

体重

30 多项研究评估 CSII 方案对于体重的影响。然而，在这篇文章中并没有体重的实际数据（均值和标准差）。Meta 分析没有评估体重指数的改变。自 2003 年以来，已发表的那些研究，只有 3 个 RCTs 研究评估了体重，且研究结果是不一致的。同样的是，匹配控制研究和纵向前后研究所报告的结果也不一致。总的来说，CSII 方案似乎并没有导致体重下降，而且大多数研究报道 CSII 表现为中等体重。然而，CSII 方案对体重的影响仍不确定。

低血糖

60 多项研究比较了 CSII 和注射疗法的低血糖事件发生频率。评估低血糖发生率的障碍是研究中如何对于低血糖进行定义的差异。例如，各种研究报告了数据，包括研究期间事件发生的频率，患者每周发生事件的频率，患者每年发生事件的频率，以及每 100 名患者每年发生事件的频率。此外，许多研究没有清晰地定义"重度低血糖"意味着什么，而且通常定义延迟了患者的自我报告。Picup 的 Meta 分析表明，与 MDI 方案相比，CSII 方案重度低血糖发生率更低；而 Pankowska 的研究表明，依据胰岛素输注方法的不同所导致的低血糖发作率并没有不同。自 2003 年发表的 6 个随机对照试验中，有两个研究报道了重度低血糖发生率降低；4 个研究报道重度低血糖发生率没有变化；3 个匹配的对照研究也同样没有定论，有 1 个显示重度低血糖发生率减少；2 个报告没有变化。纵向前后研究似乎支持了这一结论，即当从 MDI 治疗方案转变为 CSII 方案后，重度低血糖发作率降低。自 2003 年以来，14 个研究报告了这样的减少率，只有 3 个研究报告没有变化。总的来说，与 MDI 治疗方案相比，CSII 方案的低血糖事件发生风险似乎没有增高。

糖尿病酮症酸中毒（DKA）

关于使用 CSII 方案中 DKA 发生率的研究具有不确定的结果，发生率增加和降低的数据是近乎相等的。在 1993 年 DCCT 发表之前，CSII 方案发生 DKA 的风险似乎是增高的。DCCT 研究发表后，数据是不确定的，一项 Meta 分析显示 DKA 发生率没有变化；而另一项研究表明，DKA 的发生率太少了以至于不能完成一个正式的 Meta 分析。自 2003 年以来没有 RCTs 研究报道了 DKA 发作。一项匹配对照研究发现青年人中应用 CSII 方案后 DKA 风险降低，一项纵向前后研究也得出了这样的结果。其他纵向前后研究发现 DKA 风险并没有明显改变。

抑郁与焦虑

很少有研究评估使用 CSII 方案的患者中的抑郁并且没有研究评估焦虑的发生。两项研究儿童和青少年的前后纵向研究报道了抑郁症状改善。一项研究成年人使用 CSII 方案的横断面研究报道了抑郁症状的恶化。目前尚不清楚 CSII 方案对抑郁症或焦虑症的影响。

生活质量

忽略年龄和研究设计，评估使用 CSII 方案的生活质量的研究表明患者生活质量似乎有提高，特别是在过去 5 年时间里，大部分个体的生活质量都得到了明显改善。尽管有些研究没有发现明显变化，但没有研究发现生活质量的恶化。在评估生活质量中需要注意的一点就是构建的定义及用于评估构建的各种措施。

治疗的满意度

评估治疗方案满意度的所有研究表明，忽略使用者的年龄和实验设计的情况下，CSII 方案的满意度较高。RCT 研究发现与 MDI 治疗方案相比，CSII 方案能提高患者的满意度。类似的研究发现在纵向前后研究及横断面研究中均有报道。

方案的责任

6 项研究评估了治疗方案所要求责任，其中 4 项研究评估儿童患者，2 项研究评估成人。4 项研究发现，使用 CSII 方案时，受试者具有更好的依从性，更易接受糖尿病治疗方案中的责任。1 项研究没有发现责任水平的变化。Weiss-berg-Benchell 的研究评估了 CSII 任务中责任的发展轨迹，并报告了有一半的青少年患者的家长一直在分担方案责任，并且有 1/3 的家长愿意分担大龄青年的方案要求。

其他社会心理结果

一些研究已经评估了一些其他问题，如控制点、自尊、自我效能感和家庭功能等。没有研究发现 CSII 方案会导致结果恶化,但也很少有研究发现 CSII 方案能改善心理功能这方面的问题。

有 2 项研究评估育儿压力:一项是随机对照研究;另一项是纵向前后研究。这 2 项研究均发现,与 MDI 治疗方案相比,CSII 方案能够减少父母的育儿压力。

一些研究让受试者描述他们对 CSII 治疗方案优势的看法。最常见的回答是提高灵活性。其他报道的优势包括易于安排吃饭时间,睡眠和唤醒时间的灵活性,更大的自由度,减少身体限制感,减少身体的不适,以及改善血糖的控制。

3 项研究评估 CSII 方案中止的原因,其中 2 项是纵向前后设计,1 项是横断面研究。CSII 方案中断的原因包括较高的 HbA1C、忘记用药及不想时时被提醒患有糖尿病。

3 项研究评估 CSII 方案使用者的社会经济特征。这 3 项研究都评估了儿童和青少年,并且确定 CSII 方案的使用者更可能是白种人及具有更高的家庭收入和教育水平的人。

总体而言,评估这些社会心理因素的研究相对较少,有关 CSII 治疗方案对控制点、自我效能感、育儿压力、CSII 使用和中断的影响的结论是不成熟的。此外,因为大多数 CSII 的使用者是白种人,受过良好的教育,经济舒适,所以在不相同的人群组,除了要评估使用 CSII 对医疗和社会心理的影响,未来的研究还必须评估使用 CSII 技术中的这种差距的原因。

文献总结

文献研究提供了强有力的证据表明 CSII 治疗方案能够显著改善血糖控制。唯一的区别在于没有看到学龄前儿童 HbA1C 水平的改善。除了学龄前儿童,由儿童或成人患者组成的样本的研究并没有指出差别,尽管小儿糖尿病患者管理面临独特的挑战。文献研究表明,CSII 治疗导致胰岛素需求量的减少。CSII 方案似乎并没有增加低血糖事件的发生率,并且证据似乎表明 CSII 方案减少了重度低血糖的风险。CSII 对体重和 DKA 风险的影响没有确定的结论。总的来说,CSⅡ治疗似乎导致了医疗结果的提高。

　　虽然 CSII 治疗方案可能是最复杂及最精确的输注胰岛素的方法，当使用 CSII 治疗方案时，改善血糖控制只是需要考虑的众多潜在因素之一。与 100 多项评估医疗结果的研究相比，只有相对较少的研究评估社会心理结果。只有 8 项 RCT 研究同时评估医学和社会心理因素的结果。其中，7 项研究评估儿童和青少年，只有 1 项评估成年人。6 项研究只评估了生活质量，3 项研究评估治疗满意度。纵向前后研究、配对研究及横断面研究在评估了医疗、心理的同时也评估了生活质量。没有研究评估了包括抑郁或饮食失调在内的医疗结果，这两者都是糖尿病患者非常担忧的社会心理问题，因为它们与高额的医疗费用、较差的依从性及较差的代谢控制相关。

　　因此，需要更多的文献来研究社会心理功能方面的问题。胰岛素泵对重要的结果如抑郁和焦虑的影响是不确定的。胰岛素泵对生活质量的影响具有一致的研究数据，当患者将注射治疗改为胰岛素泵治疗时，生活质量这一重要的结果可得到改善。同样的是，与注射疗法相比，使用泵治疗法的患者似乎倾向于接受更多的治疗方案责任。然而，似乎高龄的青少年仍然受益于家长的参与及支持。当注射疗法转换为胰岛素泵疗法后，治疗的满意度明显提高。

临床护理建议

　　当患者及家属表现了从注射疗法转变为胰岛素泵疗法的兴趣后，建议对已知风险和随之而来获益进行讨论。讨论至少应该包括以下几点。

　　1. 胰岛素泵疗法改善所有群体的代谢控制水平（HbA1C 水平），除了学龄前儿童。

　　2. 胰岛素泵疗法减少患者每日的胰岛素用量。

　　3. 胰岛素泵疗法可以减少重度低血糖风险，并且不增加低血糖发生的风险。

　　4. 必须告知胰岛素泵疗法的潜在风险和并发症（如体重增加、DKA），并且在开始使用时应强烈关注教育和培训。胰岛素注射法和胰岛素泵疗法的选择似乎并不影响体重的增加或 DKA 风险。这些医疗结果应该定期评估并且在每一次临床访谈中讨论。

5. 关于胰岛素泵治疗的社会心理风险和获益，文献报道尚不清楚，临床医生面临着有关胰岛素泵选择的更微妙的讨论。有大量的研究表明，糖尿病增加患抑郁症的风险；因此针对抑郁症治疗似乎是一个重要的社会心理因素，包括教育项目和临床评估。不幸的是，评估使用胰岛素泵疗法的患者的抑郁或焦虑的研究相对较少，而且研究结果不确定。因此，建议临床医师继续教育和筛查患者的情绪问题，并监测患者随着时间推移的症状变化。任何抑郁症状的增加都应确保向精神卫生专业转诊以进行正式的评估。两个简单的问题即可筛选出临床抑郁症：你感觉到比平常更多的悲伤或情绪下降吗？你有注意到有些事情过去是有趣的而现在不那么有趣了么？

6. 当患者寻求胰岛素泵治疗来改善自身的生活质量时，包括灵活的时间安排，文献证据更加明确：与 MDI 治疗方法相比，CSII 治疗方法具有更好的治疗满意度和生活质量。对生活质量的简单评估可供临床使用，如糖尿病患者生活质量措施（DQOL）、糖尿病生活质量量表（DSQOLS）、成人糖尿病生活质量审计（ADDQOL）、儿童生活质量量表（PEDSQL）、糖尿病模块，以及繁忙的临床实践也只是问问患者他们从使用胰岛素泵治疗以来是否有生活质量的改变及是如何改变的。似乎在胰岛素泵使用者中所见到的治疗满意度的提高是生活质量改善的结果。

7. 最后，糖尿病不是一个"靠自己"的疾病。因此，评估分担责任和依从性行为的研究表明，家庭成员应该积极参与胰岛素泵护理的方方面面，从注射部位改变到决定监测用药时间的基础代谢率。

参 考 文 献

Alemzadeh R, Ellis J, Holzum M, Parton E, Wyatt D: Beneficial effects of continuous subcutaneous insulin infusion and flexible multiple daily insulin regimen using insulin glargine in type 1 diabetes. *Pediatrics* 114:91–95, 2004

American Diabetes Association: Economic costs of diabetes in the U.S. in 2007. *Diabetes Care* 31:596–615, 2008

Anderson RJ, Freedland K, Clouse R, Lustman P: The prevalence of comorbid depression in adults with diabetes: a meta-analysis. *Diabetes Care* 24:1069–1078, 2001

Babar G, Ali O, Parton E, Hoffman R, Alemzadeh R: Factors associated with adherence to continuous subcutaneous insulin infusion in pediatric diabetes. *Diabetes Technology and Therapeutics* 11:131–137, 2009

Barnard K, Lloyd C, Skinner T: Systematic literature review: quality of life associated with insulin pump use in type 1 diabetes. *Diabet Med* 24:607–617, 2007

Boland F, Grey M, Oesterle A, Fredrickson L, Tamborlane W: Continuous subcutaneous insulin infusion: a new way to lower risk of severe hypoglycemia, improve metabolic control, and enhance coping in adolescents with type 1 diabetes. *Diabetes Care* 22:1779–1784, 1999

Bott U, Muhlhauser I, Overmann H, Berger M: Validation of a diabetes-specific quality-of-life scale for patients with type 1 diabetes. *Diabetes Care* 21:757–769, 1998

Bradley C, Todd C, Gorton T, Symonds E, Martin A, Plowright R: The development of an individualized questionnaire measure of perceived impact of diabetes on quality of life: the ADDQoL. *Quality of Life Research* 8:79–91, 1999

Bruttomesso D, Pianta A, Crazzolara D, Scaldaferri E, Lora L, Guarneri G, Mongillo A, Gennaro R, Miola M, Moretti M, Confortin L, Beltramello G, Pais M, Baritussio A, Casiglia E, Tiengo A: Continuous subcutaneous insulin infusion (CSII) in the Veneto region: efficacy, acceptability and quality of life. *Diabet Medi* 19:628–634, 2002

Burdick J, Chase P, Slover R, Knievel K, Scrimgeour L, Maniatis A, Klingensmith G: Missed insulin meal boluses and elevated hemoglobin A1c levels in children receiving insulin pump therapy. *Pediatrics* 113:221–224, 2004

Cogen F, Henderson C, Hansen J, Streisand R: Pediatric quality of life in transitioning to insulin pump: does prior regimen make a difference? *Clinical Pediatrics* 46: 777–722, 2007

Diabetes Control and Complications Trial (DCCT) Research Group: Influence of intensive diabetes treatment on body weight and composition of adults with type 1 diabetes in the Diabetes Control and Complications Trial. *Diabetes Care* 24:1711-1721, 2001

Diabetes Control and Complications Trial (DCCT) Research Group: Adverse events and their association with treatment regimens in the Diabetes Control and Complications Trial. *Diabetes Care* 18:1415-1427, 1995

Diabetes Control and Complications Trial (DCCT) Research Group: The effect of intensive treatment of diabetes on the development and progression of long-term complications in insulin-dependent diabetes mellitus. *N Engl J Med* 329:977-985, 1993

DiMeglio L, Pottorff T, Boyd S, France L, Fineberg N, Eugster E: A randomized, controlled study of insulin pump therapy in diabetic preschoolers. *Journal of Pediatrics* 145:380-384, 2004

Doyle EA, Winzimer S, Steffen A, Ahern JA, Vincent M, Tamborlane W: A randomized, prospective trial comparing the efficacy of continuous subcutaneous insulin infusion with multiple daily injections using insulin glargine. *Diabetes Care* 27:1554-1558, 2004

Dusseldorf Study Group, Ziegler D, Dannehl K, Koschinsky T, Toeller M, Gries F: Comparison of continuous subcutaneous insulin infusion and intensified conventional therapy in the treatment of type I diabetes: a two-year randomized study. *Diabetes Nutrition and Metabolism* 3:203-213, 1990

Felsing W, Bibergeil H, Menzel R, Albrecht G, Felsing U, Dabels J, Reichel G, Luder C: Results of treatment with continuous subcutaneous insulin infusion (CSII) in insulin-dependent (type 1) diabetics. *Experimental and Clinical Endocrinology* 83:136-142, 1984

Floyd JC, Cornell RG, Jacober SJ, Griffith LE, Funnell MM, Wolf LL, Wolf FM: A prospective study identifying risk factors for discontinuance of insulin pump therapy. *Diabetes Care* 16:1470-1478, 1993

Fox L, Buckloh L, Smith S, Wysocki T, Mauras N: A randomized controlled trial of insulin pump therapy in young children with type 1 diabetes. *Diabetes Care* 28:1277-1281, 2005

Gimenez M, Congent M, Jansa M, Vidal M, Chiganer G, Levy I: Efficacy of continuous subcutaneous insulin infusion in type 1 diabetes: a 2-year perspective using the established criteria for funding from a National Health Service. *Diabet Med* 24:1419-1423, 2007

Gonzales JS, Peyrot M, McCarl L, Collins EM, et al.: Depression and diabetes treatment nonadherence: a meta-analysis. *Diabetes Care* 31:2398-2403, 2008

Hammon P, Liebl A, Grunder S: International survey of insulin pump users: impact of continuous subcutaneous insulin infusion therapy on glucose control and quality of life. *Primary Care Diabetes* 1:143-146, 2007

Hislop A, Fegan P, Schlaeppi M, Duck M, Yeap B: Prevalence and association of psychological distress in young adults with type 1 diabetes. *Diabet Med* 25:91-96, 2008

Hoogma R, Hammond P, Gomist R, Kerr D, Bruttomesso D, Bouter K, Wiefels K, de la Calle H, Schweitzer D, Pfohl M, Torlone E, Krinelke L, Bolli G: Comparison of the effects of continuous subcutaneous insulin infusion (CSII) and NPH-based multiple daily insulin injections (MDI) on glycaemic control and quality of life: results of the 5-nations trial. *Diabet Med* 23:141-147, 2005

Hoogma R, Spijker A, Van Doorn-Scheele M, Van Doorn T, Michels R, Van Doorn R, Levi M, Hoekstra J: Quality of life and metabolic control in patients with diabetes mellitus type 1 treated by continuous subcutaneous insulin infusion or multiple daily insulin injections. *The Netherlands Journal of Medicine* 62:383-387, 2004

Jacobson AM, the Diabetes Control and Complications Trial (DCCT) Research Group: The diabetes quality of life measure. In *Handbook of Psychology and Diabetes*. Bradley C, Ed. Chur, Switzerland, Harwood Academic Publishers, 1994, p. 65-87

Jakisch BI, Wagner V, Heidtmann B, Lepler R, Holterhust P, Kapellen T, Vogel C, Rosenbauer J, Holl R: Comparison of continuous subcutaneous insulin infusion (CSII) and multiple daily injections (MDI) in paediatric type 1 diabetes: a multicentre matched-pair cohort analysis over three years. *Diabet Med* 25:80-85, 2008

Jeitler K, Horvath K, Berghold A, Gratzer T, Neeser K, Pieber T, Siebenhofer A: Continuous subcutaneous insulin infusion versus multiple daily insulin injections in patients with diabetes mellitus: systematic review and meta-analysis. *Diabetologia* 51:941-951, 2008

Johannesen J, Eising S, Kohlwes S, Riis S, Beck M, Carstensen B, Bendtson I, Nerup J: Treatment of Danish adolescent diabetic patients with CSII: a matched study to MDI. *Pediatric Diabetes* 9:23-28, 2008

Kapellen T, Heidtmann B, Bachmann J, Ziegler R, Grabert M, Holl R: Indications for insulin pump therapy in different age groups: an analysis of 1,567 children and adolescents. *Diabet Med* 24:836-842, 2007

Kaufman FR, Halvorson M, Kim C, Pitukcheewanont P: Use of insulin pump therapy at nighttime only for children 7-10 years of age with type 1 diabetes. *Diabetes Care* 23:579-582, 2000

Lustman P, Anderson R, Freedland K, DeGroot M, Carney R, Clouse R: Depression and poor glycemic control: a meta-analytic review of the literature. *Diabetes Care* 23:934-942, 2000

McMahon S, Airey F, Marangou D, McElwee K, Carne C, Davis E, Jones T: Insulin pump therapy in children and adolescents: improvements in key parameters of diabetes management including quality of life. *Diabet Med* 22:92-96, 2005

Mecklenburg RS, Benson EA, Benson JW, Fredlund P, Guinn T, Metz R, Nielsen R, Sanner C: Acute complications associated with insulin infusion pump therapy: report of experience with 161 patients. *JAMA* 252:3265-3269, 1984

Muller-Godeffroy E, Treichel S, Wagner M: Investigation of quality of life and family burden issues during insulin pump therapy in children with type 1 diabetes mellitus: a large-scale multicenter pilot study. *Diabet Med* 26:493-501, 2009

Nabhan ZM, Kreher N, Greene D, Eugster E, Kronenberger W, DiMeglio L: A randomized prospective study of insulin pump vs. insulin injection therapy in very young children with type 1 diabetes: 12-month glycemic, BMI, and neurocognitive outcomes. *Pediatric Diabetes* 10:202-208, 2009

Nicolucci A, Maione A, Franciosi M, Amoretti R, Busetto E, Capani F, Bruttomesso D, Di Bartolo P, Girelli A, Leonetti F, Morviducci L, Ponzi P, Vitacolonna E: Quality of life and treatment satisfaction in adults with type 1 diabetes: a comparison between continuous subcutaneous insulin infusion and multiple daily injections. *Diabet Med* 25:213-220, 2008

Nimri R, Weintrob N, Benzaquen H, Ofan R, Fayman G, Phillip P: Insulin pump therapy in youth with type 1 diabetes: a retrospective paired study. *Pediatrics* 117:2126-2123, 2006

Nuboer R, Borsboom GJ, Zoethout J, Koot H, Bruining J: Effects of insulin pump vs. injection treatment on quality of life and impact of disease in children with type 1 diabetes mellitus in a randomized, prospective comparison. *Pediatric Diabetes* 9:291-296, 2008

Olinder AL, Kernell A, Smide B: Missed bolus doses: devastating for metabolic control in CSII-treated adolescents with type 1 diabetes. *Pediatric Diabetes* 10:142-148, 2009

Opipari-Arrigan L, Fredericks E, Burhart N, Dale L, Hodge M, Foster C: Continuous subcutaneous insulin infusion benefits quality of life in preschool-age children with type 1 diabetes. *Pediatric Diabetes* 8:377-383, 2007

Pankowska E, Blazik M, Dziechciarz P, Szypowska A, Szajewska H: Continuous subcutaneous insulin infusion vs. multiple daily injections in children with type 1 diabetes: a systematic review and meta-analysis of randomized control trials. *Pediatric Diabetes* 10:52-58, 2009

Paris C, Imperatore G, Klingensmith G, Petitti D, Rodriguez B, Anderson A, Schwartz D, Standiford D, Pihoker C: Predictors of insulin regimens and impact on outcomes in youth with type 1 diabetes: the SEARCH for Diabetes in Youth study. *Journal of Pediatrics* 155:183-189, 2009

Pickup JC, Sutton A: Severe hypoglycaemia and glycaemic control in type 1 diabetes: a meta-analysis of multiple daily insulin injections compared with continuous subcutaneous insulin infusion. *Diabet Med* 25:765-774, 2008

Rabbone I, Scaramuzza A, Bobbio A, Bonfanti R, Iafusco D, Lombardo F, Toni S, Tumini S, Cerutti F: Insulin pump therapy management in very young children with type 1 diabetes using continuous subcutaneous insulin infusion. *Diabetes Technology and Therapeutics* 11:707-709, 2009

Rodrigues I, Reid H, Ismail K, Amiel S: Indications and efficacy of continuous subcutaneous insulin infusion (CSII) therapy in type 1 diabetes mellitus: a clinical audit in a specialist service. *Diabet Med* 22:842-849, 2005

Scheidegger U, Allemann S, Scheidegger K, Diem P: Continuous subcutaneous insulin infusion therapy: effects on quality of life. *Swiss Medicine Weekly* 137:476-482, 2007

Schottenfeld-Naor Y, Galatzer A, Karp M, Josefsberg Z, Laron Z: Comparison of metabolic and psychological parameters during continuous subcutaneous insulin infusion and intensified conventional treatment in type I diabetic patients. *Israeli Journal of Medical Science* 21:822-828, 1985

Scrimgeour L, Cobry E, McFann K, Burdick P, Weimer C, Slover R, Chase P: Improved glycemic control after long-term insulin pump use in pediatric patients with type 1 diabetes. *Diabetes Technology and Therapeutics* 9:421-428, 2007

Seereiner S, Neeser K, Weber C, Schreiber K, Habacher W, Rakovac I, Beck P, Schmidt L, Pieber T: Attitudes towards insulin pump therapy among adolescents and young people. *Diabetes Technology and Therapeutics* 12:89-94, 2010

Shapiro J, Wigg D, Charles M, Perley M: Personality and family profiles of chronic insulin-dependent diabetic patients using portable insulin infusion pump therapy: a preliminary investigation. *Diabetes Care* 7:137-142, 1984

Shehadeh N, Battelino T, Galatzer A, Naveh T, Hadash A, de Vries L, Phillip M: Insulin pump therapy for 1-6 year old children with type 1 diabetes. *Israel Medical Association Journal* 6:284-286, 2004

Skogsberg L, Fors H, Hannas R, Chaplin J, Lindman E, Skogsberg J: Improved treatment satisfaction but no difference in metabolic control when using continuous subcutaneous insulin infusion versus multiple daily injections in children at onset of type 1 diabetes mellitus. *Pediatric Diabetes* 9:472-479, 2008

Slijper F, deBeaufort CE, Bruining GJ, deVisser J, Aarsen R, Dicken D, vanStrik R: Psychological impact of continuous subcutaneous insulin infusion pump therapy in non-selected newly diagnosed insulin dependent (type 1) diabetic children: evaluation after two years of therapy. *Diabetes & Métabolisme* 16:273-277, 1990

Springer D, Dziura J, Tamborlane W, Steffen A, Ahern J, Vincent M, Weinzimer S: Optimal control of type 1 diabetes mellitus in youth receiving intensive treatment. *Journal of Pediatrics* 149:227-232, 2006

Sulli N, Shashaj B: Long term benefits of continuous subcutaneous insulin infusion in children with type 1 diabetes: a 4-year follow up. *Diabet Med* 23:900-906, 2006

Tsui E, Barnie A, Ross S, Parkes R, Zinman B: Intensive insulin therapy with insulin lispro. *Diabetes Care* 24:1722-1727, 2001

UK Prospective Diabetes Study (UKPDS) Group: Intensive blood glucose control with sulphonylureas or insulin compared with conventional treatment and risk of complications in patients with type 2 diabetes (UKPDS 33). *Lancet* 352:837-853, 1998

Valenzuela J, Patino A, McCullough J, Ring C, Sanchez J, Eidson M, Nemery R, Delameter A: Insulin pump therapy and health related quality of life in children and adolescents with type 1 diabetes. *Journal of Pediatric Psychology* 31:650–660, 2006

Varni JW, Burwinkle TM, Jacobs JR, Gottschalk M, Kaufman F, Jones KL: The PedsQL in type 1 and type 2 diabetes: reliability and validity of the Pediatric Quality of Life Inventory Generic Core Scales and Type 1 Diabetes Module. *Diabetes Care* 26:631–637, 2003a

Varni JW, Burwinkle TM, Seid M, Skarr D: The PedsQL 4.0 as a pediatric population health measure: feasibility, reliability, and validity. *Ambulatory Pediatrics* 3:329–341, 2003b

Weintrob N, Benzaquen H, Galatzer A, Shalitin S, Lazar L, Fayman G, Lilos P, Dickerman Z, Phillip M: Comparison of continuous subcutaneous insulin infusion and multiple daily injection regimens in children with type 1 diabetes: a randomized open crossover trial. *Pediatrics* 112:559–564, 2006

Weinzimer S, Ahern J, Doyle E, Vincent M, Dziura J, Steffen A, Tamborlane W: Persistence of benefits of continuous subcutaneous insulin infusion in very young children with type 1 diabetes: a follow-up report. *Pediatrics* 114:1601–1605, 2004

Weissberg-Benchell J, Goodman S, Antisdel-Lomaglio J, Zebracki K: The use of continuous subcutaneous insulin infusion (CSII): parental and professional perceptions of self-care mastery and autonomy in children and adolescents. *Journal of Pediatric Psychology* 32:1196–1202, 2007

Weissberg-Benchell J, Antisdel-Lomaglio J, Seshadri R: Insulin pump therapy: a meta-analysis. *Diabetes Care* 26:1079–1087, 2003

Whittemore R, Urban AD, Tamborlane WV, Grey M: Quality of life in school-aged children with type 1 diabetes on intensive treatment and their parents. *Diabetes Educator* 29:847–854, 2003

Wilson D, Buckingham B, Kunselman E, Sullivan M, Paguntalan H, Gitelman S: A two-center randomized controlled feasibility trial of insulin pump therapy in young children with diabetes. *Diabetes Care* 28:15–19, 2005

第十一章

加强社会心理因素的管理

Lori Laffel，MD，MPH

现代社会中 1 型和 2 型糖尿病在青少年及成年人群中的比率正在增加。这种疾病如今正影响着全世界上千万的人们，到 2025 年受影响的人口数量有望上升 50%。但现代的科技水平也有了显著提高。总的来说，科技水平对我们的日常生活有着重要影响，尤其是在我们管理糖尿病的方法上。20 世纪 70 年代年末至 20 世纪 80 年代年初，也就是 30 年前，第一台家庭血糖监测（BGM）装置和胰岛素泵问世后，多学科糖尿病小组便开始致力于设计、实施和评估最佳的方法，使患者接受教育和行为支持后能成功运用这些工具来达到血糖的控制目标。

科技对糖尿病管理产生了极大的影响，不管是口服药物、胰岛素还是其他注射药物治疗都更加细致地与人体生理需求相匹配，来达到最佳的血糖控制。对 1 型和 2 型糖尿病患者而言，最佳血糖控制对降低糖尿病慢性并发症风险十分重要。

本章将阐释四种在当代糖尿病管理中广泛使用的技术方法：BGM，连续血糖监测（CGM），辅助强化胰岛素治疗的胰岛素笔使用，互联网项目或支持糖尿病自我管理的技术。本章是一个阐述胰岛素泵使用（见第十章）的独立章节。本章不是对糖尿病管理工具做一个技术性的回顾，也不会对糖尿病技术手段做彻底的评估，而是强调促使这些管理工具实施和持续使用的社会心理因素，重点关注 BGM 和 CGM。社会心理因素包括生活质量、糖尿病负担、抑郁和焦虑症状、对低血糖症的恐惧，以及坚持挑战以患者自身的努力来实现糖尿病管理目标。讨论部分将提供重要的研究例子，强调与这 4 个方法相关的社会心理问题而不是详尽所有。具体使用时可参照技术评估或荟萃分析的研究。

　　正如糖尿病管理的标准方法，治疗是根据患者的需求来个体化并由多学科治疗小组提供。本章提供信息来帮助从业者鼓励患者坚持复杂难懂、医学上规定的强化治疗方案，并讨论了患者行为对完成强化管理和血糖目标的必要性。

血糖监测

　　BGM 是糖尿病管理的基石，因为它是所有治疗方案的指路标，不论是需要更多的胰岛素来降低血糖水平还是增加糖类以提高低血糖（BG）水平。BGM 是明确治疗的第一步。实际上，糖尿病控制及并发症试验组织（DCCT）建立了重要的血糖自我监测来指导 1 型糖尿病（T1D）患者的胰岛素治疗。进行胰岛素治疗的 2 型糖尿病（T2D）患者也能从 BG 自我监测中获益。然而，接着也有文献对非胰岛素治疗的患者利用 BG 自我监测进行自我管理是否有效存在争论。尽管如此，ADA 推荐所有胰岛素治疗的患者进行 BG 自我监测，并支持口服药物或营养学治疗的患者用 BGM 作为中心方法达到血糖控制目标。

　　1 型和 2 型糖尿病患者 HbA1C 下降与日常 BMG 的使用频率增加有关。最近一项对超过 26 000 个 T1D 青年患者的研究发现，每当增加日常 BG 检查 0～10 个监测频率可使 HbA1C 下降 0.2%，增加 0～5 个监测频率可使 HbA1C 下降 0.5%。此外，这些作者报道，日常 BGM 使用频率增加使患者发生糖尿病酮症酸中毒（DKA）的概率减低。一项对非胰岛素治疗患者的回顾性研究也报道了 BGM 可使此类患者的 HbA1c 水平降低 0.4%。

　　疾病预防控制中心（CDC）分析了行为危险因素监测系统（BRFSS）1997～2006 年的数据。1997 年有 41%糖尿病成年患者每日监测 BG，到了 2006 年增加到 63%。事实上这一数据已超过 2010 健康人群上国家的糖尿病患者每日监测 BG 达 61%这一目标的 2%。并且，有 87%进行胰岛素治疗的成人患者在每日监测他们的 BG 水平。2020 健康人群计划，国家的目标包括糖尿病患者每日至少一次自我监测 BG 由在患者中由 10% 增加至 70%（目标 D-13；http：//healthypeople.gov/2020/topicsobjectives2020/objectiveslist.aspx?topicId=8）。为达成这一目标应努力确保血糖试纸在健康保险范围，围绕糖尿病自我管理的教育和以咨询服务来鼓励患者加强糖尿病医疗护理。

BGM 的障碍和克服障碍的方法

许多患者尽管承认了 BGM 使用频率与血糖控制有联系，但是仍拒绝使用 BGM。公认的监测障碍（表 11-1）包括费用、疼痛、缺乏统一的保险，需要糖尿病教育来学习正确使用方法，需要持续的咨询服务来鼓励患者加强管理，练习自我管理和避免对糖尿病的倦怠。最近几代的家庭 BGM 装备消除了一些障碍，例如，复杂性、技术依赖性，甚至是一些需要大量样本或指尖穿刺引起的不适。许多新设备使用微量的血样（小于 $1\mu l$）并认可替换部位的监测（如手臂），与指尖采血检查相比，这些设备通常被视为几乎无痛。这些设备通常提供自动日志的记忆功能和一天 BG 的平均值，提供自动下载功能，而且不需要复杂的编码。

表 11-1　BGM 障碍

指尖疼痛
低血糖检查不方便，记录结果或下载量表
中断日常事务
使用难度可能包括编码；设置日期时间；在手指尖、顶部还是侧边采血
进行低血糖结果的解读和管理变化的教育
监测的费用，尤其是血糖试纸费用
低血糖结果引发的相关态度，包括羞愧、沮丧和恐惧

T1D 患者和许多使用胰岛素治疗的 T2D 患者用该法多次检查一天中餐前和餐后，运动前中后，睡前，时常包括通宵的 BG 值。这种频率的检查会打扰患者日常活动并在 BG 水平异常时引起患者不适或受挫感。这就形成一个负反馈循环，异常水平的 BG 会使患者减少监测行为，因为患者从这个至关重要的行为管理中接收到的是消极的反馈。增加心理教育手册（即 BG 监测手册）作为标准的糖尿病教育的一种补充方法，增加了 BGM 使用频率，并减少了 BGM 对 1 型或 2 型成年糖尿病患者

在血糖控制未达到最佳时的负面影响（HbA1C≥8%为诊断标准）。有了BG 监测手册监控变成了可实现的期望，包括什么时候、为什么，以及如何监控相关的基础教育，避免异常 BG 结果经常引起的羞愧和责备，对监测的负担和由于对 BG 水平的了解引起的生活方式机动性的增加做出权衡。此外，手册还提供了一个新的词汇来帮助保持自我激励，如用"检查"一词来代替说"测试"，BG 结果描述为"BG 结果高或低"而不是"好与坏"。

　　为了进一步降低患者的负担，大多数 BG 仪器可以联通电脑并从上面直接下载血糖数据。一些设备已经通过电话或传真使用自动数据传输，以减少电脑连接所需的工作量。为了减少解释 BG 数据带来的负担，就有了基于计算机算法来检查数据并提供建议的胰岛素剂量，甚至包括其他的考虑因素，如食物的摄入、运动、压力和疾病的影响。近 12 个月，多中心的研究包括使用次优控制的胰岛素正常的成人 T2D（HbA1C≥7.5%为诊断标准），将每季结构化的自我监测 BG 的干预组与常规治疗对照组相比较。两组的季度随访集中在糖尿病管理，免费的血糖仪和试纸，和 HbA1C 的即时测试上。结构化 BGM 干预包括患者在 7 个时间点监测血糖并连续 3 天，将数据记录下来，因此试验名称为 STeP（结构测试项目）。经过 1 年的研究，结构化 BGM 的组证实了在打算做治疗分析的人中 HbA1C 显著改善了 0.3%，完成治疗分析的人中 HbA1C 改善了 0.5%。很明显两组都在健康状态上有所改善，证实了对监测行为提供积极的支持可提高药物和心理带来的效果。

　　有一个相对简单的方法来帮助卫生保健工作者和患者解释 BG 数据，方法包括测定当日时间的 BG 平均值及当日时间均值相关的变化。虽然目标血糖水平需要个性化，但是有数据表明血糖水平的变化应该是有限的，即标准偏差要小于均值或中位数的 50%。

　　一些 BG 仪器提供集成电子记录表，让患者能看到图形显示的血糖数据及时间平均血糖数据。利用这一科技结合糖尿病教育后证实了患者使用 BGM 频率增加且血糖控制改善，这一现象持续到临床试验结束 1 年之后。值得注意的是，在临床试验结束并终止额外的帮助后血糖水平仍能维持平稳。

　　已经有许多短期、随机的研究旨在鼓励患者使用电子提醒来实现

BGM 行为，或者用手机短信这种新方式来鼓励患者增加监测频率。在一项研究胰岛素治疗的青少年和成人的研究中，用短信提醒患者检查血糖比用 3 个月的试验期间的电子邮件提醒更能提高患者的日常监测频率；另一研究用手机提醒——被命名为"甜言蜜语"，旨在用 BGM 加强胰岛素治疗，也证明了坚持监测的效果。然而还不清楚的是，临床试验的极干预期之后增加的 BGM 保持不变，是否表明持续的行为改变需要积对需求的基本接受及内在动机来包含通常被视为不愉快的身体和情感活动。

BGM 相关的心理结局

上述提到 T2D 成人患者增加 BGM 频率、使用 STeP 法改善血糖控制后自我报告健康状况好转，除此之外，研究者发现患者的抑郁症状和糖尿病痛苦也有改变。12 个月后，干预组和对照组的抑郁症状和糖尿病痛苦都有显著缓解。但使用已有的 BG 自我监测工具与一般治疗相比能极大地减少处于高基线水平的抑郁症状和糖尿病痛苦。值得注意的是，这些收益独立于 HbA1C 改善和 BGM 频率之外，这表明情绪上的获益来自于血糖模式识别和自我效能感的提高。一项早期研究也证实了结构化的咨询和 BGM 在非胰岛素治疗的 T2D 成人患者的幸福感、抑郁症、自我效能感上有积极的影响。

青少年 T1D 患者中，糖尿病特异性的家庭冲突与 BGM 频率成反比。而 BGM 和糖尿病特异性家庭冲突独立地影响 HbA1C，低冲突和更频繁的监测能获得更好的血糖控制。此外，青少年频繁使用 BGM 并且达到最佳血糖控制也体现了高质量的生活。最后，患者偶尔使用 BGM 的频率过量，暗示患者心理痛苦与低血糖恐惧有关，或者是害怕高血糖和糖尿病并发症。这种患者应该转诊去糖尿病管理中的心理健康专家处就诊。因此，综上所述，增加 BGM 的频率不太可能对心理因素造成负面影响且很可能对血糖控制产生积极的影响。但是，在疾病的焦虑状态下可能会促使患者对 BGM 适应不良。

连续血糖监测

我们仍在寻求无创方法来测量血糖水平，避免测量产生的不适和减少对日常活动的干扰。糖尿病群体正等待着新技术，实时 CGM 技术就出现了，能提供前所未有的接近连续性的血糖数据。CGM 设备使用一次性血糖传感器置于患者皮下间隙 3～7 天。传感器连接着无线传输的发射器将间歇的血糖信号传给邻近的接收器，接收器每 5 分钟更新一次显示连续血糖值（图 11-1 为两种美国正在使用的 CGM 设备）。接收器以数字和图像的格式显示血糖数据，当血糖值低于或高于某一设定范围或者血糖骤降骤升时提供警报。接收器发出的警报可以设置为声音或者震动提醒。最近有两部出版物回顾了青少年和成人患者 CGM 的临床使用指南。

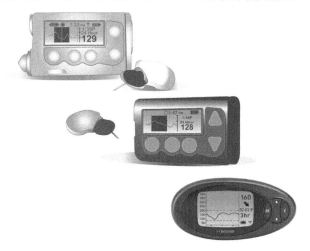

图 11-1　连续血糖监测

装置由三部分组成：一次性传感器、发射器、接收器。美国在 2012 年时有两种可用的实时 CGM 系统，生产厂家分别为 Medtronic，Inc.和 DexCom，Inc. Medtronic 的 CGM 可以单机使用也可结合胰岛素泵使用，设备更新和改良后也许能在美国境外使用，不断地研究和评估是在等美国食品药物管理局的检验和批准。两种系统都能用软件下载 CGM 数据来对葡萄糖模式进行回顾性评估，以帮助直接调整胰岛素量。

最近有许多将 CGM 用于青少年和成人 T1D 患者的临床试验研究。青少年糖尿病研究基金会（JDRF）为期 6 个月的 CGM 试验将青少年和成人 T1D 患者的CGM与传统的间断式的BGM对比,基线标准是HbA1C值 7%～10%。研究显示 CGM 与 BGM 相比能显著降低成人 T1D 患者 HbA1C 值的 0.5%。另一方面 CGM 与 BGM 相比并非能降低青少年和年青 T1D 患者的 HbA1C 均值（年龄在 8～24 岁）。有趣的是，尽管 CGM 组和 BGM 组中最年轻的参与者（年龄 8～14 岁）的 HbA1C 均值并无差异，但 CGM 相比 BGM 能改善人数比例更多的一组青少年患者（同样为 8～14 岁）HbA1C≥10%的情况或确切使 HbA1C 值减少≥0.5%。CGM 根据不同的年龄层有不同的使用,有83%的25岁以上参与者中,30%的15～24 岁参与者，50%的 8～14 岁参与者在为期 6 个月的临床试验中每周有 ≥6 天使用 CGM 技术。重要的是改善血糖控制与 CGM 的使用直接相关。也就是说，使用 CGM 的参与者通常是最大的获益者，HbA1C 的降低并不依赖于年龄。此外，HbA1C 改善并未增加严重低血糖的发生。有趣的是，能预测 CGM 使用情况的因素是在前 6 个月研究中使用 BGM 的基础频率；频繁测量 BG 水平的患者更可能频繁地使用 CGM。在青少年和成年 T1D 患者的对照研究中，入选者 HbA1C 值<7%，CGM 组与 BGM 组相比能维持目标血红蛋白水平且不增加严重低血糖发生事件。

最近公布的历时 12 个月的传感器增强泵治疗降低 HbA1C（STAR3）临床研究在青少年和成人患者中将传感器增强胰岛素泵治疗与传统 BGM 加上每日多次注射治疗做了对比，入选者 HbA1C 值 7.4%～9.5%。调查研究显示传感器增强泵治疗组的 HbA1C 显著改善，HbA1C 在成人组间差异 0.6%，青少年组间差异 0.5%。另外，传感器增强泵组和注射治疗/BGM 组在低血糖发生率和体重增加上无显著差异。值得注意的是，CGM 使用频率与 HbA1C 降低的程度也有关系。有许多短期、随机的研究也报道了患者持续携带 CGM 装置能使血糖控制获益后 HbA1C 水平改善。一些研究在 T1D 一开始就使用传感器增强泵治疗，最大限度地在疾病期内使用这些技术。

CGM 运用中的障碍和心理影响

CGM 的使用带来许多潜在的益处及障碍（表 11-2）。现今与 CGM

使用有关的挑战在于每日携带传感器带来的额外负担，这被加入到日常糖尿病管理任务中的首位。JDRF CGM 试验研究的是患者的生活质量，对低血糖的恐惧，CGM 的满意度和 CGM 使用中的障碍问题。CGM 组与 BGM 组相比成年患者对低血糖恐惧和生活质量有轻微的但相当重要的改善，生活质量是根据 12 项短期健康状况调查表（SF12）评估。CGM 组和 BGM 组中的青少年患者和他们的父母在低血糖恐惧和生活质量上并没有差异。显然，成人、青少年和他们父母都对 CGM 表示实质性的满意。不出所料，CGM 满意度与 CGM 运用有显著的关系。

表 11-2　CGM 潜在的益处和障碍

益处：

带有趋势的连续血糖数据信息提示变化的速度和方向

检测血糖水平超出正常范围过高和过低时发出警报

即时血糖数据指导胰岛素用药、饮食、运动、病中的管理等

改善血糖控制

减少低血糖发生

追溯血糖数据指导改进治疗方案

降低做指尖连续血糖监测的潜在需要

潜在增加患者意识到血糖水平异常时相关的压力

障碍：

传感器植入时的疼痛

用带子将传感器固定在身上

需要带着传感器和接收器

需要频繁校正连续血糖监测仪器

传感器操作或异常血糖水平引起的相关的"令人讨厌的警报"

不确定如何利用传感器检测到的大量的血糖数据

关于连续血糖监测和家庭血糖监测之间潜在的分歧问题

潜在降低了低血糖恐惧相关的焦虑

　　另一部由 JDRF CGM 研究小组发表的出版物中记录了在试验中得到青少年患者、他们的父母和成人患者肯定的 CGM 在使用时对感知觉的障碍和益处。血糖趋势数据的有效性、自我纠正血糖水平、检测低血糖的能力等带来共同的益处。记录最多的障碍问题包括传感器植入带来的疼痛；系统警报常被认为是"令人讨厌的警报"；身体问题带来的挫折感与不知道传感器该植入到哪里、传感器胶黏剂引起皮肤反应和如何把接收器放在身

上等有关。CGM 使用者注意到连续数据提供了先前不能利用但有价值的信息，信息分别是关于不同的食物怎样影响 BG 水平和夜间低血糖的潜在风险，尤其是饭后和午夜的数据信息。值得注意的是，成人 T1D 患者和青少年患者的父母更倾向于记录益处，而青少年患者则倾向于记录障碍问题。

最近一个出版物调查了 JDRF CGM 试验中的一个辅助研究，即 CGM 使用中的社会心理。对比了 6 个月后 CGM 组和 BGM 组中 T1D 青少年患者及他们父母和 T1D 成人患者的心理特征。青少年、青少年父母和 T1D 成人患者似乎对 CGM 的使用有不同的社会心理反应。CGM 组中的青少年患者比 BGM 组中的青少年患者存在更多的焦虑特征，而 CGM 组中的 T1D 成人患者的焦虑状态比 BGM 组的要少。父母代记录的青少年抑郁症在 CGM 组中更高。CGM 组的青少年及其父母围绕 BGM 的负面影响要多于 BGM 组。另一方面，CGM 组的成人患者被认为糖尿病相关负担比 BGM 组的要少。总的来说，该初步研究显示 CGM 使用在成人中倾向造成正面的社会心理影响而在青少年中倾向于负面的社会心理影响，提示需要进一步研究减低 CGM 使用带来的任何负面社会心理结局的方法，尤其是对青少年患者。另一项只含有 T1D 成人患者的 JDRF CGM 试验的辅助研究试验显示，有效的 CGM 使用可能需要相应的技巧、频繁地回顾数据分析和家庭的支持。

CGM 使用中的障碍可能会促进负面的社会心理反应。与 CGM 使用相关的其他的挑战包括需要时间将传感器植入，进行校准，并对真正的"扰民"警报做出应对。当前，CGM 使用者必须连续检查他们的指尖血糖水平来校正 CGM 设备，以迎合患者开始调整糖尿病的治疗，因为 CGM 设备并未被监管机构批准可以取代 BGM。然而，CGM 试验已经被证实安全和对改善血糖控制不增加低血糖有实质效果，尤其是对 T1D 成人患者。正在青少年人群中进行的研究鼓励和支持 CGM 运用，目的是为了青少年 T1D 患者能与成年患者一样从中获得同样的益处。因此，需要行为干预来帮助青少年克服 CGM 使用中的障碍。

加强胰岛素治疗：笔的使用

自糖尿病控制与并发症试验（DCCT）发布后，胰岛素强化治疗一直是 T1D 患者的主要治疗方法。此外，英国前瞻性糖尿病研究（UKPDS）也公布了调查结果，胰岛素治疗作为优化血糖控制的方法一直以来都被提倡在 HbA1C 达不到目标水平的 T2D 患者上使用。在认识早期优化血糖控制的持续健康益处之后，这些方法变得更加突出，被称为"代谢记忆"或"后续效应"。这些术语指的是每个临床试验结束后一直以来给予强化治疗的患者，持续地保护他们 10 年期间糖尿病慢性并发症的发展。此外，在 DCCT 试验中胰岛素强化治疗并没有造成任何的生活质量恶化发生。尽管如此，它仍然需要去提供患者一种易于使用和负担最少的方法来进行强化治疗。

胰岛素笔转变了胰岛素治疗方式，为 T2D 患者提供简易的胰岛素管理，尤其是对那些最初抵抗注射的患者。另一方面，胰岛素笔（如同胰岛素泵疗法，见第十章）给 T1D 患者提供了生理的胰岛素替代物，全天的基础胰岛素注射和在进餐或点心时间或 BG 水平升高时使用的速效胰岛素类似物注射。利用笔进行胰岛素注射有许多潜在的益处（表 11-3）。用胰岛素泵注射生理胰岛素替代物的方法和益处见第十章。

表 11-3 胰岛素笔使用的可能机会

避免药瓶和注射器的使用

便于胰岛素管理

剂量精准

减轻焦虑

更加便捷

社会接受度高

增加灵活性

一些笔有胰岛素剂量记忆功能

减轻自觉疼痛

潜在提高生活质量

减少低血糖发生率

对医疗保健系统的使用和成本有有利的潜在影响

胰岛素笔是一种周全的胰岛素注射装置，无论是一支预填充的一次性笔或是一支可重复使用的笔都能容纳小笔芯（3ml）的胰岛素。两种类型的笔都能独立使用，螺口式针有不同的长度和容量迎合患者不同的需求。便携和方便的胰岛素笔让 T2D 患者更容易过渡到胰岛素治疗，使 T1D 患者更快适应一天多次注射治疗或大剂量的基础治疗。速效胰岛素类似物和基础胰岛素类似物都可在胰岛素笔中使用。一些患者离家远行或是在单位、学校时，或者外出就餐，或是旅游时，更愿意使用胰岛素笔而不是胰岛素药瓶和注射器。以前的研究指出在易于使用、剂量精准、社会接受度和生活质量方面提高注射技术。最近发表的一项药物治疗满意度调查显示，在成人 T2D 患者中对药物治疗便捷性和负面事件评分上使用胰岛素笔治疗的患者的满意度要高于使用胰岛素注射的患者。美国以外的一些国家，有超过 90% 的患者在使用胰岛素笔来达到糖尿病胰岛素治疗。近几年在美国使用胰岛素笔的患者数量在增加，因为胰岛素笔是一种良好的将糖尿病胰岛素治疗变简易或者过渡到胰岛素强化治疗的工具。此外，胰岛素笔的使用可能与患者依从性增加、低血糖的发生率降低、生活质量提高及对医疗保健系统的使用和花费的有利影响等有关。

互联网项目和技术

今天的互联网几乎涉及每个人的生活。到 2011 年，北美已有 79% 的人成为互联网用户（http://www.internetworldstats.com/stats.htm）。有许多社交媒体网站都在关注糖尿病教育或者治疗，包括像 Facebook 和 YouTube 这样的网站。其他一些像糖尿病儿童网和国际糖尿病教育项目等网站则提供了更多关于糖尿病的信息（表 11-4）。匿名、便捷、广阔的浏览选项使得互联网和社交媒体有了糖尿病教育和治疗的潜在价值。当"糖尿病"被输入到浏览器搜索引擎时出现了超过 300 000 000 个的结果。不同的网站有不同方面的内容和专业知识，因此医疗服务者为患者提供知名网站的教育和支持显得尤为重要。有许多现代的交互技术也可以提高糖尿病自我管理，如 DVD 光盘，电脑的应用程序，智能手机的应用程序和短信消息提醒系统，这些有利于各年龄层的患者使用并且可在不同的环境中使用，如在诊所、工作场所、社区或者家中。最近也有许多关于互联网项目和交互技术的评论发表。接着会研究一些特定的例子。

表 11-4 互联网和交互技术管理糖尿病的可能性

患者和家庭的教育

患者和家庭的支持

预约、连续血糖监测、用药等自动提醒系统

增加连续血糖监测依从性

增加用药依从性

自动创建的血糖日志和药物使用的日期和时间

注意健康饮食和增加体力活动的生活方式

提高自我效能和心理授权

改善血糖控制和合并症

社会心理健康

提高生活质量

潜在减少医疗系统的使用和节约成本

最近一个研究是在老年 T2D 患者中用一般治疗加上基于网络的干预和只使用一般治疗的进行对比，结果发现前组患者的 HbA1C、体重、胆固醇和 HDL 水平在 6 个月后比后组的有显著的改善。干预组同时在抑郁症测量、生活质量、社会帮助和自我效能上有显著改善。6 个月基于网络的多重干预由教材、每周的网络教育课程、即时通讯、实时聊天室讨论、布告板信息、电子邮件使用目标设置和解决问题的技能等组成，从而克服障碍来改善自我管理的行为和社会心理健康。虽然该研究因为样本量少（n=62）、人群均一、时间短方面存在局限性，但是结果令人鼓舞而且支持另外的基于网络干预的研究。

在一个超过 400 名 T2D 成人患者的大样本中进行为期 4 个月的研究，将英国人或西班牙人群中基于互联网的糖尿病自我管理项目与加强常规治疗做了对比。与健康饮食、脂肪摄入和体力活动有关的行为结果在基于互联网干预组中比在常规治疗组中有显著提高，虽然在 HbA1C、体质指数、脂质、血压等生物结果上并没有区别。12 个月后，再次证实互联网干预组相比常规治疗组能显著提高健康行为。

然而，作者提出为了生物结果有意义的改善还需要更加密集和量身定制的干预。电子邮件的干预被称为有生机的！（通过电子邮件干预生活方式），目的是改善饮食规律和体力活动及与健康有关的生活质量和自我效能。接着在超过700名员工为期16周的工作场所研究中，与对照组相比，电子邮件干预组显示在饮食规律、体力活动、生活质量和自我效能感上都有显著的改善。两组改善情况的不同在于干预期结束后仍维持了4个月。

基于网络教育和情感支持讨论区的出现似乎吸引了广泛的糖尿病患者，讨论一些关于营养学、情感支持、BG水平高低和糖尿病并发症的话题。用户满意度调查显示绝大多数的受访者认为参与讨论版能积极应对糖尿病并感觉更有希望。培养BG意识也被转换成了基于网络的干预。在40例T1D患者初步研究中，用户发现基于网络的干预是有帮助的且易于使用，并支持功能的改进。另一个77例成人T1D初步研究将进行了12个月基于网络管理项目和在糖尿病专科诊所常规治疗做了对比。虽然干预组的A1C比常规治疗组只稍微改善了一点，但是糖尿病相关的自我效能在干预组中相比常规治疗组有显著提高。该作者建议需要做更大样本的研究。

有许多小的研究围绕青少年T1D使用互联网或其他干预技术。尤其是手机短信，在青少年T1D中使用可增加BGM频率，显然是因为手机短信似乎是青少年首选的联系方式。一项持续3～12个月的初步研究用手机短信来提高依从性，增加自我效能，促进行为改变和提高健康结局。这些研究表明在青少年人群中手机短信的可用性和可接受性使依从性、自我效能和HbA1C有不同的改善。一些研究表明，在学校或者诊所利用无线传输BG数据能增加BGM频率、提高自我治疗且/或能降低HbA1C。我们对40名年龄在12～25岁间的青少年和青年T1D患者试行了12周的基于电脑的电子邮件和基于手机的短信自动BGM提醒系统，并进行对比。患者渴望使用简单的试行项目，更愿意选择手机短信提醒而不是电子邮件。在开始的一个月，手机短信组的患者比邮件组的多发送了近两倍的BG结果到安全中心服务器。但是随着时间的推移两组患者对BG提醒的反应都在减退，提示青少年T1D人群需要更强的交互式干预来维持自我管理的行为。最近的一个初步研究报道，可以合并"游戏化"来奖励例行的行为，例如，iTunes®和电脑或者智能手机APP。另外需要用研究来确定奖励是否能增加并维持行为的改变和改善健康结局。

还有其他的在青少年 T1D 人群中做的基于互联网的研究。例如，随着青少年 T1D 患者训练增加自我效能和改善血糖控制等的应对技能的成功，互联网的应对技能的训练项目也开始发展并在一个初步研究中进行了评估。其他多中心研究也在进行，目的是评估互联网应对技能项目的有效性。一项对使用胰岛素泵治疗的 T1D 青少年患者的观察性研究显示使用基于互联网的胰岛素泵监测系统与改善血糖控制有显著的相关性。

许多使用互联网和交互技术的研究在样本量和研究时间上都存在局限性。但是，初步研究鼓励了 1 型和 2 型青少年和成人糖尿病患者在生物学和社会心理结局方面做出改善。

临床治疗推荐

血糖监测

1. 1 型或 2 型糖尿病患者应接受糖尿病自我管理教育，包括 BGM 训练和数据解读。

2. 应鼓励糖尿病患者配合他们的卫生保健小组，根据每日 BGM 频率增加 5～10 次使 HbA1C 有所改善这一认知来测定他们的每日 BGM 推荐频率。

3. 患者接收了加强 BGM 频率的糖尿病管理训练后应筛查心理上的问题，包括糖尿病压力、糖尿病怠倦、抑郁和焦虑症状、低血糖（或高血糖）恐惧，必要时应交付于心理健康专家诊治。

持续血糖监测

1. 实时 CGM 可以用于降低青少年和成人 T1D 患者的 HbA1C 水平或维持 HbA1C 目标水平而不增加低血糖发生的频率。

2. 患者选择使用 CGM 时应考虑当前 BGM 频率、对如何植入传感器、如何设置和对警报的反应等的学习意愿，并渴望血糖的反应趋势和下载数据。当患者想在自己孩子身上使用 CGM 时，确保父母和孩子之间对于使用 CGM 的态度达成一致这点很重要，尤其当孩子年纪大到能仔细思考他/她是否会积极地参与 CGM 的使用。当患者的配偶、伙伴或家庭成员要求他们使用 CGM 时，关于使用 CGM 的态度保持一致很重要，这样成人患者就不会没有目的地持续使用 CGM 时感觉压力过度。

3. 目前 CGM 设备与大量的患者的负担相关，需要持续的教育和心理支持来帮助患者维持 CGM 的使用。

胰岛素笔的使用

1. 胰岛素笔的使用应考虑使用笔后缓解了 T2D 患者胰岛素管理、带来了更大的方便和潜在提高生活质量造成的胰岛素治疗的变化。

2. 鉴于胰岛素笔的使用方便、易于计量精度和潜在地改善依从性，胰岛素笔的使用应考虑开始胰岛素强化治疗糖尿病患者。

3. 就像犹豫是否穿着可视性的设备，应该将胰岛素泵治疗与替代生理性胰岛素的使用注射笔为基础的基础-餐时胰岛素强化治疗进行对比，评估其成本、易用性、依从性和潜在的心理障碍。

互联网项目和交互技术

1. 互联网作为一种方法应该考虑的是 1 型和 2 型糖尿病患者接收糖尿病教育、社会支持和问题解决策略等来提高依从性、自我效能和健康结局。图书馆和社区中心等公共接入点可以帮助那些没有家庭网络的患者进入互联网。

2. 手机短信自动提醒系统应该考虑的是作为一种途径来增加青少年和成人 T1D 患者的 BGM 频率、增加依从性和自我效能。

3. 1 型和 2 型糖尿病患者应考虑通过互联网或编辑短信来传输他们的血糖数据，并通过互联网联系他们的卫生保健小组来提高健康结局。

参 考 文 献

American Diabetes Association: Standards of medical care in diabetes—2012. Diabetes Care 35 (Suppl. 1):S11–S63, 2012

Anderson BJ, Redondo MJ: What can we learn from patient-reported outcomes of insulin pen devices? J Diabetes Sci Technol 5:1563–1571, 2011

Anderson BJ, Vangsness L, Connell A, Butler D, Goebel-Fabbri A, Laffel LM: Family conflict, adherence, and glycaemic control in youth with short duration type 1 diabetes. Diabet Med 19:635–642, 2002

Asche CV, Shane-McWhorter L, Raparla S: Health economics and compliance of vials/syringes versus pen devices: a review of the evidence. Diabetes Technol Ther 12 (Suppl. 1):S101–S108, 2010

Bergenstal RM, Tamborlane WV, Ahmann A, Buse JB, Dailey G, Davis SN, et al.: Effectiveness of sensor-augmented insulin-pump therapy in type 1 diabetes. N Engl J Med 363:311–320, 2010

Block G, Sternfeld B, Block CH, Block TJ, Norris J, Hopkins D, et al.: Development of Alive! (A Lifestyle Intervention Via Email), and its effect on health-related quality of life, presenteeism, and other behavioral outcomes: randomized controlled trial. J Med Internet Res 10:e43, 2008

Blonde L, Karter AJ: Current evidence regarding the value of self-monitored blood glucose testing. Am J Med 118 (Suppl. 9A):20S–26S, 2005

Bond GE, Burr RL, Wolf FM, Feldt K: The effects of a web-based intervention on psychosocial well-being among adults aged 60 and older with diabetes: a randomized trial. Diabetes Educ 36:446–456, 2010

Bond GE, Burr R, Wolf FM, Price M, McCurry SM, Teri L: The effects of a web-based intervention on the physical outcomes associated with diabetes among adults age 60 and older: a randomized trial. Diabetes Technol Ther 9:52–59, 2007

Cafazzo JA, Casselman M, Hamming N, Katzman DK, Palmert MR: Design of an mHealth app for the self-management of adolescent type 1 diabetes: a pilot study. J Med Internet Res 14:e70, 2012

Centers for Disease Control and Prevention: Self-monitoring of blood glucose among adults with diabetes: United States, 1997–2006. MMWR Morb Mortal Wkly Rep 56:1133–1137, 2007

Corriveau EA, Durso PJ, Kaufman FD, Skipper BJ, Laskaratos LA, Heintzman KB: Effect of Carelink, an internet-based insulin pump monitoring system, on glycemic control in rural and urban children with type 1 diabetes mellitus. Pediatr Diabetes 9:360–366, 2008

Cox D, Ritterband L, Magee J, Clarke W, Gonder-Frederick L: Blood glucose awareness training delivered over the Internet. Diabetes Care 31:1527–1528, 2008

Cox DJ, Irvine A, Gonder-Frederick L, Nowacek G, Butterfield J: Fear of hypoglycemia: quantification, validation, and utilization. Diabetes Care 10:617–621, 1987

Dailey G: Assessing glycemic control with self-monitoring of blood glucose and hemoglobin A(1c) measurements. Mayo Clin Proc 82:229–235, 2007

Dang DK, Lee J: Analysis of symposium articles on insulin pen devices and alternative insulin delivery methods. J Diabetes Sci Technol 4:558–561, 2010

DCCT Research Group: Influence of intensive diabetes treatment on quality-of-life outcomes in the Diabetes Control and Complications Trial. Diabetes Care 19:195–203, 1996

DCCT Research Group: The effect of intensive treatment of diabetes on the development and progression of long-term complications in insulin-dependent diabetes mellitus. N Engl J Med 329:977–986, 1993

Deiss D, Bolinder J, Riveline JP, Battelino T, Bosi E, Tubiana-Rufi N, et al.: Improved glycemic control in poorly controlled patients with type 1 diabetes using real-time continuous glucose monitoring. Diabetes Care 29:2730–2732, 2006

Farmer AJ, Wade AN, French DP, Simon J, Yudkin P, Gray A, et al.: Blood glucose self-monitoring in type 2 diabetes: a randomised controlled trial. Health Technol Assess 13:iii–iv, ix-xi, 1-50, 2009

Fisher L, Polonsky W, Parkin CG, Jelsovsky Z, Amstutz L, Wagner RS: The impact of blood glucose monitoring on depression and distress in insulin-naive patients with type 2 diabetes. Curr Med Res Opin 27 (Suppl. 3):39-46, 2011

Franklin VL, Greene A, Waller A, Greene SA, Pagliari C: Patients' engagement with "Sweet Talk": a text messaging support system for young people with diabetes. J Med Internet Res 10:e20, 2008

Franklin VL, Waller A, Pagliari C, Greene SA: A randomized controlled trial of Sweet Talk, a text-messaging system to support young people with diabetes. Diabet Med 23:1332–1338, 2006

Franklin V, Waller A, Pagliari C, Greene S: "Sweet Talk": text messaging support for intensive insulin therapy for young people with diabetes. Diabetes Technol Ther 5:991–996, 2003

Garg SK, Bookout TR, McFann KK, Kelly WC, Beatson C, Ellis SL, et al.: Improved glycemic control in intensively treated adult subjects with type 1 diabetes using insulin guidance software. Diabetes Technol Ther 10:369–375, 2008

Glasgow RE, Kurz D, King D, Dickman JM, Faber AJ, Halterman E, et al.: Twelve-month outcomes of an Internet-based diabetes self-management support program. Patient Educ Couns 87:81–92, 2012

Glasgow RE, Kurz D, King D, Dickman JM, Faber AJ, Halterman E, et al.: Outcomes of minimal and moderate support versions of an internet-based diabetes self-management support program. J Gen Intern Med 25:1315–1322, 2010

Glasgow RE: Using interactive technology in diabetes self-management. In Practical Psychology for Diabetes Clinicians. 2nd ed. Anderson BJ, Rubin RR, Eds. Alexandria, VA, American Diabetes Association, 2002, p. 51–62

Goyder E: Should we stop patients with non-insulin treated diabetes using self monitoring of blood glucose? The implications of the Diabetes Glycaemic Education and Monitoring (DiGEM) trial 2. Prim Care Diabetes 2:91–93, 2008

Grey M, Boland EA, Davidson M, Li J, Tamborlane WV: Coping skills training for youth with diabetes mellitus has long-lasting effects on metabolic control and quality of life. J Pediatr 137:107–113, 2000

Hanas R, de Beaufort C., Hoey H., Anderson B: Insulin delivery by injection in children and adolescents with diabetes. Pediatr Diabetes 12:518–526, 2011

Hanauer DA, Wentzell K, Laffel N, Laffel LM: Computerized Automated Reminder Diabetes System (CARDS): e-mail and SMS call phone text messaging reminders to support diabetes management. Diabetes Technol Ther 11:99–106, 2009

Harris MA, Hood KK, Mulvaney SA: Pumpers, skypers, surfers and texters: technology to improve the management of diabetes in teenagers. Diabetes Obes Metab. doi: 10.1111/j.1463-1326.2012.01599.x.

Hirsch IB, Bode BW, Childs BP, Close KL, Fisher WA, Gavin JR, et al.: Self-Monitoring of Blood Glucose (SMBG) in insulin- and non-insulin-using adults with diabetes: consensus recommendations for improving SMBG accuracy, utilization, and research. Diabetes Technol Ther 10:419–439, 2008

Holman RR, Paul SK, Bethel MA, Matthews DR, Neil HA: 10-year follow-up of intensive glucose control in type 2 diabetes. N Engl J Med 359:1577–1589, 2008

Ingerski LM, Laffel L, Drotar D, Repaske D, Hood KK: Correlates of glycemic control and quality of life outcomes in adolescents with type 1 diabetes. Pediatr Diabetes 11:563–571, 2010

Juvenile Diabetes Research Foundation Continuous Glucose Monitoring Study Group: Validation of measures of satisfaction with and impact of continuous and conventional glucose monitoring. Diabetes Technol Ther 12:679–684, 2010a

Juvenile Diabetes Research Foundation Continuous Glucose Monitoring Study Group, Beck RW, Lawrence JM, Laffel L, Wysocki T, Xing D, et al.: Quality-of-life measures in children and adults with type 1 diabetes: Juvenile Diabetes Research Foundation Continuous Glucose Monitoring randomized trial. Diabetes Care 33:2175–2177, 2010b

Juvenile Diabetes Research Foundation Continuous Glucose Monitoring Study Group: Factors predictive of use and of benefit from continuous glucose monitoring in type 1 diabetes. Diabetes Care 32:1947–1953, 2009a

Juvenile Diabetes Research Foundation Continuous Glucose Monitoring Study Group: The effect of continuous glucose monitoring in well-controlled type 1 diabetes. Diabetes Care 32:1378–1383, 2009b

Juvenile Diabetes Research Foundation Continuous Glucose Monitoring Study Group, Tamborlane WV, Beck RW, Bode BW, et al.: Continuous glucose monitoring and intensive treatment of type 1 diabetes. N Engl J Med 359:1464–1476, 2008

Kaufman N: Internet and information technology use in treatment of diabetes. Int J Clin Pract Suppl, 41–46, 2010

Klonoff DC, Buckingham B, Christiansen JS, Montori VM, Tamborlane WV, Vigersky RA, et al.: Continuous glucose monitoring: an Endocrine Society Clinical Practice Guideline. J Clin Endocrinol Metab 96:2968–2979, 2011

Kordonouri O, Pankowska E, Rami B, Kapellen T, Coutant R, Hartmann R, et al.: Sensor-augmented pump therapy from the diagnosis of childhood type 1 diabetes: results of the Paediatric Onset Study (ONSET) after 12 months of treatment. Diabetologia 53:2487–2495, 2010

Kumar VS, Wentzell KJ, Mikkelsen T, Pentland A, Laffel LM: The DAILY (Daily Automated Intensive Log for Youth) trial: a wireless, portable system to improve adherence and glycemic control in youth with diabetes. Diabetes Technol Ther 6:445–453, 2004

Laffel LM, Hsu W, McGill JB, Meneghini L, Volkening LK: Continued use of an integrated meter with electronic logbook maintains improvements in glycemic control beyond a randomized, controlled trial. Diabetes Technol Ther 9:254–264, 2007

Laffel L, Volkening L, Hood K, Lochrie A, Nansel T, Anderson B, et al.: Optimizing glycemic control in youth with T1DM: importance of BG monitoring and supportive family communication [Abstract]. Diabetes 55:A197, 2006

Lawlor MT, Laffel L, Anderson BJ: Blood Sugar Monitoring Owner's Manual. Boston, Joslin Diabetes Center, 1997

Lenhart A, Ling R, Campbell S, Purcell K, Pew Internet & American Life Project: Teens and mobile phones, 2010. Available at http://pewinternet.org/reports/2010/teens-and-mobile-phones.aspx. Accessed 21 June 2012

Levine BS, Anderson BJ, Butler DA, Brackett J, Laffel L: Predictors of glycemic control and short-term adverse outcomes in youth with type 1 diabetes. J Pediatr 139:197–203, 2001

Luijf YM, DeVries JH: Dosing accuracy of insulin pens versus conventional syringes and vials. Diabetes Technol Ther 12 (Suppl. 1):S73–S77, 2010

Magwire ML: Addressing barriers to insulin therapy: the role of insulin pens. Am J Ther 18:392–402, 2011

Markowitz JT, Pratt K, Aggarwal J, Volkening LK, Laffel LM: Psychosocial correlates of continuous glucose monitoring use in youth and adults with type 1 diabetes and parents of youth. Diabetes Technol Ther 14:523-526, 2012

McCarrier KP, Ralston JD, Hirsch IB, Lewis G, Martin DP, Zimmerman FJ, et al.: Web-based collaborative care for type 1 diabetes: a pilot randomized trial. Diabetes Technol Ther 11:211–217, 2009

Misono AS, Cutrona SL, Choudhry NK, Fischer MA, Stedman MR, Liberman JN, et al.: Healthcare information technology interventions to improve cardiovascular and diabetes medication adherence. Am J Manag Care 16 (12 Suppl. HIT):SP82–SP92, 2010

Moreland EC, Volkening LK, Lawlor MT, Chalmers KA, Anderson BJ, Laffel LM: Use of a blood glucose monitoring manual to enhance monitoring adherence in adults with diabetes: a randomized controlled trial. Arch Intern Med 166:689–695, 2006

Mulvaney SA, Anders S, Smith AK, Pittel EJ, Johnson KB: A pilot test of a tailored mobile and web-based diabetes messaging system for adolescents. J Telemed Telecare 18:115–118, 2012

Mulvaney SA, Ritterband LM, Bosslet L: Mobile intervention design in diabetes: review and recommendations. Curr Diab Rep 11:486–493, 2011

Nathan DM, Cleary PA, Backlund JY, Genuth SM, Lachin JM, Orchard TJ, et al.: Intensive diabetes treatment and cardiovascular disease in patients with type 1 diabetes. N Engl J Med 353:2643–2653, 2005

Nathan DM, McKitrick C, Larkin M, Schaffran R, Singer DE: Glycemic control in diabetes mellitus: have changes in therapy made a difference? Am J Med 100:157–163, 1996

Nationwide Children's Hospital: Pilot study supports adolescent diabetes patients through personalized text messages. *ScienceDaily* 10 Aug 2010. Available from http://www.sciencedaily.com/releases/2010/07/100730191628.htm. Accessed 20 July 2012

Nguyen TM, Mason KJ, Sanders CG, Yazdani P, Heptulla RA: Targeting blood glucose management in school improves glycemic control in children with poorly controlled type 1 diabetes mellitus. *J Pediatr* 153:575-578, 2008

Pearson TL: Practical aspects of insulin pen devices. *J Diabetes Sci Technol* 4:522-531, 2010

Peyrot M, Harshaw Q, Shillington AC, Xu Y, Rubin RR: Validation of a tool to assess medication treatment satisfaction in patients with type 2 diabetes: the Diabetes Medication System Rating Questionnaire (DMSRQ). *Diabet Med.* doi: 10.1111/j.1464-5491.2011.03558.x.

Phillip M, Danne T, Shalitin S, Buckingham B, Laffel L, Tamborlane W, et al.: Use of continuous glucose monitoring in children and adolescents (*). *Pediatr Diabetes* 13:215-228, 2012

Pistrosch F, Koehler C, Wildbrett J, Hanefeld M: Relationship between diurnal glucose levels and HbA1c in type 2 diabetes. *Horm Metab Res* 38:455-459, 2006

Polonsky WH, Fisher L, Schikman CH, Hinnen DA, Parkin CG, Jelsovsky Z, et al.: Structured self-monitoring of blood glucose significantly reduces A1C levels in poorly controlled, noninsulin-treated type 2 diabetes: results from the Structured Testing Program study. *Diabetes Care* 34:262-267, 2011

Raccah D, Sulmont V, Reznik Y, Guerci B, Renard E, Hanaire H, et al.: Incremental value of continuous glucose monitoring when starting pump therapy in patients with poorly controlled type 1 diabetes: the RealTrend study. *Diabetes Care* 32:2245-2250, 2009

Ritholz MD, Atakov-Castillo A, Beste M, Beverly EA, Leighton A, Weinger K, et al.: Psychosocial factors associated with use of continuous glucose monitoring. *Diabet Med* 27:1060-1065, 2010

Russell-Minda E, Jutai J, Speechley M, Bradley K, Chudyk A, Petrella R: Health technologies for monitoring and managing diabetes: a systematic review. *J Diabetes Sci Technol* 3:1460-1471, 2009

Siebolds M, Gaedeke O, Schwedes U: Self-monitoring of blood glucose: psychological aspects relevant to changes in HbA1c in type 2 diabetic patients treated with diet or diet plus oral antidiabetic medication. *Patient Educ Couns* 62:104-110, 2006

Siminerio LM: The role of technology and the chronic care model. *J Diabetes Sci Technol* 4:470-475, 2010

Sternfeld B, Block C, Quesenberry CP Jr, Block TJ, Husson G, Norris JC, et al.: Improving diet and physical activity with ALIVE: a worksite randomized trial. *Am J Prev Med* 36:475-483, 2009

Tansey M, Laffel L, Cheng J, Beck R, Coffey J, Huang E, et al.: Satisfaction with continuous glucose monitoring in adults and youths with type 1 diabetes. *Diabet Med* 28:1118-1122, 2011

Toscos TR, Ponder SW, Anderson BJ, Davidson MB, Lee ML, Montemayor-Gonzalez E, et al.: Integrating an automated diabetes management system into the family management of children with type 1 diabetes: results from a 12-month randomized controlled technology trial. *Diabetes Care* 35:498-502, 2012

UK Prospective Diabetes Study (UKPDS) Group: Intensive blood-glucose control with sulphonylureas or insulin compared with conventional treatment and risk of complications in patients with type 2 diabetes (UKPDS 33). *Lancet* 352:837-853, 1998

Webb TL, Joseph J, Yardley L, Michie S: Using the internet to promote health behavior change: a systematic review and meta-analysis of the impact of theoretical basis, use of behavior change techniques, and mode of delivery on efficacy. *J Med Internet Res* 12:e4, 2010

Welschen LM, Bloemendal E, Nijpels G, Dekker JM, Heine RJ, Stalman WA, et al.: Self-monitoring of blood glucose in patients with type 2 diabetes who are not using insulin: a systematic review. *Diabetes Care* 28:1510-1517, 2005

Wen L, Parchman ML, Linn WD, Lee S: Association between self-monitoring of blood glucose and glycemic control in patients with type 2 diabetes mellitus. *Am J Health Syst Pharm* 61:2401-2405, 2004

White NH, Sun W, Cleary PA, Tamborlane WV, Danis RP, Hainsworth DP, et al.: Effect of prior intensive therapy in type 1 diabetes on 10-year progression of retinopathy in the DCCT/EDIC: comparison of adults and adolescents. *Diabetes* 59:1244-1253, 2010

Whittemore R, Grey M, Lindemann E, Ambrosino J, Jaser S: Development of an internet coping skills training program for teenagers with type 1 diabetes. *Comput Inform Nurs* 28:103-111, 2010

Williams AS, Schnarrenberger PA: A comparison of dosing accuracy: visually impaired and sighted people using insulin pens. *J Diabetes Sci Technol* 4:514-521, 2010

Wood JR, Laffel LMB: Technology and intensive management in youth with type 1 diabetes: state of the art. *Curr Diab Rep* 7:104-113, 2007

Ziegler R, Heidtmann B, Hilgard D, Hofer S, Rosenbauer J, Holl R, et al.: Frequency of SMBG correlates with HbA1c and acute complications in children and adolescents with type 1 diabetes. *Pediatr Diabetes* 12:11-17, 2011

Zrebiec JF: Internet communities: do they improve coping with diabetes? *Diabetes Educ* 31:825-828, 830-832, 834, 836, 2005

Zrebiec JF, Jacobson AM: What attracts patients with diabetes to an Internet support group? A 21-month longitudinal website study. *Diabet Med* 18:154-158, 2001

第十二章

减 重 手 术

Brooke A. Bailer，PhD，Thomas A. Wadden，PhD，
Lucy F. Faulconbridge，PhD， and David B. Sarwer，PhD

　　极度肥胖，定义为 BMI＞40kg/m^2，如今影响了美国 5.7% 的成人。这种情况与逐渐增长的死亡率相关，尤其是心血管疾病，2 型糖尿病及一些肿瘤。它也与精神疾病增长的风险和生活质量的显著损害相关。对于那些使用行为和药物方法减肥失败的极度肥胖者，手术介入是最有效的治疗方法。Roux-en-Y 胃旁路术（RYGB）可长期（即 10 年）减少原始体重的 25%，然而腹腔镜下可调节胃束带术可达到 15%～20% 的减重效果。这些干预手段所达到的减重效果与身体健康的显著改善相关，尤其是 2 型糖尿病患者。

　　寻求减重手术的人必须经过大量的医学评估，由此决定他们是否适合医疗手术。他们通常需要完成一个行为社会心理评估，这个评估由国立卫生研究院（NIH）在 1991 年所举行的关于重度肥胖的胃肠手术的共识发展大会及最近的一个专家小组推荐。这一章描述了寻求减重手术的肥胖患者的行为状况，心情、饮食行为的改变及术后可预期的生活质量。这一章结合了一些研究成果的综述，这些研究成果是通过观察长期与这些患者相处的临床经验所得。

术前精神状态

　　减重手术申请者的精神状态有显著的不同。在手术评估的时候，大多数个体基本上拥有正常的心理功能。因此，心理保健和其他执业医师应该准备好迎接那些拥有良好的自尊并且享受工作和个人生活的申请者。然

而，有不少人报告有显著的心理困扰。例如，Kalarchian 等人使用定式临床会谈量表（SCID）检查了 288 名连续候选人的精神状态，他们发现在手术评估时有 37.8%的样本符合轴 I 障碍的标准，66.3%的人有轴 I 障碍的病史。其他调查者已经使用定式临床会谈量表报道了相似的发现。

情感障碍

在手术申请者的观察中，最常见的精神状况是重度抑郁症（MDD）和轻度抑郁症。MDD 的终身患病率为 5%～50%，然而 MDD 的现患率为 3%～25%。轻度抑郁症是一种程度较轻的抑郁症，估计其终身患病率为 5%，比率比其现患率低（见第一章抑郁症的诊断标准）。

导致肥胖患者抑郁的几个危险因素已经明确，首先是高 BMI。Onyike 等在国家健康与营养调查研究的数据中发现在过去的一个月中，BMI $\geqslant 40kg/m^2$ 的个体患重度抑郁症的风险比平均体重的人群高 4.6 倍。相比之下，BMI 在 35～39.9kg/m^2 范围的个体其风险只增加 1.9 倍。高 BMI 与受损的机体功能和身体疼痛相关，而这些又转而与抑郁症相关。高 BMI 的人也可能经历更大的体重相关耻辱和体像不满，这两种体会都与高水平的抑郁症状相关。年轻的手术申请者和女人也会出现情绪紊乱的高风险。

焦虑症

在减重手术申请者中也可频繁地观察到焦虑症，尤其是特定恐惧症、社交恐惧症、恐慌症和创伤后应激障碍。使用半结构性临床面谈的研究表明 15%～40%的手术患者有终身焦虑症病史。现患焦虑症，即在评估时定义的焦虑症，在 12%～24%的申请者中可被观察到。

药物滥用

药物滥用的终身患病率，包括酒精和毒品滥用，在手术申请者中估计是 1%～35%，大多数估计在 15%以下。药物滥用的现患率更低，波动在 1%～2%的范围。Kalarchian 等猜测终身患病率和现患率的差别可能是由于在心理访谈过程中申请者们试图从正面的角度表现自己，以便不被取消手术资格。或者，一些患者已经停止使用酒精或其他药物，并以过度饱食替代。

人格障碍

根据定式临床会谈量表，20%～30%的手术申请者被评估符合轴Ⅱ障碍的标准。这些障碍包括了一系列与长期社会功能障碍相关的人格特征。在手术申请者中最常见的人格障碍包括强迫型、回避型、偏执型、边缘型人格障碍。在许多案例中，有人格障碍的个体不会给自身带来麻烦，取而代之的是，他们以自我为中心和好操纵他人的人际行为模式给朋友、家人和同事带来了困难。

评估中方法的变化

对于目前所描述的所有诊断分类，评估方法的不同似乎是造成评估患病率范围差异的原因。诊断程序已经从结构化的临床会谈（即最理想的研究评估方法）扩展到半结构化以执业医师为基准的评估，再到自我报告衡量法，这种方法倾向于高估精神障碍的患病率。最近的一项研究调查了半结构化以执业医师为基准的评估与定式临床会谈量表（SCID）对于精神病诊断的现患率和终身患病率的频数符合度，结果发现目前诊断轴Ⅰ障碍的一致性很低。另外一种方法，即对精神病症状追溯性回忆，也不能很好地解决诊断的准确性问题。

术前精神障碍评估的临床意义和治疗

调查者们最初期望术前的精神障碍与术后不理想的减重有关。然而，在这个领域的研究并不一致。例如，最近的一项研究发现，有终身情绪障碍或焦虑症病史的个体与那些无此病史的个体相比，术后体重减轻更少，然而现患轴Ⅰ障碍和轴Ⅱ障碍的个体并不能预测受损的减肥。另一项调查发现对于较重的精神障碍者（即多种精神障碍），与那些较轻的精神障碍者（即只有一种或无精神障碍）相比，其减肥效果欠佳。然而，一些研究已报道抑郁症患者和有精神病治疗史的患者可减掉更多体重。通过对文献进行综合归纳，Hepertz等得出结论患者与肥胖苦恼相关的负面影响可能促进术后体重减轻。相比之下，与体重无关的重度抑郁和其他精神障碍的患者可能与欠佳的术后结果相关，包括医学并发症。这是一个有趣的假说，值得进一步研究。

对于术前精神状态能否预测减重的研究结果并不一致，这导致一些人质疑是否需要心理评估。鉴于临床上重度抑郁和其他精神障碍的频繁出现，这些疾病可采用行为或药物干预减轻患者的痛苦，故彻底的术前治疗应包括重症精神障碍的治疗，以及重度高血压、睡眠呼吸暂停和其他疾病的管理。不必惊讶，不少减重手术的申请者有精神病治疗的病史。接近 15%～40% 的患者接受了精神疗法，大约 40% 的人指出在他们术前行为评估时正在进行精神药物治疗。最常见的精神药物是抗抑郁药，接着是抗焦虑药，一小部分申请者使用安定药。Sarwer 等发现在 90 名减重手术申请者的样本中，只有 3% 的人使用安定药，与之相比，30% 的人使用抗抑郁药。

术前饮食行为

极度肥胖患者与普通体重的人相比有更高的能量需求（由间接测热法决定）。因此，极度肥胖的个体比平均体重者消耗更多的卡路里。尽管这些卡路里只相当于每日多出几百卡路里，但这些能量需要来维持过度肥胖。因此，执业医师可能惊奇地发现许多减重手术的患者并没有消耗过多的食物。然而，一部分手术申请者遭受了暴食症或其他饮食障碍。

暴食症的患病率

暴食症（BED）以短期内（如 2 小时）客观地消耗大量的食物为特征，在吃的时候伴随着一种不可控制感。它也与其他精神疾病的增长风险相关，包括抑郁症和焦虑症。BED 不同于在暴食后缺乏补偿性行为的暴食症，如呕吐、使用泻药或者过量运动。手术申请者中，BED 整体患病率估计是 2%～50%。

自我报告衡量法，与由经验丰富的评估者执行的结构化或半结构化临床访谈相比，倾向于高估 BED 的患病率。与之矛盾的是，过重或者肥胖患者倾向于低估必须要吃的符合客观大量的食物总量，客观大量的值定义为接近大多数人在对照情况下食量的两倍。依据是否使用 DSM-IV

规定的每两周（持续6个月）至少发生一次暴食的频率，或者使用由DSM-V提出的每周一次的暴食频率，其患病率的评估有所不同。结构化临床访谈，使用严格的DSM-Ⅳ诊断标准，评估BED的患病率为4%～25%。

术前BED患者的术后减重效果已经是一个讨论热题。一些早期的报道表明BED与术后欠佳的减重效果有关，致使一些调查者建议这些患者在术前接受暴食症的认知行为治疗。然而，这些早期的研究，许多都有重大的研究方法的限制。更多的近期调查已经发现，对于有或者无术前BED的患者，对术后1～2年的减重效果影响很小或者没有影响。例如，Wadden等发现有BED的患者在第一年体重减轻原始体重的22.1%，与之相比，那些没有现患饮食障碍且优先手术的患者，其体重减轻原始体重的24.1%（$P>0.30$）。患者在术后对饮食不可控制的体验（不管是现在还是非术前）似乎与欠佳的减重有关。主观的饮食失控感的评估应该在手术前和术后重大回访时被监测。如果需要，向认知行为治疗转诊的患者也应该做这项监测。

夜食综合征

手术申请者的夜食综合征（NES）患病率为2%～55%。NES以在傍晚或夜间不正常的摄入大量的食物为特征。NES患者至少在晚饭后摄取日摄食量的25%，并且他们至少每周经历两次与饮食有关的夜间觉醒。为使诊断有意义，患者必须对夜间进食发作是有意识的，这使得NES与睡眠相关的饮食失调症（SRED）不同。为使患者符合NES的标准，他们的饮食行为必须与痛苦或机体功能损坏有关。

Allison等使用自我报告衡量与半结构化临床访谈结合的方法，发现在手术前访谈时有5%的手术患者符合NES的诊断标准。这种不一致的NES患病率似乎是由于使用不同的诊断标准和不同的评估方法造成的。关于术前NES的患者其术后减重效果的信息很少。

术前生活质量

正如前面提到的，在手术评估的时候，大多数申请者基本上精神状态正常。尽管如此，这些个体可能由于过度肥胖遭遇生活质量受损。

与健康相关的生活质量

过度肥胖的压力能妨碍最基本的身体功能和个人护理任务。许多调查已经发现极度肥胖的个体在进行走路、爬楼梯、洗澡和穿衣服等活动时有身体功能的损伤，在肥胖患者最痛苦的事情中就存在这些困难。健康相关的生活质量（HRQoL）是一个宽泛的名词，用以描述跨越众多方面的个体功能状态，如身体、精神的及社交的表现。由于过度肥胖进行减重手术的人最容易受损的方面是身体功能和疼痛。与肥胖相关的情况，包括睡眠呼吸暂停、2型糖尿病和骨关节炎似乎能进一步加剧生活质量的损害。

近期的一项54个研究的荟萃分析在1980～2006年调查了三组人的 HRQoL：①减肥手术申请者；②寻求非手术治疗的肥胖个体；③未寻求治疗的超重或肥胖参与者。这项分析发现与其他两组肥胖个体相比，那些寻求手术治疗的个体在跨越众多方面的 HRQOL 有更显著的损害，包括机体功能和身体作用的限制。对未寻求治疗的个体的研究表明，高 BMI 水平与最大的生活质量损害相关。

一些研究已经调查了 BMI、HRQoL 及情绪间的联系。Kalarchian 等发现与没有身体状况异常的手术患者相比，有严重身体疼痛和多种功能限制的肥胖手术患者增加了患轴Ⅰ障碍的风险——典型的是情绪障碍（如重度抑郁症）或焦虑症（如惊恐发作）。Fabricatore 等也在 306 名手术申请者中调查了 BMI、HRQoL 及抑郁症状之间的关系。患者们依据有无生活质量的损害被分成三个 BMI 等级组（40～49.9kg/m^2，50～59.9kg/m^2 和＞60kg/m^2）。贝克抑郁量表（BDI）的抑郁症分数一般因HRQoL 损害而变化，而不因 BMI 分级变化。例如，没有身体功能损伤，身体疼痛或身体作用限制的Ⅱ级和Ⅲ级肥胖个体与那些在相同 BMI 等级并且没有这些身体障碍的人相比，其抑郁分数更低，如图 12-1 和图12-2 所示。而且，对于没有 HRQoL 损害的个体其 BDI 分数并没有随 BMI 分级而增加（因为小样本的限制，对于每一种 BMI 等级，不是所有 HRQoL 的差别都具有统计学意义，但是所有结果指向同一方向）。这些发现表明HRQoL 在 BMI 水平和抑郁症之间扮演中介者的角色。

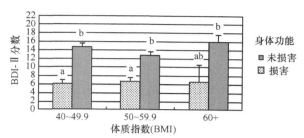

图 12-1　以 BMI 分组的手术申请者中平均抑郁症得分及针对个体是否提示了有意义或无意义的 SF-36 量表中身体功能损害水平

不同字母的条形图彼此间的差异很大，它由 Tukey 的显著差异比较决定（$P<0.05$）。水平线表明抑郁症状的水平有临床意义。

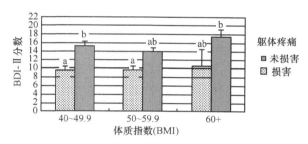

图 12-2　以 BMI 分组的手术申请者中平均抑郁症得分及针对个体是否提示了有意义或无意义的 SF-36 量表中躯体疼痛障碍

不同字母的条形图彼此间的差异很大，它由 Tukey 的显著差异比较决定（$P<0.05$）。水平线表明抑郁症状的水平有临床意义。

体像和性功能

体像。不少肥胖患者经历了显著的体像不满。早在 1967 年，Stunkard 和 Mendelson 描述了一群有着体像"蔑视"的肥胖患者，他们认为他们的身体是"丑陋而卑劣"的，其他人对他们是"敌对而蔑视"的。他们的体像蔑视以压倒性的形式占据肥胖，通常将其他的性格特征排除在外。近来，Sarwer 等观察到 8% 的参加临床试验的肥胖个体有类似的现象。这一群体符合身体畸形恐惧症的标准。身体畸形恐惧症被定义为患者过度关注自己的体像并对轻微的体貌缺陷进行臆想，从而引起临床上或社交、工作和其他领域的功能障碍。有这种障碍的患者其 BDI 分数平均为 13.2（指示为轻度抑郁），而有体像不满但未达身体畸形恐惧症标准的患者其分数正常（如平均 7.2）。Stunkard 和 Sarwer 研究的患者都不是减肥手术的申请者，而且只有小部分手术申请者表现出了这个程度的体像蔑视。

Adami 等调查了 30 名手术申请者的体像不满，并以 30 名从未有肥胖的患者作对照组。手术申请者与从未有肥胖的对照组相比，对体像的关注更甚，尤其是在整体肥胖及下半身肥胖的体像不满的领域，这个数据由饮食障碍库存体像不满分量表、体型问卷和身体自我态度问卷测量所得。Grilo 等发现在手术申请者中自卑及 BED 患者预测有更大的体像不满，这样的结果在非手术肥胖个体中也有报道。在一项 131 名女性手术申请者的研究中，Rosenberger 等发现，抑郁症、自卑、高度完美主义的存在可预测重度的体像不满。

性功能。手术申请者性功能障碍是常见的问题。Bond 等报道 60% 的女性手术申请者符合性功能障碍（FSD）的标准，在这些样本中老年妇女和更年期妇女预测了 FSD。与健康对照组相比，对这些个体所有性过程的评估（如性欲望、性兴奋，体液分泌，性高潮，满足感及疼痛）表明了其有更严重的性功能障碍。与普通群体相比，男性手术申请者也发现有更严重的性功能障碍。所有性过程都观察到有损害，包括性冲动、勃起功能、射精功能和性满足感。

减重手术后精神状态的改变

情感障碍

大量的研究已经得出结论，极度肥胖的患者实行减肥手术使体重减轻后，其精神状态得到了改善。瑞典肥胖主题（SOS）研究提供了术后情绪障碍和焦虑症改变的评估，这可能是一项最好的研究。这项实验包括了严谨的对照组，该对照组接受了传统饮食和运动咨询服务。与对照组相比，手术患者的自我报告的抑郁症分数在一年内下降的更显著（40%vs.10% 的减少，分别）。类似的分数下降在焦虑症患者中也能被观察到。在第 2 年，主要由垂直捆绑胃成形术所致的平均体重减少是原始体重的 23%。在这两个时间及 4 年的随访评估中，情绪障碍和焦虑水平在第一年从最低值开始增长。然而，在这两个时间段里，体重减少的增多与抑郁和焦虑显著改善有关。在亚组患者的 10 年随访中，手术患者的抑郁症改善仍比对照组显著，但是焦虑症的改善并没有显著的差别。

在一项无对照的研究中，Dixon 等报道，使用腹腔镜下可调节胃束带术减轻原始体重的20%后，患者获得了良好的抑郁症改善。在一组评估的患者中，术前平均 17.7 分的 BDI 值指示了轻微的抑郁症状，术后 1 年，这个值下降到 7.8 并在第 4 年保持在 9.0。后续的这些值指示了极小的抑郁症症状。

许多患者在术后 1～2 年经常发生抑郁症和焦虑症症状的反弹，故需要其他的长期研究来确定与之相关的因素。如果患者停止减重或者开始重增一点体重，后者在术后 18～24 个月很常见，那么患者的情感障碍可能回到基线水平。而且，手术前有情绪障碍和焦虑症病史的人可能在术后持续存在这些问题，尽管术后他们获得了很大的减重效果。

术后自杀的风险

一些队列研究已经指出，在经历了减重手术的个体中，其自杀率比预期的更高。Higa 等报道了在调查术后患者的全因死亡率中，1040 名手术者中有 1 名自杀死亡。在文献回顾中，Hsu 等报道，在随访的 14 年期间，1785 名减重手术患者中有 8 名自杀死亡。Waters 等报道，在 3 年期间，队列研究的 157 名减重手术患者中有 3 名自杀死亡。Omalu 等描述了肥胖患者减重手术后的 3 个自杀案例（没有描述他们的样本量）。美国人口的自杀率是每年 11/10 万（ww.cdc.gov/ncipc/wisqars）

一个大的病例对照研究表明，实行减重手段的极度肥胖患者的自杀率比预期更好。Adams 等调查了同一地理位置以驾照确定个人身份的 10000 名手术治疗患者和 9600 名未寻求手术治疗的肥胖患者。研究对象以年龄、性别和 BMI 进行匹配，并且评估了特因死亡率（如心血管疾病、癌症）和全因死亡率的差别。在平均 7 年的随访期间，进行自杀的手术患者（n=43）比对照组（n=24）大约多 50%。这个差别没有显著的统计学意义但是表明了有必要进一步研究的趋势。

如果减重手术患者的自杀率比预期高，何种因素可以解释？有限的数据表明减重手术后有最大自杀风险的患者可能是术前有抑郁症或其他精神障碍的人。Waters 等描述的 3 例自杀死亡案例中，这三个人都有术前情绪障碍（如焦虑症和抑郁症）。减重手术后的最初 6～12 个月的精神并发症有改善，但经过一段时间又会反弹。类似的情况出现在了 Omalu 等的案例报告中，术后进行自杀的 3 个人都有术前周期性重度抑郁的病史。案例报告中的 3 个人在术后平均 21.6 个月结束他们的生命，同时维持体重减轻是原始体重的 25%～41%。

与体重匹配的对照对象相比，Adams 等发现了他们的患者术后更高的自杀率，但是他们的研究并没有包括手术治疗者和对照者的术前精神障碍的信息。因此，不管他们是否经历了手术，寻求手术治疗的个体很可能比对照组有更高的抑郁症和自杀观念的发生率，并且有增加了自杀死亡的风险率。

术后饮食行为的改变

暴食症

一些研究已经报道了减重手术后暴食症的显著改善。例如，Kalarchian 等调查了术后 4 个月的患者并且观察到暴食活动完全终止。Wadden 等同样观察到术后 6 个月的患者其暴食活动的完全停止，这些人在术前 28 天暴食症平均值是 9.5。这些发现可能是由于胃体积的骤然缩减，从而限制了患者可消耗的食物量。

尽管在减重手术后短期内暴食症患者降低，不少患者继续报告经历着吃东西的不可控感。一些研究报道这种经历预测了术后 2 年或更多年欠佳的减重效果。其他的调查者已经报道了真正的暴食活动（患者消耗客观大量的食物）经常在长期随访中复发。一项近期研究术后 8.5 年患者的发现表明，在先前的几个月有 51%的患者报道了不规律的暴食活动。

减重手术患者中夜食综合征的患病率

很少的研究调查了 NES 患者的减重手术效果，这些研究获得了不一致的结果。Rand 等得出结论，在术后 32 个月，NES 的患病率从 31%到

27%轻微的下降。另外的研究报道了术后 NES 患病率未改变。这两个研究都有研究方法的缺陷（如回顾性设计、小样本），因而限制了结果的完整性。最近，Colles 等评估了 129 名手术患者的预期的 NES，使用了自我报告调查问卷和半结构化访谈两种方式（用电话调查）。NES 的患病率在术前是 17.1%，在术后 12 个月显著下降到了 7.8%。值得注意的是，多于一半的患者在术前没有此诊断，在术后 1 年符合 NES 标准。更多的研究表明，阐明减重手术对 NES 症状的效果有明显的必要性。而且，那些不想对术后影响减肥轨迹的行为引起关注的患者很可能呈现一个偏倚的饮食习惯自我报告。

饮食依从性

在术后第一年，多达 20% 的患者被观察到欠佳的减重效果，这通常与较差的饮食和行为建议的依从性相关，包括进行低能量的饮食。Sarwer 等查了术后减重的预测因子并且发现（还有男性和认知约束），与那些最低饮食依从性的患者相比，有最高依从性的患者（利开特式量表 9 分）可多减 28% 的体重。Kruseman 等对患者随访了 8 年并且发现，术后的饮食依从性，低能量饮食在术后第一年显著的降低。作者根据患者减掉的超重的体重将患者分成两组，减重受损的组别比成功组（超重部分减掉＞50% 的重量）每日多吃 300kcal 的能量。

呕吐和梗阻。接近 1/3 的手术患者报道有呕吐。它在术后最初的几个月发生最频繁，而后随着时间流逝频率降低。然而，一些个体报道在术后几年发生呕吐。术后呕吐似乎并不是一种清除行为，即便它是自我诱导的。相反的，他似乎是一种对过度饮食的反射性反应或者是对不可忍受食物的反应。呕吐可能也发生在食物卡在手术凹陷或者上消化道。后者的发生指的是梗阻或者口吐白沫。这通常是对进食像面包、意大利面和干硬肉类这些食物的反应。

胃倾倒综合征。胃倾倒综合征，是行 RYGB 手术患者的一种并发症，以恶心、严重的腹泻、心悸、眩晕和疲乏为特征。它通常发生在进食糖类食物之后，并且可在 50%～70% 行 RYGB 手术的患者中观察到。随着时间流逝倾倒综合征的发生频率下降。胃倾倒综合征的不愉快症状加强了患者逃避进食糖类食物。

术后生活质量

与健康相关的生活质量

由减重手术达到的较大的减肥效果显著提高了身体功能和其他方面的生活质量，包括走路、爬楼梯、洗澡和穿衣。例如，Nguyen 等研究了术前 BMI 平均为 $48kg/m^2$ 的患者并且在 3 个月和 6 个月的术前评估中发现，他们的身体功能已经提高到了普通人水平。O'Brien 等研究了较轻的肥胖患者（平均 BMI=33.7 kg/m^2），他们进行了腹腔镜下可调节胃束带术。患者的所有 SF-36® 量表分数在基线水平下降到了显著受损范围，但是在术后 2 年，伴随原始体重减少 22%，此分数上升至符合或超出标准的水平。与那些被随机分配到生活方式干预加药物治疗的此项研究的参与者相比，那些手术治疗的患者其身体功能分数提高的更显著。

减重及身体功能提高也可能与体重相关疼痛的显著减少、限制活动的体重相关姿势异常的改正（或提高）有关。SOS 研究发现位于颈部、后背、臀部、膝盖和脚踝的"工作限制性"疼痛，以及与力相关的小腿疼痛，肥胖患者比普通人更常见。与使用非手术方法减重并具有相近体重的对照组相比，那些实行了减重手术的患者 2 年来这些类型的疼痛有显著的改善（或者解决）。手术治疗的患者也不太可能得这样的疼痛。承重关节疼痛的减轻，如膝盖和脚踝，似乎比患者之前报道的在下背部和非承重部位的缓解更加持久。减重术后至少 6 年能观察到前面那些部位疼痛的改善。

HRQoL 的改善与减重密切相关。一项近期的研究调查了 SOS 研究中 HRQoL 的 10 年趋势，发现 HRQoL 的改善在术后 6 个月到 1 年之间达到高峰。此后，HRQoL 从 1～6 年下降，在这期间患者重增了一些体重。作者报道了体重重增的稳定性和 6～10 年的 HRQoL，表明 HRQoL 的改变反映了体重重增。这一趋势在其他研究中已经被重复。

体像和性功能

体像。由减重手术所达到的体重减轻也与体像的改善有关。一项对 200 名患者的近期研究中，Sarwer 等在术后第 20、40 和 92 周观察到体型问卷分数提高了 30%。参与者也报道了与体像相关的生活质量（BIQoL）的提高，这是一种构建，用以评估积极或消极体像对生活质量的几个方面的影响。在第 40 周 BIQoL 持续提高并在第 40～92 周之间稳定。根据临床报告这些积极的长期发现是重要的，即当手术患者开始关注他们胸部、腹部、大腿及手臂的松弛而下垂的皮肤时，体像不满可能随着时间流逝而增加。

性功能。大量的研究报道了手术后性功能的提高。例如，Bond 等在评估术后 6 个月的 54 名女性手术患者时发现其 FSD 显著提高。几乎 2/3 的患者报告他们的 FSD 已经解决。在男性中类似的改善也已被报道。Dallal 等调查了术后 19 个月 97 名男性的性功能，并且观察到评估的所有性过程都有改善（如性冲动、勃起功能、射精功能和性满足感）。在这个样本中减重预测了性功能提高的程度，减重越大，性功能改善越明显。

小结

如前所述，减重手术申请者的精神评估首次由 NIH 在 1991 年所举行的关于重度肥胖的胃肠手术的共识发展大会，以及 2008 年的一个专家小组推荐，当前几乎实践于所有的减重手术程序。对术前评估和术后护理的近期推荐代表了一种临床观点共识，这个共识由美国临床内分泌医师学会（AACE），肥胖协会（TOS）及美国代谢和肥胖症外科协会（ASMBS）达成。如这一章前面所描述，临床观点由相关性和观察性研究的结果所指导。然而，没有或者很少的随机对照试验陈述了这些问题，例如对申请者进行初始行为评估的益处，或者为了提高术后减重欠佳患者的饮食和行为习惯，为其提供术后 12～24 个月的的行为咨询服务。对于这些问题的对照实验是需要的，但是他们如今的缺失并不应阻碍患者获得能陈述患者需求的适当的临床干预。

一些调查者描述了行为评估的内容和结构。目前没有统一的方法，尽管所有的评估目的都是为了确定被认为是手术禁忌证（如药物滥用和暴食症）或者能导致减重欠佳的行为和精神因素，也是为了确定可能妨碍长期体重管理的潜在障碍。3 项近期研究报道了 3% 的手术申请者被认为不适合手术，8%～32% 被建议在术前进行精神护理和营养咨询。为了精神和营养咨询而推迟手术是罕见的，而且这样做的益处并没有得到充分的研究。

临床护理的建议

1. 不可控的精神并发症，如重度抑郁，应该在术前被治疗以便缓解患者的痛苦。术后抑郁和自杀的有限的证据表明，对于慢性的精神状况，由手术引起的体重减轻似乎并不能得到充分的治疗。术前有精神疾病的患者在术后常规的间歇期也应该进行评估，以确保他们达到了精神状况的最佳控制。如果需要，所有进行减重手术的患者应该有机会获得心理健康专家的帮助，以便适应术后身体和精神功能的改变。在大量手术治疗的个体中，这样的改变是相当积极的。

2. 心理健康专家应该对减重手术的申请者进行评估，这些专家也应有肥胖方面的专业知识并且是术前小组的一员。正如在其他地方所描述的，执业医师可以通过访谈筛查抑郁症，辅以纸笔问卷，如患者健康问卷中抑郁症状群量表（PHQ-9）。尽管体重减轻普遍提高了情绪，对于重度抑郁和其他精神疾病来说这不是一种主要的治疗。因此，对于期望减重能解决重大精神健康问题的情况，精神护理不应该被延迟。

3. HRQoL 应该是术前社会心理评估的基本组成部分，在术后也应该被监测。这个评估成分可能确定与抑郁情绪和减重结果相关的问题。

4. 与其他方面的精神痛苦一样，术前和术后检查的临床上重大体像的问题，包括性功能，也应该被评估和监测。

5. 鉴于 Omalu 等的发现，大量的减重本身并不能缓解抑郁症和自杀行为，减重手术患者增长的自杀风险凸显了申请者应该进行一次彻底的术前行为评估的需要，并且应该为抑郁症和其他精神疾病患者提供合适的精神护理，这样的护理也该在术后继续提供。

6. 在定期医疗管理访问中，饮食习惯和紊乱的饮食行为（见第二章）病史应该在术前和术后被评估和监测。

7. 与其他饮食习惯障碍一样，NES 应该在术前被评估，在术后被监测。

8. 减重受损的患者也许能从提高对饮食建议依赖性的术后咨询中获益。

参 考 文 献

Adami GF, Meneghelli A, Bressani A, Scopinaro N: Body image in obese patients before and after stable weight reduction following bariatric surgery. *J Psychosomatic Res* 46:275–281, 1999

Adami GF, Gandolfo P, Campostano A, Meneghelli A, Ravera G, Scopinaro N: Body image and body weight in obese patients. *Int J Eat Disord* 24:299–306, 1998

Adami GF, Gandolfo BB, Scopinaro N: Binge eating in massively obese patients undergoing bariatric surgery. *Int J Eat Disord* 17:45–50, 1995

Adams TD, Gress RE, Smith SC, Halverson RC, et al.: Long-term mortality after gastric bypass surgery. *N Engl J Med* 357:753–761, 2007

Alger-Mayer S, Rosati C, Polimeni JM, Malone M: Preoperative binge eating status and gastric bypass surgery: a long-term outcome study. *Obes Surg* 19:139–145, 2009

Allison DB, Fontaine KR, Manson JE, Stevens J, VanItallie TB: Annual deaths attributable to obesity in the United States. *JAMA* 282:1530–1538, 1999

Allison KC, Lundgren JD, O'Reardon JP, Galiehter A, et al.: Proposed diagnostic criteria for night eating syndrome. *Int J Eat Disord* 43:241–247, 2010

Allison KC, Wadden TA, Sarwer DB, Fabricatore AN, et al.: Night eating syndrome and binge eating disorder among persons seeking bariatric surgery: prevalence and related features. *Obesity (Silver Spring)* 14 (Suppl. 2):S77–S82, 2006

Allison KC, Stunkard AJ: Obesity and eating disorders. *Psychiatr Clin North Am* 28:55–67, 2005

American Psychiatric Association: *Diagnostic and Statistical Manual of Mental Disorders (DSM-IV-TR).* 4th ed. Washington, DC, American Psychiatric Association, 2000

Ashton K, Drerup M, Windover A, Heinberg L: Brief, four-session group CBT reduces binge eating behaviors among bariatric surgery candidates. *Surg Obes Relat Dis* 5:257–262, 2009

Assimakopoulos K, Karaivazoglou K, Panayiotopoulos S, Hyphantis T, Iconomou G, Kalfarentzos F: Bariatric surgery is associated with reduced depressive symptoms and better sexual function in obese female patients: a one-year follow-up study. *Obes Surg* 21:362–366, 2010

Assimakopoulos K, Panayiotopoulos S, Iconomou G, Karaivazoglou K, et al.: Assessing sexual function in obese women preparing for bariatric surgery. *Obes Surg* 16:1087–1091, 2006

Averbukh Y, Heshka S, El-Shoreya H, Flancbaum L, et al.: Depression score predicts weight loss following Roux-en-Y gastric bypass. *Obes Surg* 13:833–836, 2003

Balsiger BM, Poggio JL, Mai J, Kelly KA, Sam MG: Ten and more years after vertical banded gastroplasty as primary operation for morbid obesity. *J Gastrointest Surg* 4:598–605, 2000

Barry DT, Grilo CM, Masheb RM: Comparison of patients with bulimia nervosa, obese patients with binge eating disorder, and nonobese patients with binge eating disorder. *J Nerv Ment Dis* 191:589–594, 2003

Batsis JA, Lopez-Jimenez F, Collazo-Clavell ML, Clark MM, Somers VK, Sarr MG: Quality of life after bariatric surgery: a population-based cohort study. *Am J Med* 122:1055.e1–1055.e10, 2009

Black DW, Goldstein RB, Mason EE: Prevalence of mental disorder in 88 morbidly obese bariatric clinic patients. *Am J Psychiatry* 149:227–234, 1992

Bloomston M, Zervos EE, Camps MA, Goode SE, Rosemurgy AS: Outcome following bariatric surgery in super versus morbidly obese patients: does weight matter? *Obes Surg* 7:414–419, 1997

Bond DS, Wing RR, Vithiananthan S, Sax HC, et al.: Significant resolution of female sexual dysfunction after bariatric surgery. *Surg Obes Relat Dis* 7:1–7, 2011

Bond DS, Vithiananthan S, Leahey TM, Thomas JG, et al.: Prevalence and degree of sexual dysfunction in a sample of women seeking bariatric surgery. *Surg Obes Relat Dis* 5:698–704, 2009

Brolin RE, Robertson LB, Kenler HA, Cody RP: Weight loss and dietary intake after vertical banded gastroplasty and Roux-en-Y gastric bypass. *Ann Surg* 220:782–790, 1994

Brolin RE: Gastric restrictive surgery. *JAMA* 262:1188, 1989

Buchwald H, Consensus Conference Panel: Consensus conference statement bariatric surgery for morbid obesity: health implications for patients, health professionals, and third-party payers. *Surg Obes Relat Dis* 1:371–381, 2005

Buchwald H, Avidor Y, Braunwald E, Jensen MD, et al.: Bariatric surgery: a systematic review and meta-analysis. *JAMA* 292:1724–1737, 2004

Burgmer R, Grigutsch K, Zipfel S, Wolf AM, et al.: The influence of eating behavior and eating pathology on weight loss after gastric restriction operations. *Obes Surg* 15:684–691, 2005

Calle EE, Rodriguez C, Walker-Thurmond K, Thun MJ: Overweight, obesity, and mortality from cancer in a prospectively studied cohort of U.S. adults. *N Engl J Med* 348:1625–1638, 2003

Camps MA, Zervos E, Goode S, Rosemurgy AS: Impact of bariatric surgery on body image perception and sexuality in morbidly obese patients and their partners. *Obes Surg* 6:356–360, 1996

Carmichael AR, Sue-Ling HM, Johnston D: Quality of life after the Magenstrasse and Mill procedure for morbid obesity. *Obes Surg* 11:708–715, 2001

Centers for Disease Control and Prevention, National Center for Injury Prevention and Control: Web-based Injury Statistics Query and Reporting System (WISQARS™). Available at www.cdc.gov/ncipc/wisqars. Accessed 25 June 2012

Choban PS, Onyejekwe J, Burge JC, Flancbaum L: A health status assessment of the impact of weight loss following Roux-en-Y gastric bypass for clinically severe obesity. *J Am Coll Surg* 188:491–497, 1999

Clark MM, Balsiger BM, Sletten CD, Dahlman KL, et al.: Psychosocial factors and 2-year outcome following bariatric surgery for weight loss. *Obes Surg* 13:739–745, 2003

Colles SL, Dixon JB, O'Brien PE: Grazing and loss of control related to eating: two high-risk factors following bariatric surgery. *Obesity (Silver Spring)* 16:615–622, 2008

Colles SL, Dixon JB: Night eating syndrome: impact on bariatric surgery. *Obes Surg* 16:811–820, 2006

Crémieux PY, Ledoux S, Clerici C, Crémieux F, Buessing M: The impact of bariatric surgery on comorbidities and medication use among obese patients. *Obes Surg* 20:861–870, 2010

Dallal RM, Chernoff A, O'Leary MP, Smith JA, Braverman JD, Quebbermann BB: Sexual dysfunction is common in the morbidly obese male and improves after gastric bypass surgery. *J Am Coll Surg* 207:859–864, 2008

de Zwaan M, Mitchell JE, Howell LM, Monson N, et al.: Characteristics of morbidly obese patients before gastric bypass surgery. *Compr Psychiatry* 44:428–434, 2003

de Zwaan M, Lancaster KL, Mitchell JE, Howell LM, et al.: Health-related quality of life in morbidly obese patients: effect of gastric bypass surgery. *Obes Surg* 12:773–780, 2002

Devlin MJ, Goldfein JA, Flancbaum L, Bessler M, Eisenstadt R: Surgical management of obese patients with eating disorders: a survey of current practice. *Obes Surg* 14:1252–1257, 2004

Dixon JB, Dixon ME, O'Brien PE: Depression in association with severe obesity: changes with weight loss. *Arch Intern Med* 163:2058–2065, 2003

Dixon JB, Dixon ME, O'Brien PE: Quality of life after lap-band placement: influence of time, weight loss, and comorbidities. *Obes Res* 9:713–721, 2001

Duval K, Marceau P, Lescelleur O, Hould FS, et al.: Health-related quality of life in morbid obesity. *Obes Surg* 16:574–579, 2006

Dymek MP, le Grange D, Neven K, Alverdy J: Quality of life and psychosocial adjustment in patients after Roux-en-Y gastric bypass: a brief report. *Obes Surg* 11:32–39, 2001

Dymek-Valentine M, Rienecke-Hoste R, Alverdy J: Assessment of binge eating disorder in morbidly obese patients evaluated for gastric bypass: SCID versus QEWP-R. *Eat Weight Disord* 9:211–216, 2004

Fabricatore AN, Crerand CE, Wadden TA, Sarwer DB, Krasucki JL: How do mental health professionals evaluate candidates for bariatric surgery? Survey results. *Obes Surg* 16:567–573, 2006

Fabricatore AN, Wadden TA, Sarwer DB, Faith M: Health-related quality of life and symptoms of depression in extremely obese persons seeking bariatric surgery. *Obes Surg* 15:304–309, 2005

Flegal KM, Carroll MD, Ogden CL, Curtin LR: Prevalence and trends in obesity among US adults, 1999–2008. *JAMA* 303:235–241, 2010

Friedman KE, Applegate KL, Grant J: Who is adherent with preoperative psychological treatment recommendations among weight loss surgery candidates? *Surg Obes Relat Dis* 3:376–382, 2007

Fujioka K, Yan E, Wang HJ, Li Z: Evaluating preoperative weight loss, binge eating disorder, and sexual abuse history on Roux-en-Y gastric bypass outcome. *Surg Obes Relat Dis* 4:137–143, 2008

Gentry K, Halverson JD, Heisler S: Psychologic assessment of morbidly obese patients undergoing gastric bypass: a comparison of preoperative and postoperative adjustment. *Surgery* 95:215–220, 1984

Glinski J, Wetzler S, Goodman E: The psychology of gastric bypass surgery. *Obes Surg* 11:581–588, 2001

Greenberg I, Sogg S, M Perna F: Behavioral and psychological care in weight loss surgery: best practice update. *Obesity (Silver Spring)* 17:880–884, 2009

Grilo CM, Masheb RM, Brody M, Burke-Martindale CH, Rothschild BS: Binge eating and self-esteem predict body image dissatisfaction among obese men and women seeking bariatric surgery. *Int J Eat Disord* 37:347–351, 2005

Guisado JA, Vaz FJ, Lopez-Ibor JJ, Rubio MA: Eating behavior in morbidly obese patients undergoing gastric surgery: differences between obese people with and without psychiatric disorders. *Obes Surg* 11:576–580, 2001

Hell E, Miller KA, Moorehead MK, Samuels N: Evaluation of health status and quality of life after bariatric surgery: comparison of standard Roux-en-Y gastric bypass, vertical banded gastroplasty and laparoscopic adjustable silicone gastric banding. *Obes Surg* 10:214–219, 2000

Herpertz S, Kielmann R, Wolf AM, Hebebrand J, Senf W: Do psychosocial variables predict weight loss or mental health after obesity surgery? A systematic review. *Obes Res* 12:1554-1569, 2004

Higa KD, Boone KB, Ho T: Complications of the laparoscopic Roux-en-Y gastric bypass: 1040 patients—what have we learned? *Obes Surg* 10:509-513, 2000

Hörchner R, Tuinebreijer W: Improvement of physical functioning of morbidly obese patients who have undergone a lap-band operation: one-year study. *Obes Surg* 9:399-402, 1999

Hsu LK, Benotti PN, Dwyer J, Roberts SB, et al.: Nonsurgical factors that influence the outcome of bariatric surgery: a review. *Psychosom Med* 60:338-346, 1998

Hsu LK, Sullivan SP, Benotti PN: Eating disturbances and outcome of gastric bypass surgery: a pilot study. *Int J Eat Disord* 21:385-390, 1997

Hsu LK, Betancourt S, Sullivan SP: Eating disturbances before and after vertical banded gastroplasty: a pilot study. *Int J Eat Disord* 19:23-34, 1996

James WP, Davies HL, Bailes J, Dauncey MJ: Elevated metabolic rates in obesity. *Lancet* 1:1122-1125, 1978

Jia H, Lubetkin E: The impact of obesity on health-related quality-of-life in the general adult US population. *J Pub Health* 27:156-164, 2005

Jones-Corneille LR, Wadden TA, Sarwer DB, Faulconbridge LF, et al.: Axis I psychopathology in bariatric surgery candidates with and without binge eating disorder: results of structured clinical interviews. *Obesity* 22:389-397, 2010

Kalarchian MA, Marcus MD, Levine MD: Relationship of psychiatric disorders to 6-month outcomes after gastric bypass. *Surg Obes Relat Dis* 4:544-549, 2008

Kalarchian MA, Marcus MD, Levine MD, Courcoulas AP, et al.: Psychiatric disorders among bariatric surgery candidates: relationship to obesity and functional health status. *Am J Psychiatry* 164:328-334, 2007

Kalarchian MA, Marcus MD, Wilson GT, Labouvie EW, Brolin RE, LaMarca LB: Binge eating among gastric bypass patients at long-term follow-up. *Obes Surg* 12:270-275, 2002

Kalarchian MA, Wilson GT, Brolin RE, Bradley L: The effects of bariatric surgery on binge eating and related psychopathology. *Eat Weight Disord* 4:1-5, 1999

Karason K, Peltonen M, Lindroos AK, Sjostrom L, Lonn L, Torgerson JS: Effort-related calf pain in the obese and long-term changes after surgical obesity treatment. *Obes Res* 13:137-145, 2005

Karlsson J, Taft C, Rydén A, Sjostrom L, Sullivan M: Ten-year trends in health-related quality of life after surgical and conventional treatment for severe obesity: the SOS intervention study. *Int J Obes* 31:1248-1261, 2007

Karlsson J, Sjostrom L, Sullivan M: Swedish Obese Subjects (SOS): an intervention study of obesity: two-year follow-up of health-related quality of life (HRQL) and eating behavior after gastric surgery for severe obesity. *Int J Obes* 22:112-126, 1998

Kinzl JF, Schrattenecker M, Traweger C, Mattesich M, Fiala M, Biebl W: Psychosocial predictors of weight loss after bariatric surgery. *Obesity Surgery* 16:1609-1614, 2006

Kinzl JF, Trefalt E, Fiala M, Biebl W: Psychotherapeutic treatment of morbidly obese patients after gastric banding. *Obes Surg* 12:292-294, 2002

Kinzl JF, Trefalt E, Fiala M, Hotter A, Biebl W, Aiger F: Partnership, sexuality, and sexual disorders in morbidly obese women: consequences of weight loss after gastric banding. *Obes Surg* 11:455-458, 2001

Kolotkin RL, Crosby RD, Gress RE, Hunt SC, Adams TD: Two-year changes in health-related quality of life in gastric bypass patients compared with severely obese controls. *Surg Obes Relat Dis* 5:250-256, 2009

Kolotkin RL, Binks M, Crosby RD, Ostbye T, Mitchell JE, Hartley G: Improvements in sexual quality of life after moderate weight loss. *Int J Impot Res* 20:487-492, 2008

Kolotkin RL, Binks M, Crosby RD, Ostbye T, Gress RE, Adams TD: Obesity and sexual quality of life. *Obesity (Silver Spring)* 14:472-479, 2006

Kolotkin RL, Crosby RD, Williams GR, Hartley GG, Nicol S: The relationship between health-related quality of life and weight loss. *Obes Res* 9:564-571, 2001

Kral JG, Naslund E: Surgical treatment of obesity. *Nature Clin Practice Endocrinology & Metabolism* 3:574-583, 2007

Kral JG, Sjöström LV, Sullivan MB: Assessment of quality of life before and after surgery for severe obesity. *Am J Clin Nutr* 55 (2 Suppl.):S611-S614, 1992

Kruseman M, Leimgruber A, Zumbach F, Golay A: Dietary, weight, and psychological changes among patients with obesity, 8 years after gastric bypass. *J Am Diet Assoc* 110:527-534, 2010

Larsen F: Psychosocial function before and after gastric banding surgery for morbid obesity: a prospective psychiatric study. *Acta Psychiatr Scan Suppl* 359:1-57, 1990

Larsen JK, Geenen R, van Ramshorst B, Brand N, et al.: Psychosocial functioning before and after laparoscopic adjustable gastric banding: a cross-sectional study. *Obes Surg* 13:629-636, 2003

Larsson UE, Mattsson E: Functional limitations linked to high body mass index, age and current pain in obese women. *Int J Obes Relat Metab Disord* 25:893-899, 2001a

Larsson UE, Mattsson E: Perceived disability and observed functional limitation in obese women. *Int J Obes Relat Metab Disord* 25:1705-1712, 2001b

Ma Y, Pagoto SL, Olendzki BC, Hafner AR, et al.: Predictors of weight status following laparoscopic gastric bypass. *Obes Surg* 16:1227-1231, 2006

Mamplekou E, Komesidou V, Bissias C, Papakonstantinou A, Melissas J: Psychological condition and quality of life in patients with morbid obesity before and after surgical weight loss. *Obes Surg* 15:1177-1184, 2005

Mauri M, Rucci P, Calderone A, Santini F, et al.: Axis I and II disorders and quality of life in bariatric surgery candidates. *J Clin Psychiatry* 69:295-301, 2008

Mechanick JI, Kushner RF, Sugerman HJ, Gonzalez-Campoy JM, et al.: American Association of Clinical Endocrinologists, The Obesity Society, and American Society for Metabolic & Bariatric Surgery medical guidelines for clinical practice for the perioperative nutritional, metabolic, and nonsurgical support of the bariatric surgery patient. *Obesity (Silver Spring)* 17 (Suppl. 1):S1-S70, v, 2009

Millon T, Davis RD: *Disorders of Personality: DSM-IV and Beyond.* New York, John Wiley & Sons, 1996

Mitchell JE, Steffen KJ, de Zwaan M, Ertelt TW, Marino JM, Mueller A: Congruence between clinical and research-based psychiatric assessment in bariatric surgical candidates. *Surg Obes Relat Dis* 6:628-634, 2010

Mitchell JE, Lancaster KL, Burgard MA, Howell LM, et al.: Long-term follow-up of patients' status after gastric bypass. *Obes Surg* 11:464-468, 2001

Muhlhans B, Horbach T, de Zwaan M: Psychiatric disorders in bariatric surgery candidates: a review of the literature and results of a German prebariatric surgery sample. *General Hospital Psychiatry* 31:414-421, 2009

Müller MK, Wenger C, Schiesser M, Clavien PA, Weber M: Quality of life after bariatric surgery: a comparative study of laparoscopic banding vs. bypass. *Obes Surg* 18:1551-1557, 2008

Myers A, Rosen J: Obesity stigmatization and coping: relation to mental health symptoms, body image, and self-esteem. *Int J Obes Relat Metab Disord* 23:221-230, 1999

Nguyen NT, Slone JA, Nguyen XM, Hartman JS, Hoyt DB: A prospective randomized trial of laparoscopic gastric bypass versus laparoscopic adjustable gastric banding for the treatment of morbid obesity: outcomes, quality of life, and costs. *Ann Surg* 250:631-641, 2009

Niego SH, Kofman MD, Weiss JJ, Geliebter A: Binge eating in the bariatric surgery population: a review of the literature. *Int J Eat Disord* 40:349-359, 2007

NIH conference: Gastrointestinal surgery for severe obesity: Consensus Development Conference Panel. *Ann Intern Med* 115:956-961, 1991

O'Brien PE, Dixon JB, Laurie C, Skinner S, et al.: Treatment of mild to moderate obesity with laparoscopic adjustable gastric banding or an intensive medical program. *Ann Intern Med* 144:625-633, 2006

Omalu B, Cho P, Shakir A, Agumadu UH, et al.: Suicides following bariatric surgery for the treatment of obesity. *Surg Obes Relat Dis* 1:447-449, 2005

Onyike CU, Crum RM, Lee HB, Lyketsos CG, Eaton WW: Is obesity associated with major depression? Results from the Third National Health and Nutrition Examination Survey. *Am J Epidemiol* 158:1139-1147, 2003

O'Reardon JP, Ringel BL, Dinges DF, Allison KC, et al.: Circadian eating and sleeping patterns in the night eating syndrome. *Obes Res* 12:1789-1796, 2004

Pawlow LA, O'Neil PM, White MA, Byrne TK: Findings and outcomes of psychological evaluations of gastric bypass applicants. *Surg Obes Relat Dis* 1:523-527, discussion 528-529, 2005

Pekkarinen T, Koskela K, Huikuri K, Mustajoki: Long-term results of gastroplasty for morbid obesity: binge-eating as a predictor of poor outcome. *Obes Surg* 4:248-255, 1994

Peltonen M, Lindroos AK, Torgerson JS: Musculoskeletal pain in the obese: a comparison with a general population and long-term changes after conventional and surgical obesity treatment. *Pain* 104:549-557, 2003

Pories WJ, Swanson MS, MacDonald KG, Long SB, et al.: Who would have thought it? An operation proves to be the most effective therapy for adult-onset diabetes mellitus. *Ann Surg* 222:339-350, discussion 350-352, 1995

Pories WJ, Caro JF, Flickinger EG, Meelheim HD, Swanson MS: The control of diabetes mellitus (NIDDM) in the morbidly obese with the Greenville Gastric Bypass. *Ann Surg* 206:316-323, 1987

Powers PS, Perez A, Boyd F, Rosemurgy A: Eating pathology before and after bariatric surgery: a prospective study. *Int J Eat Disord* 25:293-300, 1999

Powers PS, Rosemurgy A, Boyd F, Perez A: Outcome of gastric restriction procedures: weight, psychiatric diagnoses, and satisfaction. *Obes Surg* 7:471-477, 1997

Rand CSW, Macgregor AMC, Stunkard AJ: The night eating syndrome in the general population and among postoperative obesity surgery patients. *Int J Eat Disord* 22:65-69, 1997

Rosenberger PH, Henderson KE, Grilo CM: Psychiatric disorder comorbidity and association with eating disorders in bariatric surgery patients: a cross-sectional study using structured interview-based diagnosis. *J Clin Psychiatry* 67:1080-1085, 2006

Rosik CH: Psychiatric symptoms among prospective bariatric surgery patients: rates of prevalence and their relation to social desirability, pursuit of surgery, and follow-up attendance. *Obes Surg* 15:677-683, 2005

Sallet PC, Sallet JA, Dixon JB, Collis E, et al.: Eating behavior as a prognostic factor for weight loss after bariatric bypass. *Obes Surg* 17:445-451, 2007

Sanchez-Santos R, Del Barrio MJ, Gonzalez C, Madico C, et al.: Long-term health-related quality of life following gastric bypass: influence of depression. *Obes Surg* 16:580-585, 2006

Sarwer DB, Wadden TA, Moore RH, Eisenberg MH, et al.: Changes in quality of life and body image after gastric bypass surgery. Surg Obes Relat Dis 6:608–614, 2010

Sarwer DB, Wadden TA, Moore RH, Baker AW, et al.: Preoperative eating behavior, postoperative dietary adherence, and weight loss after gastric bypass surgery. Surg Obes Relat Dis 4:640–646, 2008

Sarwer DB, Thompson JK, Cash TF: Body image and obesity in adulthood. Psychiatr Clin North Am 28:69–87, 2005a

Sarwer DB, Wadden TA, Fabricatore AN: Psychosocial and behavioral aspects of bariatric surgery. Obes Res 13:639–648, 2005b

Sarwer DB, Cohn NI, Gibbons LM, Magee L, et al.: Psychiatric diagnoses and psychiatric treatment among bariatric surgery candidates. Obes Surg 14:1148–1156, 2004

Sarwer DB, Wadden TA, Foster GD: Assessment of body image dissatisfaction in obese women: specificity, severity, and clinical significance. J Consult Clin Psychol 66:651–654, 1998

Saunders R: Binge eating in gastric bypass patients before surgery. Obes Surg 9:72–76, 1999

Schok M, Geenen R, de Wit P, Brand N, van Antwerpen T, van Ramshorst B: Quality of life after laparoscopic adjustable gastric banding for severe obesity: postoperative and retrospective preoperative evaluations. Obes Surg 10:502–508, 2000

Sears D, Fillmore G, Bui M, Rodriquez J: Evaluation of gastric bypass patients 1 year after surgery: changes in quality of life and obesity-related conditions. Obes Surg 18:1522–1525, 2008

Sjostrom L, Narbro K, Sjostrom D, Karason K, et al.: Effects of bariatric surgery on mortality in Swedish obese subjects. N Engl J Med 357:741–752, 2007

Solow C, Silberfarb PM, Swift K: Psychosocial effects of intestinal bypass surgery for severe obesity. N Engl J Med 290:300–304, 1974

Spitzer RL, Kroenke K, Williams JB: Validation and utility of a self-report version of PRIME-MD: the PHQ primary care study. JAMA 282:1737–1744, 1999

Spitzer RL, Devlin M, Walsh TB, Hasin D, et al.: Binge eating disorder: a multisite field trial of the diagnostic criteria. Int J Eat Disord 11:191–203, 1992

Stunkard A, Foster GD, Glassman J, Rosato E: Retrospective exaggeration of symptoms: vomiting after gastric surgery for obesity. Psychosom Med 47:150–155, 1985

Stunkard A, Mendelson M: Obesity and body image: characteristics of disturbances in the body image of some obese persons. Am J Psychiatry 123:1296–1300, 1967

Sugarman HJ, Londrey GL, Kellum JM: Weight loss with vertical banded gastroplasty and Roux-Y gastric bypass for morbid obesity with selective vs. random assignment. Am J Surg 157:93–102, 1989

Sugarman HJ, Starkey JV, Birkenhauer R: A randomized prospective trial of gastric bypass versus vertical banded gastroplasty for morbid obesity and their effects on sweets versus non-sweets eaters. Ann Surg 205:613–624, 1987

Sullivan M, Karlsson J, Sjostrom L, et al.: Why quality of life measures should be used in the treatment of patients with obesity. In International Textbook of Obesity. Bjorntrop P, Ed. London, John Wiley and Sons, 2001

Sullivan M, Karlsson J, Sjostrom L, Backman L, et al.: Swedish Obese Subjects (SOS): an intervention study of obesity: baseline evaluation of health and psychosocial functioning in the first 1743 subjects examined. Int J Obes Relat Metab Disord 17:503–512, 1993

van Gemert WG, Adang EM, Greve JW, Soeters PB: Quality of life assessment of morbidly obese patients: effect of weight-reducing surgery. Am J Clin Nutr 67:197–201, 1998

van Hout GC, Fortuin FA, Pelle AJ, van Heck GL: Psychosocial functioning, personality, and body image following vertical banded gastroplasty. Obes Surg 18:115–120, 2008

van Hout G, Verschure SK, van Heck G: Psychosocial predictors of success following bariatric surgery. Obes Surg 15:553–560, 2005

van Nunen A, Wouters E, Vingerhoets A, Hox JJ, Geenen R: The health-related quality of life of obese persons seeking or not seeking surgical or non-surgical treatment: a meta-analysis. Obes Surg 17:1357–1366, 2007

Wadden TA, Faulconbridge LF, Jones-Corneille LR, Sarwer DB, et al.: Binge eating disorder and the outcome of bariatric surgery at one year: a prospective, observational study. Obesity (Silver Spring) 19:1220–1228, 2011

Wadden TA, Sarwer DB, Fabricatore AN, Jones L, Stack R, Williams NS: Psychosocial and behavioral status of patients undergoing bariatric surgery: what to expect before and after surgery. Med Clin North Am 9:451–469, 2007

Wadden TA, Butryn ML, Sarwer DB, Fabricatore AN, et al.: Comparison of psychosocial status in treatment-seeking women with class III vs. class I-II obesity. Obesity (Silver Spring) 14 (Suppl. 2):S90–S98, 2006a

Wadden TA, Foster GD: Weight and Lifestyle Inventory (WALI). Obesity (Silver Spring) 14 (Suppl. 2):S99–S118, 2006b

Wadden TA, Sarwer DB: Behavioral assessment of candidates for bariatric surgery: a patient-oriented approach. Obesity (Silver Spring) 14 (Suppl 2):S53–S62, 2006c

Wadden TA, Foster GD, Sarwer BD, Anderson DA, et al.: Dieting and the development of eating disorders in obese women: results of a randomized controlled trial. Am J Clin Nutr 80:560–568, 2004

Wadden, TA, Phelan S: Assessment of quality of life in obese individuals. Obesity Research 10 (Suppl. 1):S50–S7, 2002

Waters GS, Pories WJ, Swanson MS, Meelheim HD, Flickinger EG, May HJ: Long-term studies of mental health after the Greenville gastric bypass operation for morbid obesity. Am J Surg 161:154–158, 1991

Weiner R, Datz M, Wagner D, Bockhorn H: Quality-of-life outcome after laparoscopic adjustable gastric banding for morbid obesity. Obes Surg 9:539–545, 1999

White MA, Kalarchian MA, Masheb RM, Marcus MD, Grilo CM: Loss of control over eating predicts outcomes in bariatric surgery patients: a prospective, 24-month follow-up study. J Clin Psychiatry 71:175–184, 2010

White MA, Masheb RM, Rothschild BS, Burke-Martindale CH, Grilo CM: The prognostic significance of regular binge eating in extremely obese gastric bypass patients: 12-month postoperative outcomes. J Clin Psychiatry 67:1928–1935, 2006

White MA, O'Neil PM, Kolotkin RL, Byrne TK: Gender, race, and obesity-related quality of life at extreme levels of obesity. Obes Res 12:949–955, 2004

Wyss C, Laurent-Jaccard A, Burckhardt P, Jayet A, Gazzola L: Long-term results on quality of life of surgical treatment of obesity with vertical banded gastroplasty. Obes Surg 5:387–392, 1995

Zimmerman M, Francione-Witt C, Chelminski I, Young D, et al.: Presurgical psychiatric evaluations of candidates for bariatric surgery, part 1: reliability and reasons for and frequency of exclusion. J Clin Psychiatry 68:1557–1562, 2007

第四篇

生命相关问题

第十三章

糖尿病的社会心理适应和社会心理风险的关键时期

Richard R. Rubin，PhD，Mark Peyrot，PhD

Hamburg 和 Inoff 是众多学者中，首先意识到存在糖尿病相关的社会心理压力的人，包括：①糖尿病的诊断；②并发症的出现；③治疗方案的转变。在这一章中，我们将讨论每一阶段的社会心理结果都是什么，以及旨在改善这些结果所涉及的干预措施，为临床医生提供了筛选和重点干预的建议。

诊断

儿童与父母

一些研究表明，罹患 1 型糖尿病（T1D）的儿童会出现与糖尿病诊断相关的社会心理问题，但其他一些研究并没有发现儿童在诊断 1 型糖尿病后出现社会心理状态的改变。甚至发现与诊断相关的社会心理问题（主要是适应障碍和抑郁）的研究报道，这些问题具有一定的时限性，基本上所有的儿童在确诊一年后即可恢复过来。另一方面，Kovacs 研究表明，对糖尿病诊断有适应障碍的儿童，新发的精神障碍 5 年累积概率为 0.48，而该研究的其他儿童仅为 0.16。

Kovacs 研究发现，母亲（通常承担大部分照顾糖尿病儿童的责任）与儿童类似，也有一个适应糖尿病诊断的模式，而父亲似乎在任何时候都只有很小的压力。

1 型糖尿病儿童与诊断相关的社会心理问题的风险因素包括女性、家庭压力、不完整的家庭结构及逃避型处理方式。2 型糖尿病儿童对诊断后的社会心理适应还没被研究，因为直到现在，2 型糖尿病儿童也并不是很常见以至于无法确保系统地调查。

Grey 等对 8～14 岁新诊断为糖尿病的儿童及非糖尿病同龄儿童进行了对比研究。儿童对诊断的适应问题在诊断一年后消失，但在诊断后的第二年又再次出现，这与 Kovacs 和他的同事们发现的模式类似。Grey 认为，尽管诊断后的即时适应是非常重要的，但他们的数据表明，适应的第二个"关键时期"发生在诊断后的第二年，在糖尿病生活关键的第二年进行干预以防止发生社会心理恶化是重要的。最近一项研究比较了 1 型糖尿病儿童的父母与癌症儿童的父母的适应经验，在病程的早期和以后学龄儿童在青春期面临新的发展挑战时，干预的时期是很重要的。

成人

对糖尿病诊断的社会心理适应，很少有正式的研究，特别是与精神紊乱相关的适应和糖尿病诊断对配偶及患者的其他社交网成员的影响。一项大型的国际研究让患者（有 2/3 被诊断为 2 型糖尿病）回忆被诊断为糖尿病的反应。85%的患者反映在那时有强烈的负面情绪（包括震惊、愤怒、焦虑、抑郁和无助感）。另一项研究表明这些反应在 1 型糖尿病患者中可能更强烈一点。成人对诊断的情绪反应也可能受到社会支持、个人资源和处事风格的影响。

诊断时体会的强烈负面情绪可能预测随后的问题，包括较差的自我报告治疗方案的依从性，糖尿病的控制和生活质量，以及更高水平的糖尿病相关社会心理痛苦，尤其是当无效处理时，这些问题可能更明显。另一方面，虽然糖尿病的诊断可能需要经历个人身份的攻击，但很多患者正努力解决这些身份问题，并将患有糖尿病的新身份整合到他们的生活当中。

干预措施

糖尿病诊断的社会心理干预研究非常少并且限于儿童。Laron 描述了新诊断儿童患者的特殊社会心理危机临床干预，Galatzer 报告了 3～15 年干预时间内的积极效果，包括方案依从性的改善和社会心理适应，以及与在诊断时没有进行特殊干预的儿童相比，心理干预的需要减少了

2/3。另一项随机临床试验对诊断后 2 年的常规护理组与心理咨询组进行来对比，但没有任何发现。

小结

糖尿病诊断时的社会心理问题在成人、儿童及确诊儿童的父母中都很常见。另外，这些问题，虽然可以迅速解决，但预示了长期的临床和社会心理的负面结果。最后，急性的和长期的社会心理问题的危险因素已经确定，包括女性、缺少支持、家庭压力和逃避型处理方式。

糖尿病并发症

糖尿病并发症的存在（尤其是两个或两个以上并发症）和并发症的严重程度似乎与心理压力有关，包括临床有意义的抑郁或焦虑症状及较低的生活质量评分。Polonsky 等研究发现，糖尿病相关的痛苦在那些具有短期和长期的糖尿病并发症患者中具有很高的发生率。

另外，对糖尿病并发症的研究发现，神经病变、心血管疾病或终末期肾病（ESRD）与患者的健康生活质量的下降密切相关。ESRD 的存在显著增加了功能障碍；肾病的存在与更大的健康担忧相关，并可使 1 型糖尿病患者的健康感知下降。另一项研究发现，胃轻瘫患者（糖尿病的神经并发症）的健康相关的生活质量降低。

一些研究人员发现在增殖性糖尿病视网膜病变诊断后的 2 年内，抑郁和消极的生活经历会增加。不论视力损害的严重程度如何，这些社会心理困扰都会存在，即使失明后患者重获视力，这些困扰仍会持续存在。这些视力损害引起的社会心理后果不是糖尿病患者独有的。有趣的是，一项研究发现，精神疾病病史是糖尿病视网膜病变发展的一个危险因素，原因可能与之相关的是 HbA1C 水平的升高。

糖尿病神经病变似乎也与社会心理痛苦有关。一项研究发现，神经病变的症状与抑郁症状评分之间的关系由两组社会心理变量介导：①对糖尿病神经病变症状感知的不可预测性和缺乏治疗控制；②日常活动的受限和社交的自我认知的改变。另一项研究发现，截肢患者的社会心理状态比糖尿病足溃疡的患者要好一点，但是比未截肢和未患足部溃疡的患者要差。

不论男性还是女性糖尿病患者均出现性功能障碍。大约有 50%合并阳痿问题的糖尿病男性有显著的情感叠加，如抑郁或焦虑，导致勃起功能障碍。其他研究人员在男性和女性患者中发现性问题和抑郁显著的联系。这些社会心理因素可能会加剧性功能障碍同时被性功能障碍所加剧。

小结

在糖尿病并发症患者中社会心理问题是很常见的。这些心理问题可能导致发生其他并发症或加剧现有并发症（通过不积极的糖尿病管理及血糖水平升高）的一个危险因素，所以有效地治疗社会心理问题是有益处的。

治疗方案的转变

2 型糖尿病患者治疗方案的转变（如增加新种类的治疗药物）与社会心理问题相关。大量研究发现不用药物治疗的糖尿病患者与使用口服降糖药的患者相比，其糖尿病生活质量量表的评分更高，整体的生活质量更好。类似的是，与使用胰岛素的患者相比，口服降糖药物的患者具有更好的生活质量，而且那些转变为使用胰岛素治疗的患者幸福感也下降。相比之下，一些研究发现，治疗类型和 2 型糖尿病患者的生活质量没有显著相关性，使用胰岛素与不使用胰岛素的糖尿病患者的抑郁或焦虑状态也没有显著差异。

使用胰岛素强化治疗的 1 型糖尿病患者在糖尿病控制和并发症试验中似乎并没有出现幸福感降低。事实上，其他研究发现，使用胰岛素强化治疗的糖尿病患者在生活满意度、焦虑、抑郁症方面有改善，并且当糖尿病患者他们把每日的注射次数增加或改用持续皮下胰岛素输注（CSII）时，其治疗满意度和糖尿病负担也提高。还有其他研究表明，胰岛素注射方式的改变，即从注射器转换到胰岛素笔或 CSII，与健康相关的生活质量提高相关。与使用胰岛素注射器相比，使用胰岛素笔或 CSII 患者的社会心理结果更好。

小结

2 型糖尿病患者因为胰岛 B 细胞功能的恶化而转变治疗方案可能与患者的社会心理问题有关。

临床护理建议

诊断

1. 诊断时解决心理问题本身就是一个值得追求的目标；它可以通过减少负面的神经内分泌和生理压力来直接改善健康状况；或者间接地重建一种情绪状态来促进学习糖尿病自我管理的积极模式。在糖尿病诊断时，临床医生应该确定那些抑郁和家庭适应性差的患者，为他们提供适当的社会心理支持，尤其是高危个体。

2. 使用一般的情绪或精神症状的测量方法可能无法确定糖尿病特定的心理问题。因此，糖尿病相关的检测方法如糖尿病区域检测方法（PAID-Revised）应该被纳入所有的评估过程中。

糖尿病并发症

1. 当并发症发生时，临床医生应该执行常规的社会心理评估。内容应该包括情绪、幸福的生活质量（常规的和糖尿病相关的）、医疗、社会和经济资源。

2. 因为症状的不可预测性和自我认知的变化可以通过并发症影响抑郁症状，临床医生应该设计干预措施来帮助患者了解并发症的过程，并且设计培养和保持积极的自我意识的干预，因为这些干预措施可能会对社会心理健康产生积极的影响。

3. 性功能问题在糖尿病患者中常见，既然这些问题影响心理健康，临床医生应该常规询问性功能和幸福感，并讨论改善性功能的社会心理方法和医学方法。

治疗方案的转变

1. 临床医生应该帮助患者理解 2 型糖尿病的进展特性（如胰岛素分

泌自然的下降）来减轻开始需要用口服药物或胰岛素治疗患者的内疚感和伴随而来的心理问题。

2. 建议临床医生不要威胁患者使用口服药物或胰岛素等措施，以鼓励更积极的自我管理，因为这些可能会导致心理问题，并且增加开启适宜治疗措施的抵抗情绪。

3. 为了减少治疗负担和提高治疗的满意度及生活质量，临床医生应该识别和开具患者能够简便使用的治疗处方和药物输送系统（如胰岛素笔和胰岛素泵）。

参 考 文 献

Ahroni JH, Boyko EJ, Davignon DR, Pecaro RE: The health and functional status of veterans with diabetes. *Diabetes Care* 17:318–321, 1994

Amer KS: Children's adaptation to insulin-dependent diabetes mellitus: a critical review of the literature. *Pediatr Nurs* 25:627–631, 1999

Anderson RM, Fitzgerald JT, Wisdom K, Davis WK, Hiss RG: A comparison of global versus disease-specific quality-of-life measures in patients with NIDDM. *Diabetes Care* 20:299–305, 1997

Boman KK, Viksten J, Kogner P, Samuelsson U: Serious illness in childhood: the different threats of cancer and diabetes from a parent perspective. *J Pediatr* 145:373–379, 2004

Brown SA: Diabetes and grief. *Diabetes Educ* 6:409–416, 1985

Carrington AL, Mawdsley SK, Morley M, Kincey J, Boulton AJ: Psychological status of diabetic people with and without lower limb disability. *Diabetes Res Clin Pract* 32:19–25, 1996

Cavan DA, Barnett AH, Leatherdale BA: Diabetic impotence: risk factors in a clinic population. *Diab Res* 5:145–148, 1987

Chantelau E, Schiffers T, Schutze J, Hansen B: Effect of patient-selected intensive insulin therapy on quality of life. *Patient Educ Couns* 30:167–173, 1997

Cohen ST, Welch G, Jacobson AM, de Groot M, Samson J: The association of lifetime psychiatric illness and increased retinopathy in patients with type 1 diabetes mellitus. *Psychosomatics* 38:98–108, 1997

DeVries JH, Snoek FJ, Kostense PJ, Masurel N, Heine RJ: A randomized trial of continuous subcutaneous insulin infusion and intensive injection therapy in type 1 diabetes for patients with long-standing poor glycemic control. *Diabetes Care* 25:2074–2080, 2002

Diabetes Control and Complications Trial Research Group: Influence of intensive diabetes treatment on quality-of-life outcomes in the Diabetes Control and Complications Trial. *Diabetes Care* 19:195–203, 1996

Enzlin P, Mathieu C, Van den Bruel A, Vanderschueren D, Demyttenaere K: Prevalence and predictors of sexual dysfunction in patients with type 1 diabetes. *Diabetes Care* 26:409–414, 2003

Enzlin P, Mathieu C, Van den Bruel A, Bosteels J, Vanderschueren D, Demyttenaere K: Sexual dysfunction in women with type 1 diabetes: a controlled study. *Diabetes Care* 25:672–677, 2002

Farup CE, Leidy NK, Murray M, Williams GR, Helbers L, Quigley EM: Effect of domperidone on the health-related quality of life of patients with symptoms of diabetic gastroparesis. *Diabetes Care* 21:1699–1706, 1998

Galatzer A, Amir S, Gil R, Karp M, Laron Z: Crisis intervention program in newly diagnosed diabetic children. *Diabetes Care* 5:414–419, 1982

Glasgow RE, Ruggiero L, Eakin EG, Dryfoos J, Chobanian L: Quality of life and associated characteristics in a large national sample of adults with diabetes. *Diabetes Care* 20:562–567, 1997

Goldman JB, MacLean HM: The significance of identity in the adjustment to diabetes among insulin users. *Diabetes Educ* 24:741–748, 1998

Grey M, Lipman T, Cameron ME, Thurber FW: Coping behaviors at diagnosis and in adjustment one year later in children with diabetes. *Nurs Res* 46:312–317, 1997

Grey M, Cameron ME, Lipman TH, Thurber FW: Psychosocial status of children with diabetes in the first 2 years after diagnosis. *Diabetes Care* 18:1330–1336, 1995

Hamburg BA, Inoff GE: Coping with predictable crises of diabetes. *Diabetes Care* 6:409–416, 1983

Holmes DM: The person and diabetes in psychosocial context. *Diabetes Care* 9:194–206, 1986

Hornquist JO, Wikby A, Stenstrom U, Andersson PO: Change in quality of life among type 1 diabetes. *Diab Res Clin Pract* 28:63–72, 1995

Jacobson AM, Hauser ST, Willett JB, Wolfsdorf JI, Dvorak R, Herman L, de Groot M: Psychological adjustment to IDDM: 10-year follow-up of an onset cohort of child and adolescent patients. *Diabetes Care* 20:811–818, 1997

Jacobson AM, de Groot M, Samson JA: The evaluation of two measures of quality of life in patients with type I and type II diabetes. *Diabetes Care* 17:267–274, 1994

Keinanen-Kiukaanniemi S, Ohinmaa A, Pajunpaa H, Koivukangas P: Health related quality of life in diabetic patients measured by the Nottingham Health Profile. *Diabet Med* 13:382–388, 1996

Klein BE, Klein R, Moss SE: Self-rated health and diabetes of long duration. The Wisconsin Epidemiologic Study of Diabetic Retinopathy. *Diabetes Care* 21:236–240, 1998

Kovacs M, Goldston D, Obrosky DS, Bonar LK: Psychiatric disorders in youths with IDDM: rates and risk factors. *Diabetes Care* 20:36–44, 1997a

Kovacs M, Obrosky DS, Goldston D, Drash A: Major depressive disorder in youths with IDDM: a controlled prospective study of course and outcome. *Diabetes Care* 20:45–51, 1997b

Kovacs M, Ho V, Pollock MH: Criterion and predictive validity of the diagnosis of adjustment disorder: a prospective study of youths with new-onset insulin-dependent diabetes mellitus. *Am J Psychiatry* 152:523–528, 1995

Kovacs M, Iyengar S, Goldston D, Obrosky DS, Marsh J: Psychological functioning among mothers of children with insulin-dependent diabetes mellitus: a longitudinal study. *J Consult Clin Psychol* 58:189–195, 1990a

Kovacs M, Iyengar S, Goldston D, Stewart J, Obrosky DS, Marsh J: Psychological functioning of children with insulin-dependent diabetes mellitus: a longitudinal study. *J Pediatr Psychol* 15: 619–632, 1990b

Kovacs M, Feinberg TL, Paulauskas S, Finkelstein R, Pollock M, Crouse-Novak M: Initial coping responses and psychosocial characteristics of children with insulin-dependent diabetes mellitus. *J Pediatr* 106:827–834, 1985a

Kovacs M, Finkelstein R, Feinberg TL, Crouse-Novak M, Paulauskas S, Pollock M: Initial psychologic responses of parents to the diagnosis of insulin-dependent diabetes mellitus in their children. *Diabetes Care* 8:568–575, 1985b

Langewitz W, Wossmer B, Iseli J, Berger W: Psychological and metabolic improvement after an outpatient teaching program for functional intensified insulin therapy (FIT). *Diab Res Clin Pract* 37:157–164, 1997

Laron Z, Galatzer A, Amir S, Gil R, Karp M, Minouni M: A multidisciplinary, comprehensive, ambulatory treatment scheme for diabetes mellitus in children. *Diabetes Care* 2:342–348, 1979

Leedom LJ, Procci WP, Don D, Meehan WP: Sexual dysfunction and depression in diabetic women (Abstract). *Diabetes* 35 (Suppl. 1):23A, 1986

Linkeschova R, Raoul M, Bott U, Berger M, Spraul M: Less severe hypoglycemia, better metabolic control, and improved quality of life in type 1 diabetes mellitus with continuous subcutaneous insulin infusion (CSII) therapy: an observational study of 100 consecutive patients followed for a mean of 2 years. *Diabet Med* 19:746–751, 2002

Lo R, MacLean D: The dynamics of coping and adapting to the impact when diagnosed with diabetes. *Aust J Adv Nurs* 19:26–32, 2001

Lustman PJ, Clouse RE: Relationship of psychiatric illness to impotence in men with diabetes. *Diabetes Care* 13:893–95, 1990

Mayou R, Bryant B, Turner R: Quality of life in non-insulin-dependent diabetes and a comparison with insulin-dependent diabetes. *Journal of Psychosomatic Research* 34:1–11, 1990

Northam E, Anderson P, Adler R, Werther G, Warne G: Psychosocial and family functioning in children with insulin-dependent diabetes at diagnosis and one year later. *J Pediatr Psychol* 21:699–717, 1996

Parkerson GR, Connis RT, Broadhead WE, Patrick DL, Taylor TR, Chiu-Kit JT: Disease-specific versus generic measurement of health-related quality of life in insulin-dependent diabetic patients. *Medical Care* 31:629–639, 1993

Peyrot M, Rubin RR: Levels and risks of depression and anxiety symptomatology among diabetic adults. *Diabetes Care* 20:585–590, 1997

Pibernik-Okanovic M, Roglic G, Prasek M, Metelko Z: Emotional adjustment and metabolic control in newly diagnosed diabetic persons. *Diab Res Clin Pract* 34:99–105, 1996

Polonsky WH, Anderson BJ, Lohrer, PA, Welch G, Jacobson AM, Aponte JE, Schwartz CE: Assessment of diabetes-related distress. *Diabetes Care* 18:754–760, 1995

Robertson N, Burden ML, Burden AC: Psychological morbidity and problems of daily living in people with visual loss and diabetes: do they differ from people without diabetes? *Diabet Med* 23:1110–1116, 2006

Rodin G: Quality of life in adults with insulin-dependent diabetes mellitus. *Psychotherapy Psychosomatics* 54:132–139, 1990

Schiavi PC, Hogan B: Sexual problems in diabetes mellitus: psychological aspects. *Diabetes Care* 2:9–17, 1979

Skovlund SE, Peyrot M: The Diabetes Attitudes, Wishes, and Needs (DAWN) Program: a new approach to improving outcomes of diabetes care. *Diabetes Spectrum* 18:136–142, 2005

Sundelin J, Forsandfer G, Mattson SE: Family-oriented support at the outset of diabetes mellitus: a comparison of two group conditions during 2 years following diagnosis. *Acta Paediatr* 85:49–55, 1996

Trief PM, Grant W, Elbert K, Weinstock RS: Family environment, glycemic control, and the psychosocial adaptation of adults with diabetes. *Diabetes Care* 21:241–245, 1998

Van der Does FE, De Neeling JN, Snoek FJ, Kostense PJ, Grootenhuis PA, Bouter LM, Heine RJ: Randomized study of two different levels of glycemic control within the acceptable range in type 2 diabetes. *Diabetes Care* 21:2085–2093, 1998

Vileikyte L, Leventhal H, Gonzalez JS, Peyrot M, Rubin RR, Ulbrecht JS, Garrow A, Waterman C, Cavanagh PR, Boulton AJ: Diabetic peripheral neuropathy and depressive symptoms: the association revisited. *Diabetes Care* 28:2378–2383, 2005

Watson-Miller S: Living with a diabetic foot ulcer: a phenomenological study. *J Clin Nurs* 15:1336–1337, 2006

Whitehead ED, Klyde BJ, Zussman S, Wayne N, Shinbach K, Davis D: Male sexual dysfunction and diabetes mellitus. *New York State J Med* 83:1174–1179, 1983

Willoughby DF, Kee C, Demi A: Women's psychosocial adjustment to diabetes. *J Adv Nurs* 32:1422–1430, 2000

Wuslin LR: Visual and psychological function in PDR (Abstract). *Diabetes* 38 (Suppl. 1):242A, 1989

Wuslin LR, Jacobson AM, Rand LI: Psychosocial aspects of diabetic retinopathy. *Diabetes Care* 10:367–373, 1987

Wysocki T, Huxtable K, Linscheid TR, Wayne W: Adjustment to diabetes mellitus in preschoolers and their mothers. *Diabetes Care* 12:524–529, 1989

第十四章

儿童和青少年的特殊问题

Tim Wysocki，PhD，Barbara J.Anderson，PhD

糖尿病日常复杂的操作规程影响整个儿童时期儿童的发展及其家庭生活。本章节主要讨论糖尿病在婴儿（0～2 岁）、幼儿及学龄前儿童（2～5 岁）、学龄儿童（6～11 岁）、青少年（12～18 岁）人群中的正常发展及研究。尽管全球 1 型糖尿病在婴幼儿及学龄前儿童中的患病率逐年攀升，但仍然缺乏研究 6 岁以下的糖尿病儿童及其家庭的大型多中心临床试验。因此，本章前两部分（婴儿及幼儿/学龄前儿童）的证据相对不足。

婴儿与糖尿病

在生命的最初两年，社会心理任务的中心便是在婴儿与其照护者之间建立一种强烈、相互信任的情感纽带关系。在婴儿糖尿病方面尽管缺乏大型的研究或者临床试验，但是仍有一些小型的临床研究阐述糖尿病对于母婴关系的影响。在一项定性研究当中，糖尿病患儿的母亲曾报道与孩子联系减弱并且丢失了理想的母婴关系。在另一项小型、描述性研究当中，母亲感觉"持续性警觉"，因为其孩子过于依赖她们来管理疾病及识别危险的血糖波动。由于日常糖尿病管理的复杂性，许多父母报告找到一个称职、有经验的照护者照顾孩子相当困难。一项研究指出这种慢性压力及社会支持的缺乏很容易导致母亲身体上、情绪上的问题。这就强调了帮助糖尿病患儿的父母确定支持系统来降低 1 型糖尿病诊断给家庭带来的压力的重要性。

幼儿及学龄前儿童与糖尿病

幼儿有两个中心发展任务：①与父母或者照护者分离，建立一种自主性；②建立一种对周围环境的控制感及能够影响身体及社会环境的自信感。学龄前儿童依赖这种新建立的自主性来探索家庭外的世界。

基于这个年龄段的大型经验研究还比较缺乏，但仍有一些研究指出幼儿及学龄前儿童患糖尿病对亲子关系会有深远影响。在 Powers 等的研究当中，糖尿病患儿的父母报告，与健康对照组的父母相比，他们在进餐时间有更多的行为上的及喂养的问题。该团队之后实施的观察性研究揭示了尽管会增加父母的担忧，但患 1 型糖尿病的学龄前儿童并不比那些年龄相匹配的对照着者有更多的富有挑战性的进餐时行为。最后，在一项有关家庭进餐时互动的大型临床对照研究当中，1 型糖尿病患儿的父母需要对孩子做更多的叮嘱及在控制进餐时间上要做出更多的努力，虽然孩子吃的更少。很显然，对于 1 型糖尿病患儿的父母来说，喂养孩子的正常任务就变得更有挑战性。

Wysocki 等报道了 20 名 2～6 岁的糖尿病患者的心理调查报告。与正常对照组相比，糖尿病儿童显示更多的"内在化"行为问题（参见儿童行为目录，CBCL），如抑郁、焦虑、睡眠问题、抱怨不适抑或退学。相反，Northam 等发现与对照组相比，18 例 4 岁以下儿童在诊断时或者 1 年以后 CBCL 中任何一项的评分都没有差异。没有研究评估过儿童行为的独立性。Wysocki 等同样指出与非糖尿病人群相比，糖尿病患儿的父母面临更多的亲子压力。Powers 等也发现与非糖尿病儿童的父母相比，糖尿病患儿的父母面临更高的压力。Eiser、Garrison 和 McQuiston 都建议当学龄前儿童患任何慢性疾病时，期望儿童的行为及父母经验都能改变。因此，不要轻易从这些研究当中下定结论，认为是糖尿病本身导致了行为调整问题或者学龄前糖尿病患儿的母亲认为其家庭承受过多的压力。

与年龄更大的糖尿病患儿相比，幼儿糖尿病患者的母亲报告更加担忧低血糖的发生。越来越多的证据表明糖尿病患儿中任何的负面后果或者轻度认知缺陷都可能是源于低血糖。Ryan 团队展开的一系列研究，进行了一连串的神经行为测试来观察糖尿病患儿与对照组之间的不同。此外，5 岁以下诊断为糖尿病的患儿在青少年时期接受评估，结果显示出显著的认知缺陷，可能是由于在中枢神经系统尚未发育成熟之前有症状性或无症状性的低血糖发作。在另一项 Rovet 等的研究当中，4 岁以下诊断为糖尿病的患儿在视觉-空间定位测试中比其他在童年稍晚时期诊断的儿童评分更低，而且比那些非糖尿病兄弟姐妹对照组更低，但是语言能力评分不低。与更大年龄诊断为糖尿病的患儿相比，4 岁以下诊断为糖尿病的患儿其低血糖发作的频率更高，提示严重的低血糖可能影响之后的认知功能。Golden 等收集了 23 例 5 岁以下诊断为糖尿病的患儿从诊断之日起低血糖发生频率的横断面数据。这些研究者认为无症状性或轻微症状性的低血糖与较低的抽象/视觉推理评分呈显著相关，提示即使是轻微的或者无症状性的低血糖发作也会对认知功能有负面累积效应。

　　在之前描述过的研究当中，在诊断时没有任何神经认知功能的检测排除糖尿病代谢失代偿会影响这些功能的可能性。有两项研究从诊断时就应用神经心理学评估前瞻性随访了糖尿病患儿。Rovet 等初步的结论是在这些糖尿病患儿诊断时及 1 年以后没有发现神经认知损伤的证据，但是作者报告也许是没有达到足够的随访时间以发现任何损伤。Northam 等比较了 1 型糖尿病患儿与对照组在智力、专注力、思维速度、记忆力、学习能力、操作技能方面的表现。在诊断后的第 3 个月，两组没有差异，而在诊断后 2 年内，糖尿病患儿显示出进步更小，尤其是在信息处理速度、接受新知识及概念性推理技巧方面。随后表现最差的糖尿病患儿是那些在生命早期即患糖尿病的患者，这就进一步证实了早期的影响效应。然而，还有其他方面的证据，在一项有关瑞典新发 1 型糖尿病患儿的前瞻性、横断面研究当中，诊断时的代谢状态及长期的代谢控制是智力发展受阻的风险因素，而不是重度低血糖发生的频率。

　　鉴于研究结果报道认知缺陷与重度低血糖相关，预防重度低血糖的复发对于幼儿及学龄前儿童相当重要。因此，糖尿病控制及并发症研究（DCCT 研究）提倡对于 13 岁以上的儿童应谨慎应用强化胰岛素治疗方案。这个年龄段挑剔的饮食习惯、不稳定的身体锻炼及快速成长使之达到最适血糖控制水平更加复杂。因此，治疗目标必须个体化来保证安全有效，同时也使得儿童掌握相应年龄段正常的学习发展任务。

　　持续皮下胰岛素输注（CSII）治疗或者胰岛素泵治疗在儿童中的应用越来越广泛。许多研究已经证实了胰岛素泵治疗是每日多次胰岛素注射的安全替代治疗方案，而且可以降低低血糖的发生率、改善糖尿病患儿家庭的生活质量。基于这些研究结果，对于儿童来说CSII治疗是一种安全有效的替代，假如他们的家庭有教育和支持资源来应用这个复杂的技术。正如所有的管理问题一样，起始胰岛素泵治疗必须个体化，考虑每个家庭的生活方式及能力水平。

　　如果每日多次应用胰岛素注射，甘精胰岛素（一种长效胰岛素类似物，没有明显峰值）能够降低儿童低血糖的发生率，尤其是夜间低血糖。降低低血糖的发生率便会降低糖尿病患儿的家庭压力，这些新的管理手段能够改善这些家庭的生活质量。

学龄儿童与糖尿病

　　学龄儿童的首要发展任务包括：从家庭到学校环境的平稳过渡；与同性儿童建立亲密的友谊；学习新的智力、运动及艺术方面的技能；形成一种积极的自我意识。

　　有关学龄期糖尿病患儿的研究将自卑和社会-情感调整能力低下与糖尿病控制不佳相关联。Dumont等发现自诊断之日起，超过8年以上反复的糖尿病酮症酸中毒（DKA）与行为问题更高的发生率及社会竞争力低下有关。Liss等发现那些在年幼时发生过DKA的儿童比没发生过DKA的儿童更易自卑，社会竞争力更低。在DKA组更多的儿童至少有一项精神障碍可以达到诊断标准（88%vs.28%）。

　　儿童血糖控制不佳会影响孩子入学，导致教育过程受阻、与同龄人交流减少及自尊心培养受限。研究认为即使低血糖的身体症状已经减退，记忆及注意力也许会持续受损，据此，使低血糖的发生率最小化是很重要的。

　　相比幼儿糖尿病大型研究的缺乏现状，在学龄儿童中家庭环境如何影响血糖控制的研究更加多见。Waller等进行了一项有关12岁以下糖尿病患儿家庭的经验性描述性研究。在糖尿病患儿的家庭当中，更多的糖尿病相关家庭指导和控制与更好的代谢结果相关，糖尿病相关的父母的温暖和关怀对于优化结果很重要。Liss 等同样发现住院期间发生过 DKA 的糖尿病患儿，其亲子亲密度更低。非糖尿病相关的家庭因素，如竞争、压力、家庭凝聚力也与血糖控制、依从性相联系。例如，在 12 岁以下儿童中高水平的家庭压力与血糖控制不佳相关。相反，Kovacs 等在一项有关学龄期儿童的纵向研究当中没有发现一般家庭因素与代谢控制或者治疗依从性有关系。然而，Jacobson 及其同事进行的有关新诊断的学龄期儿童的二次纵向研究指出，在 4 年的随访中，在诊断时测量的孩子对家庭冲突的看法是胰岛素管理、饮食计划、锻炼及血糖监测依从性降低最强烈的预测因子。

Miller-Johnson 等也研究了冲突、依从性及血糖控制之间的关系。亲子冲突与依从性及血糖控制之间显著相关。作者认为冲突通过扰乱治疗的依从性，从而影响血糖控制。一项有关 4～10 岁的 1 型糖尿病患儿及其父母的教养方式、治疗依从性及血糖控制的研究当中，"权威型教养"父母的支持和爱与更好的治疗依从性及血糖控制相关。权威型教养方式的特点是将冲突最小化，例如，父母对孩子的行为设置持续的、实际的限制，同时又表现出温暖的爱及对孩子的需求及感受灵敏快速的回应，这样就改善了糖尿病患儿的行为方式。最后，在 1 型糖尿病患儿中，结构化、严格规则化的家庭环境与更好的血糖控制相关。

经验研究支持这一结论，即给予更多的糖尿病管理责任的大龄的学龄期儿童在自我管理中会犯更多的错误，依从性更低，比那些父母参与的孩子代谢控制情况更差。从这些研究结果看，整个学龄期都需要父母参与孩子的糖尿病管理。

青少年与糖尿病

青少年时期的中心发展任务是逐渐成为一个个体，在心理上与父母分开，表现为形成受父母影响或者有别于父母想法的人生目标、价值观、偏好及观念。糖尿病患儿家庭管理的大环境使得这些问题更加复杂。尽管很多家庭能够处理好这种微妙的平衡关系，但仍有一些家庭做起来很吃力，在处理糖尿病及其管理的过程中面临严重、长期的问题。本章节总结了当前有关影响青少年时期糖尿病家庭管理有效性的心理变化的知识并评估了旨在指导青少年及其家庭如何适应糖尿病的心理干预对照试验。

　　由于胰岛素敏感性降低，在青少年群体中达到并维持严格的血糖控制更加困难。加上这一正常生理现象的代谢影响，青少年的许多行为及心理特点也会影响糖尿病结局，如叛逆、冒险、同龄人的影响及父母监督的下降。尽管青少年的糖尿病知识和技能在稳步增长，对糖尿病管理具有越来越多的责任，但从儿童到青少年治疗的依从性倾向于降低。与此同时，家庭沟通及问题解决技巧成为家庭糖尿病管理有效性的决定因素。那些有更多的父母参与、监督指导下合作管理糖尿病的患儿倾向于达到和维持更好的糖尿病结局。来自同龄人及兄弟姐妹的社会支持对青少年适应糖尿病也有重要影响。伴随神经病理学症状的青少年，尤其是焦虑、抑郁及饮食紊乱，面临更大的糖尿病管理不佳的挑战及过度医疗。如前所述，糖尿病增加了认知和学习功能障碍的风险，尤其是学龄前诊断为糖尿病的患儿，但是还没有对这些症状紊乱影响糖尿病管理的程度进行研究。严重低血糖及慢性高血糖都会与 1 型糖尿病相关的认知及神经解剖学变化相关。最后，有研究证实，青少年时期糖尿病管理方面消极的发展轨迹会持续到成年早期，增加了长期糖尿病医学及心理学方面并发症的风险，强调心理干预的重要性，使得家庭在这一不断变化的发展阶段更有效地处理糖尿病。

　　许多针对青少年及其家庭糖尿病管理的干预措施已经被评估。各种各样的心理-教育策略都会有益处，包括行为改变技巧，有关糖尿病特异性社会技能的团体或者个人训练，处理技巧，问题解决及压力管理技巧。最初的几个临床试验已经证实动机性访谈的有效性。应用远程医疗来进行糖尿病管理同样也显示出其可行性。不同的家庭治疗模式会对糖尿病结局产生有益的影响，尤其是评估行为导向型的家庭干预如行为家庭系统治疗及多系统治疗。许多研究也已经证实预防策略的益处，包括一项在新诊断糖尿病患儿家庭中为期 8 周的自我管理训练项目及一项旨在促进家庭糖尿病管理的亲子合作的临床干预试验。

　　总体上，在 1 型糖尿病青少年患者中进行的行为学和心理学干预研究显示，很容易达到行为学及心理学方面显著的临床疗效，然而对血糖的效果比较很难获得。这些研究都没有涉及大型、多中心样本，很少达到随机对照试验的严格标准。同样，还有其他大量的干预研究，其中不乏其他研究团队的相同研究结果。需要更多的大型、多样本研究来证实这些干预措施的有效性，探索影响干预措施有效性的因素，分析成本-效益及将这些方法转化为临床实践的可行性。

2 型糖尿病在儿童中的发病率越来越高，"混合型"的糖尿病也越来越多（例如，青少年中的成年发病型糖尿病；1.5 型糖尿病），这些都带来全新的临床及科研挑战。在青少年时期，这与 1 型糖尿病的管理有许多相似之处，但 2 型糖尿病有特殊的社会心理问题需要考虑，可能阻碍了科研对这些状况的研究。与 1 型糖尿病相比，2 型糖尿病发病更晚，更易在不同种族和少数民族中及那些较低的社会经济状态的人群中不成比例的发生，更易与有阳性家族史的一级亲属、肥胖、缺乏运动相关。不幸的是，与 1 型糖尿病相比，2 型糖尿病尤其是儿童和青少年中的 2 型糖尿病，行为科学家们几乎没有关注。

有大量的文献证实行为干预能够有效促进青少年的体重控制并增加体育活动，但是这些研究大多数是自主挑选的受试者。需要在那些已经诊断为 2 型糖尿病或者有高风险的青少年中进行诸如此类的对照试验来识别预测治疗结局的风险因素。

美国国立卫生研究院进行的治疗或者预防青少年 2 型糖尿病研究（STOPP-T2D）是 2 个青少年 2 型糖尿病队列研究中的第一个大型研究。首先，HEALTHY 研究是一项基于学校的多因素干预试验，研究人群为少数民族、低社会经济状态（SES）的学生，研究目标为降低糖尿病风险。全国 42 所学校随机分配到全面以学校为基础的干预组，或者作为对照组只进行评估，选择 6～8 年级的青少年。研究结果显示超重和肥胖的发病率在干预组和对照组都降低了，两者没有显著性差异。然而，以学校为基础的干预组其 BMI、腰围、空腹胰岛素水平更低。研究者认为这些肥胖指标的变化也许会降低 2 型糖尿病的发病率；然而，这些假设有待进一步研究。

第二项 STOPP-T2D 研究是最近完成的 TODAY 研究（青少年 2 型糖尿病患者的治疗选择），为新诊断为 2 型糖尿病的患者，在 BMI 大于第85 百分位数的 10～17 岁青少年中比较了 3 种治疗方法——单用二甲双胍，二甲双胍加严格生活方式干预，二甲双胍加罗格列酮。大多数研究对象是少数民族或者处于低社会经济状态，90%有阳性家族史，常常有糖尿病并发症。这项随机对照试验的结果显示，在超过平均 3.8 年的随访时间中，在单用二甲双胍治疗组，51%的患者治疗失败。加上罗格列酮治疗，而没有严格生活方式干预，有效率比单用二甲双胍稍高，39%的患者治疗失败；二甲双胍加严格生活方式干预组47%的患者治疗失败。这些治疗结果令人沮丧，提示青少年 2 型糖尿病很难控制，大多数 2 型糖尿病患者在诊断的最初几年中都需要多种口服药和（或）胰岛素治疗。这两项大型研究提供了重要信息来指导已患或者有 2 型糖尿病风险的青少年高危人群的临床治疗及研究。

临床护理的建议

基于广泛的研究文献综述，推荐以下针对儿童及青少年的临床糖尿病管理策略。

1. 促进家庭合作、交流及良好的问题解决能力　临床医生应鼓励家庭成员之间交流糖尿病的知识并帮助家庭成员养成有效的问题解决能力与技巧，父母与孩子之间形成富有成效的合作关系更有助于成功管理糖尿病。

2. 察觉并早期调整问题　早期识别抑郁、焦虑、饮食失调及学习障碍有助于改进治疗方案，并且将不良反应最小化。

3. 寻求适当的服务并鼓励合理应用这些服务　介绍患者及其家属寻求专业化的糖尿病相关的心理学或者精神方面的服务。如果没有条件，可以与那些有资质的儿童心理健康专业人员培养转诊关系。.

4. 在社区水平倡导保健　在学校及社区鼓励健康饮食、规律的体育活动及体重控制可能预防 2 型糖尿病的发生并更有效地管理 1 型糖尿病。

5. 建议患者及其家属关注医疗水平的进步　胰岛素泵、持续血糖监控、糖类计量、更精确的胰岛素治疗方案等正逐渐变为现实（第十一章）。谨慎的选择这些备选方案可能会促进患者更好的控制血糖，提高生活质量。

6. 接受糖尿病心理学方面的继续教育　有关糖尿病心理学及行为学方面的经验研究越来越广泛。那些能够对这些研究非常熟悉的临床医师会更好地传达这些建议。

参 考 文 献

Achenbach TM, Edelbrock CS: *Manual for the Child Behavior Checklist and Revised Child Behavior Profile.* Burlington, VT, University of Vermont Press, 1983

Adams GR, Berzonsky MD: *The Blackwell Handbook of Adolescence.* New York, Blackwell Publishing, 2005

American Diabetes Association: Type 2 diabetes in children and adolescents. *Pediatrics* 105:671–680, 2000

Amiel SA, Sherwin RS, Simonson DC, Lauritano AA, Tamborlane WV: Impaired insulin action in puberty: a contributing factor to poor glycemic control in adolescents with diabetes. *N Engl J Med* 315:215–219, 1986

Anderson B, Ho J, Brackett J, Finkelstein D, Laffel L: Parental involvement in diabetes management tasks: relationships to blood glucose monitoring adherence and metabolic control in young adolescents with insulin-dependent diabetes mellitus. *J Pediatr* 130:257–265, 1997

Anderson BJ: Family conflict and diabetes management in youth: clinical lessons from child development and diabetes research. *Diabetes Spectrum* 17:22–26, 2004

Anderson BJ, Loughlin C, Goldberg E, Laffel L: Comprehensive, family-focused outpatient care for very young children living with chronic disease: lessons from a program in pediatric diabetes. *Child Serv Soc Policy Res Pract* 4:235–250, 2001

Anderson BJ, Brackett J, Ho J, Laffel LM: An office-based intervention to maintain parent-adolescent teamwork in diabetes management. *Diabetes Care* 22:713–721, 1999

Anderson BJ, Auslander WF, Jung KC, Miller JP, Santiago JV: Assessing family sharing of diabetes responsibilities. *J Pediatr Psychol* 15:477–492, 1990

Anderson BJ, Wolf FM, Burkhart MT, Cornell RG, Bacon GE: Effects of a peer group intervention on metabolic control of adolescents with IDDM: randomized outpatient study. *Diabetes Care* 12:184–188, 1989

Anderson BJ, Auslander WF: Research on diabetes management and the family: a critique. *Diabetes Care* 3:696–702, 1980

Arnett J: *Adolescence and Emerging Adulthood: A Multicultural Approach.* 4th ed. Boston, Prentice Hall, 2010

Auslander WF, Bubb J, Rogge M, Santiago JV: Family stress and resources: potential areas of intervention in children recently diagnosed with diabetes. *Health Soc Work* 18:101–113, 1993

Balik B, Haig B, Moynihan PM: Diabetes and the school-aged child. *MCN Am J Matern Child Nurs* 11:324–330, 1986

Banion CR, Miles MS, Carter MC: Problems of mothers in management of children with diabetes. *Diabetes Care* 6:548–551, 1983

Bearman KJ, La Greca AM: Assessing friend support of adolescents' diabetes care: the diabetes social support questionnaire—friends version. *J Pediatr Psychol* 27:417–428, 2002

Boardway RH, Delamater AM, Tomakowsky J, Gutai JP: Stress management training for adolescents with diabetes. *J Pediatr Psychol* 18:29–45, 1993

Bobrow ES, AvRuskin TW, Siller J: Mother-daughter interactions and adherence to diabetes regimens. *Diabetes Care* 8:146–151, 1985

Brink SJ, Moltz K: The message of the DCCT for children and adolescents. *Diabetes Spectrum* 10:259–267, 1997

Brownell KD, Kelman JH, Stunkard AJ: Treatment of obese children with and without their mothers: changes in weight and blood pressure. *Pediatr* 71:515–523, 1983

Bryden KS, Dunger DB, Mayou RA, Peveler RC, Neil HA: Poor prognosis of young adults with type 1 diabetes: a longitudinal study. *Diabetes Care* 26:1052–1057, 2003

Bryden KS, Peveler RC, Stein A, Neil A, Mayou RA, Dunger DB: Clinical and psychological course of diabetes from adolescence to young adulthood. *Diabetes Care* 24:1536–1540, 2001

Bryden KS, Neil A, Mayou RA, Peveler RC, Fairburn CG, Dunger DB: Eating habits, body weight, and insulin misuse. *Diabetes Care* 22:1956–1960, 1999

Burns KL, Green P, Chase HP: Psychosocial correlates of glycemic control as a function of age in youth with IDDM. *J Adoles Health Care* 7:311–319, 1986

Burroughs TE, Harris MA, Pontious SL, Santiago JV: Research on social support in adolescents with IDDM: a critical review. *Diabetes Educ* 23:438–440, 1997

Carney RM, Schechter K, Davis T: Improving adherence to blood glucose monitoring in insulin-dependent diabetic children. *Behav Ther* 14:247–254, 1983

Chambless DL, Ollendick TH: Empirically supported psychological interventions: controversies and evidence. *Ann Rev Psychol* 52:685–716, 2001

Channon SJ, Huws-Thomas M, Rollnick S, Hood K, Cannings-John R, Rogers C, Gregory JW: A multicenter randomized controlled trial of motivational interviewing in teenagers with diabetes. *Diabetes Care* 30:1390–1395, 2007

Channon S, Huws-Thomas MV, Gregory JW, Rollnick S: Motivational interviewing with teenagers with diabetes. *Clin Child Psychol Psychiatr* 10:43–51, 2005

Cohen DM, Lumley MA, Naar-King S, Partridge T, Cakan N: Child behavior problems and family functioning as predictors of adherence and glycemic control in economically disadvantaged children with type 1 diabetes: a prospective study. *J Pediatr Psychol* 29:171–184, 2004

Colas C, Mathieu P, Techobroutsky G: Eating disorders and retinal lesions in type 1 (insulin-dependent) diabetic women. *Diabetologia* 34:288, 1991

Colton P, Olmsted M, Daneman D, Rydall A, Rodin G: Disturbed eating behavior and eating disorders in preteen and early teenage girls with type 1 diabetes. *Diabetes Care* 27:1654–1659, 2004

Colton PA, Olmsted MP, Daneman D, Rydall AC, Rodin G: Five-year prevalence and persistence of disturbed eating behavior and eating disorders in girls with type 1 diabetes. *Diabetes Care* 30:2861–2862, 2007

Cook S, Herold K, Edidin DV, Briars R: Increasing problem solving in adolescents with type 1 diabetes: the choices diabetes program. *Diabetes Educ* 28:115–123, 2002

Daneman D, Frank M, Perlman K, Wittenberg J: The infant and toddler with diabetes: challenges of diagnosis and management. *Paediatr Child Health* 4:57–63, 1999

Davis CL, Delamater AM, Shaw KH, LaGreca AM, Eidson MS, Perez-Rodriguez JE: Parenting styles, regimen adherence, and glycemic control in 4-10-year-old children with diabetes. *J Pediatr Psychol* 26:123–129, 2001

Delamater AM, Jacobson AM, Anderson B, Cox D, Fisher L, Lustman P, Rubin R, Wysocki T: Psychosocial therapies in diabetes: report of the psychosocial therapies working group. *Diabetes Care* 24:1286–1292, 2001

Delamater AM, Bubb J, Davis SG, Smith JA, Schmidt L, White NH: Randomized prospective study of self-management training with newly diagnosed diabetic children. *Diabetes Care* 13:492–498, 1990

Delamater AM, Davis S, Bubb J, Smith J, White NH, Santiago JV: Self-monitoring of blood glucose by adolescents with diabetes: technical skills and utilization of data. *Diabetes Educ* 15:56–61, 1989

Delamater AM, Smith JA, Kurtz SM, White NH: Dietary skills and adherence in children with type 1 diabetes mellitus. *Diabetes Educ* 14:33–36, 1988

Diabetes Control and Complications Trial Research Group: Effect of intensive diabetes treatment on the development and progression of long-term complications in adolescents with insulin-dependent diabetes mellitus: Diabetes Control and Complications Trial. *J Pediatr* 125:177–188, 1994

DiMeglio LA, Pottorff TM, Boyd SR, France L, Fineberg N, Eugster EA: A randomized, controlled study of insulin pump therapy in diabetic preschoolers. *J Pediatr* 145:380–384, 2004

Drash AL: The child, the adolescent, and the Diabetes Control and Complications Trial. *Diabetes Care* 16:1515–1516, 1993

Dubbert PM, King AC, Marcus BH, Sallis JF: Promotion of physical activity through the life span. In *Handbook of Clinical Health Psychology. Volume 2: Disorders of Behavior and Health.* Boll TJ, Raczynski JM, Leviton LC, Eds. Washington, DC, American Psychological Association, 2004, p. 147–181

Dumont RH, Jacobson AM, Cole C, Hauser ST, Wolfsdorf JI, Willett JB, Milley JF, Wertlieb D: Psychosocial predictors of acute complications of diabetes in youth. *Diabet Med* 12:612–618, 1995

Eastman BG, Johnson SB, Silverstein J, Spillar R, McCallum M: Understanding of hypo- and hyperglycemia by youngsters with diabetes and their parents. *J Pediatr Psychol* 8:229–243, 1983

Eiser C: *Chronic Childhood Disease: An Introduction to Psychological Theory and Research.* New York, Cambridge University Press, 1990

Ellis DA, Templin T, Podolski CL, Frey M, Naar-King S, Moltz K: The Parental Monitoring of Diabetes Care scale: development, reliability and validity of a scale to evaluate parental supervision of adolescent illness management. *J Adol Health* 42:146–153, 2008

Ellis DA, Podolski CL, Frey M, Naar-King S, Wang B, Moltz K: The role of parental monitoring in adolescent health outcomes: impact on regimen adherence in youth with type 1 diabetes. *J Pediatr Psychol* 32:907–917, 2007

Ellis DA, Frey M, Naar-King S, Templin T, Cunningham P, Cakan N: Use of multi-systemic therapy to improve regimen adherence among adolescents with type 1 diabetes in chronic poor metabolic control: a randomized controlled trial. *Diabetes Care* 28:1604–1610, 2005

Ellis DA, Naar-King S, Frey M, Templin T, Rowland M, Greger N: Use of multisystemic therapy to improve regimen adherence among adolescents with type 1 diabetes in poor metabolic control: a pilot investigation. *J Clin Psychol Med Settings* 11:315–324, 2004

Epstein LH, Valoski A, Wing RR, McCurley J: Ten-year outcomes of behavioral family-based treatment for childhood obesity. *Health Psychol* 13:373–383, 1994

Epstein LH, Beck S, Figueroa J, Farkas G, Kazdin AE, Daneman D, Becker DJ: The effects of targeting improvement in urine glucose on metabolic control in children with insulin-dependent diabetes mellitus. *J App Behav Anal* 14:365–375, 1981

Erikson EH: *Identity: Youth and Crisis.* New York, W. W. Norton, 1968

Erikson EH: *Childhood and Society.* New York, W. W. Norton, 1950

Farmer AJ, Gibson OJ, Dudley C, Bryden KS, Hayton PM, Tarasenko L, Neil A:

A randomized controlled trial of the effect of real-time telemedicine support on glycemic control in young adults with type 1 diabetes (ISRCTN 46889446). *Diabetes Care* 28:2697–2702, 2005

Ferguson SC, Blane A, Wardlaw J, Frier BM, Perros P, McCrimmon RJ, Deary IJ: Influence of early onset age of type 1 diabetes on cerebral structure and cognitive function. *Diabetes Care* 28:1431–1437, 2005

Fowler J, Budzynski T, Vandebergh R: Effects of an EMG biofeedback relaxation program on control of diabetes: a case study. *Biofeedback Self Regul* 1:105–112, 1976

Gardner SG, Bingley PJ, Sawtell PA, Weeks S, Gale EA: Rising incidence of insulin-dependent diabetes in children aged under 5 years in the Oxford region: time trend analysis. The Bart's Oxford Study Group. *BMJ* 315:712–717, 1997

Garrison WT, McQuiston S: *Chronic Illness during Childhood and Adolescence.* Newbury Park, CA, Sage Publications, 1989

Golden MP, Ingersoll GM, Brack CJ, Russell BA, Wright JC, Huberty TJ: Longitudinal relationship of asymptomatic hypoglycemia to cognitive function in IDDM. *Diabetes Care* 12:89–93, 1989

Golden MP, Russell BP, Ingersoll GM, Gray DL, Hummer KM: Management of diabetes in children younger than 5 years of age. *Am J Dis Child* 139:448–452, 1985

Goldston DB, Kovacs M, Obrosky S, Iyengar S: A longitudinal study of life events and metabolic control among youths with insulin-dependent diabetes mellitus. *Health Psychol* 14:409–414, 1995

Greco P, Pendley JS, McDonell K, Reeves G: A peer group intervention for adolescents with type 1 diabetes and their best friends. *J Pediatr Psychol* 26:485–490, 2001

Grey M, Boland E, Davidson M, Li J, Tamborlane W: Coping skills training for youth on intensive therapy has long-lasting effects on metabolic control and quality of life. *J Pediatr* 137:107–113, 2000

Grey M, Boland E, Davidson M, Yu C, Tamborlane W: Coping skills training for youth with diabetes on intensive therapy. *Appl Nurs Res* 12:3–12, 1999

Grey M, Boland E, Davidson M, Yu C, Sullivan-Bolyai S, Tamborlane WV: Short-term effects of coping skills training as adjunct to intensive therapy in adolescents. *Diabetes Care* 21:902–908, 1998

Gross AM, Magalnick LJ, Richardson P: Self management training with families of insulin-dependent diabetic children: a long term controlled investigation. *Child Fam Behav Ther* 3:141–153, 1985

Gross AM, Heimann L, Shapiro R, Schultz RM: Children with diabetes: social skills training and HbA1c levels. *Behav Modif* 7:151–163, 1983

Grylli V, Hafferl-Gattermayer A, Wagner G, Schober E, Karwautz A: Eating disorders and eating problems among adolescents with type 1 diabetes: exploring relationships with temperament and character. *J Pediatr Psychol* 30:197–206, 2005

Hains AA, Davies WH, Parton E, Silverman AH: Brief report: a cognitive behavioral intervention for distressed adolescents with type 1 diabetes. *J Pediatr Psychol* 26:61–66, 2001

Hampson SE, Skinner TC, Hart J, Storey L, Gage H, Foxcroft D, Kimber A, Shaw K, Walker J: Effects of educational and psychosocial interventions for adolescents with diabetes mellitus: a systematic review. *Health Technol Assess* 5:1–79, 2001

Hanson CL, Rodrigue J, Henggeler SW, Harris MA, Klesges R, Carle D: The perceived self-competence of adolescents with insulin-dependent diabetes mellitus: deficit or strength? *J Pediatr Psychol* 15:605–618, 1990

Harris MA, Wysocki T, Sadler M, Wilkinson K, Harvey LM, Buckloh LM, Mauras N, White NH: Validation of a structured interview for the assessment of diabetes self management. *Diabetes Care* 23:1301–1304, 2000

Hathout EH, Fujishige L, Geach J, Ischandar M, Mauro S, Mace JW: Effect of therapy with insulin glargine (Lantus) on glycemic control in toddlers, children, and adolescents with diabetes. *Diabetes Technol Ther* 5:801–806, 2003

Hatton DL, Canam C, Thorne S, Hughes AM: Parents' perceptions of caring for an infant or toddler with diabetes. *J Adv Nurs* 22:569–577, 1995

Hauser ST, Jacobson AM, Lavori P, Wolfsdorf JI, Herskowitz RD, Milley JE, Bliss R, Gelfand E, Wertlieb D, Stein J: Adherence among children and adolescents with insulin-dependent diabetes mellitus over four-year longitudinal follow-up: II. Immediate and long-term linkages with the family milieu. *J Pediatr Psychol* 15:527–542, 1990

HEALTHY Study Group, Foster GD, Linder B, Baranowski T, Cooper DM, Goldberg L, et al.: A school-based intervention for diabetes risk reduction. *N Engl J Med* 363:443–453, 2010

Helgeson VS, Lopez LC, Kamarck T: Peer relationship and diabetes: retrospective and ecological momentary assessment approaches. *Health Psychol* 28:273–282, 2009a

Helgeson VS, Siminerio L, Escobar O, Becker D: Predictors of metabolic control among adolescents with diabetes: a 4-year longitudinal study. *J Pediatr Psychol* 34:254–270, 2009b

Helgeson VS, Reynolds K, Siminerio L, Escobar O, Becker D: Parent and adolescent distribution of responsibility for self-care: links to health outcome. *J Pediatr Psychol* 33:497–508, 2008

Hershey T, Perantic DC, Wu J, Weaver PM, Black KJ, White NH: Hippocampal volumes in youth with type 1 diabetes. *Diabetes* 59:236–241, 2010

Herzer M, Hood KK: Anxiety symptoms in adolescents with type 1 diabetes: association with blood glucose monitoring and glycemic control. *J Pediatr Psychol* 35:415–425, 2010

Holmes CS, Cant M, Fox MA, Lampert NL, Greer T: Disease and demographic risk factors for disrupted cognitive functioning in children with insulin-dependent diabetes mellitus (IDDM). *Sch Psychol Rev* 28:215–227, 1999

Hood KK, Huestis S, Maher A, Butler D, Volkening LA, Laffel LM: Depressive symptoms in children and adolescents with type 1 diabetes: association with diabetes-specific characteristics. *Diabetes Care* 29:1389–1391, 2006

Iannotti RJ, Nansel TR, Schneider S, Haynie DL, Simons-Morton B, Sobel DO, Zeitzoff L, Plotnick LP, Clark L: Assessing regimen adherence of adolescents with type 1 diabetes. *Diabetes Care* 29:2263–2267, 2006

Jacobson AM, Hauser ST, Lavori P, Willett JB, Cole CF, Wolfsdorf JI, Dumont RH, Wertlieb D: Family environment and glycemic control: a four-year prospective study of children and adolescents with insulin-dependent diabetes mellitus. *Psychosom Med* 56:401–409, 1994

Jacobson AM, Hauser ST, Lavori P, Wolfsdorf JI, Herskowitz RD, Milley JE, Bliss R, Gelfand E, Wertlieb D, Stein J: Adherence among children and adolescents with insulin-dependent diabetes mellitus over four-year longitudinal follow-up: I. The influence of patient coping and adjustment. *J Pediatr Psychol* 15:511–526, 1990

Jeffrey RW, Epstein LH, Wilson GT, Drewnowski A, Stunkard AJ, Wing RR: Long-term maintenance of weight loss: current status. *Health Psychol* 19:5–16, 2000

Jelalian E, Saelens B: Empirically supported treatments in pediatric psychology: pediatric obesity. *J Pediatr Psychol* 24:223–248, 1999

Johnson SB, Silverstein J, Rosenbloom A, Carter R, Cunningham W: Assessing daily management of childhood diabetes. *Health Psychol* 5:545–564, 1986

Johnson SB: Knowledge, attitudes and behavior: correlates of health in childhood diabetes. *Clinical Psychology Review* 5:545–564, 1984

Johnson SB, Pollak R, Silverstein J, Rosenbloom A, Spillar R, McCallum M, Harkavy J: Cognitive and behavioral knowledge about insulin-dependent diabetes among children and parents. *Pediatr* 69:708–713, 1982

Johnson SB: Psychological factors in juvenile diabetes: a review. *J Behav Med* 3:95–102, 1980

Jones JM, Lawson ML, Daneman D, Olmsted MP, Rodin G: Eating disorders in adolescent females with and without type 1 diabetes: cross sectional study. *BMJ* 320:1563–1566, 2000

Kaplan RM, Chadwick MW, Schimmel LE: Social learning intervention to promote metabolic control in type 1 diabetes mellitus: pilot experiment results. *Diabetes Care* 8:152–155, 1985

Kovacs M, Goldston D, Obrosky DS, Bonar LK: Psychiatric disorders in youths with IDDM: rates and risk factors. *Diabetes Care* 20:36–44, 1997a

Kovacs M, Goldston D, Obrosky DS, Drash A: Major depressive disorder in youths with IDDM. *Diabetes Care* 20:45–51, 1997b

Kovacs M, Mukerji P, Iyengar S, Drash A: Psychiatric disorder and metabolic control among youths with IDDM. A longitudinal study. *Diabetes Care* 19:318–323, 1996

Kovacs M, Kass RE, Schnell TM, Goldston D, Marsh J: Family functioning and metabolic control of school-aged children with IDDM. *Diabetes Care* 12:409–414, 1989

Kushion W, Salisbury PJ, Seitz KW, Wilson BE: Issues in the care of infants and toddlers with insulin dependent diabetes mellitus. *Diabetes Educ* 17:107–110, 1991

La Greca AM, Bearman KJ: The diabetes social support questionnaire-family version: evaluating adolescents' diabetes-specific support from family members. *J Pediatr Psychol* 27:665–676, 2002

La Greca AM, Auslander WF, Greco P, Spetter D, Fisher EB, Santiago JV: I get by with a little help from my family and friends: adolescents' support for diabetes care. *J Pediatr Psychol* 26:279–282, 1995

La Greca AM, Follansbee DM, Skyler JS: Developmental and behavioral aspects of diabetes management in youngsters. *Children's Health Care* 19:132–139, 1990

Laffel LM, Vangsness L, Connell A, Goebel-Fabri A, Butler D, Anderson BJ: Impact of ambulatory, family-focused teamwork intervention on glycemic control in youth with type 1 diabetes. *J Pediatr* 142:409–416, 2003

Lerner RM, Steinberg L: *Handbook of Adolescent Psychology.* 2nd ed. New York: Wiley, 2004

Lewin AB, Storch E, Wiliams LB, Duke DC, Silverstein J, Geffken GR: Brief report: normative data on a structured interview for diabetes adherence in childhood. *J Pediatr Psychol* 35:177–182, 2010

Liss DS, Waller DA, Kennard BD, McIntire D, Capra P, Stephens J: Psychiatric illness and family support in children and adolescents with diabetic ketoacidosis: a controlled study. *J Am Acad Child Adolesc Psychiatry* 37:536–544, 1998

Litton J, Rice A, Friedman N, Oden J, Lee MM, Freemark M: Insulin pump therapy in toddlers and preschool children with type 1 diabetes mellitus. *J Pediatr* 141:490–495, 2002

Lowe K, Lutzker J: Increasing compliance to a medical regimen with a juvenile diabetic. *Behav Ther* 10:57–64, 1979

Marteau TM, Bloch S, Baum JD: Family life and diabetic control. *J Child Psychol Psychiat* 28:823–833, 1987

McGrady ME, Laffel L, Drotar D, Repaske D, Hood KK: Depressive symptoms and glycemic control in adolescents with type 1 diabetes: mediational role of blood glucose monitoring. *Diabetes Care* 32:804–806, 2009

McNabb W, Quinn M, Murphy D, Thorp F, Cook S: Increasing children's responsibility for self-care: the in-control study. *Diabetes Educ* 20:121-124, 1994

Mendez FJ, Belendez M: Effects of a behavioral intervention on treatment adherence and stress management in adolescents with IDDM. *Diabetes Care* 20:1370-1375, 1997

Miller-Johnson S, Emery RE, Marvin RS, Clarke W, Lovinger R, Martin M: Parent-child relationships and the management of diabetes mellitus. *J Consult Clin Psychol* 62:603-610, 1994

Mulvaney S, Rothman RL, Wallston KA, Lybarger C, Dietrich MS: An Internet-based program to improve self-management in adolescents with type 1 diabetes. *Diabetes Care* 33:602-604, 2010

Northam EA, Anderson PJ, Jacobs R, Hughes M, Warne GL, Werther GA: Neuropsychological profiles of children with type 1 diabetes 6 years after disease onset. *Diabetes Care* 24:1541-1546, 2001

Northam EA, Anderson PJ, Werther GA, Warne GL, Adler RG, Andrewes D: Neuropsychological complications of IDDM in children 2 years after disease onset. *Diabetes Care* 21:379-384, 1998

Northam E, Anderson P, Adler R, Werther G, Warne G: Psychosocial and family functioning in children with insulin-dependent diabetes at diagnosis and one year later. *J Pediatr Psychol* 21:699-717, 1996

Palmer D, Berg CA, Wiebe DJ, Beveridge R, Korbel CD, Upchurch R, Swinyard M, Lindsay R, Donaldson D: The role of autonomy and pubertal status in understanding age differences in maternal involvement in diabetes responsibility across adolescence. *J Pediatr Psychol* 29:35-46, 2004

Patton SR, Dolan LM, Powers SW: Differences in family mealtime interactions between young children with type 1 diabetes and controls: implications for behavioral intervention. *J Pediatr Psychol* 33:885-893, 2008

Patton SR, Dolan LM, Mitchell MJ, Byars KC, Standiford D, Powers SW: Mealtime interactions in families of pre-schoolers with type 1 diabetes. *Pediatr Diabetes* 5:190-198, 2004

Pendley JS, Kasmen LJ, Miller DL, Donze J, Swenson C, Reeves G: Peer and family support in children and adolescents with type 1 diabetes. *J Pediatr Psychol* 27:429-438, 2002

Peveler RC, Bryden KS, Neil HA, Fairburn CG, Mayou RA, Dunger DB, Turner HM: The relationship of disordered eating habits and attitudes to clinical outcomes in young adult females with type 1 diabetes. *Diabetes Care* 28:84-88, 2005

Pond JS, Peters ML, Pannell DL, Rogers CS: Psychosocial challenges for children with insulin-dependent diabetes mellitus. *Diabetes Educ* 21:297-299, 1995

Powers SW, Byars KC, Mitchell MJ, Patton SR, Standiford DA, Dolan LM: Parent report of mealtime behavior and parenting stress in young children with type 1 diabetes and in healthy control subjects. *Diabetes Care* 25:313-318, 2002

Puczynski MS, Puczynski SS, Reich J, Kaspar JC, Emanuele M: Mental efficiency and hypoglycemia. *J Dev Behav Pediatr* 11:170-174, 1990

Rose MI, Firestone P, Heick HM, Faught AK: The effect of anxiety management training on the control of juvenile diabetes. *J Behav Med* 6:381-395, 1983

Rosenbloom AL, Silverstein JH: *Type 2 Diabetes in Children and Adolescents: A Guide to Diagnosis, Epidemiology, Pathogenesis, Prevention, and Treatment.* Alexandria, VA, American Diabetes Association, 2003

Rosenbloom AL, Joe JR, Winter WE: Emerging epidemic of type 2 diabetes in youth. *Diabetes Care* 22:345-354, 1999

Rovet JF, Ehrlich RM, Czuchta D, Akler M: Psychoeducational characteristics of children and adolescents with insulin-dependent diabetes mellitus. *J Learn Disabil* 26:7-22, 1993

Rovet JF, Ehrlich RM, Czuchta D: Intellectual characteristics of diabetic children at diagnosis and one year later. *J Pediatr Psychol* 15:775-788, 1990

Rovet JF, Ehrlich RM, Hoppe M: Intellectual deficits associated with early onset of insulin-dependent diabetes mellitus in children. *Diabetes Care* 10:510-515, 1987

Rubin RR, Peyrot M: Psychological issues and treatments for people with diabetes. *J Clin Psychol* 57:457-478, 2001

Ryan CM, Becker DJ: Hypoglycemia in children with type 1 diabetes mellitus. Risk factors, cognitive function, and management. *Endocrinol Metab Clin North Am* 28:883-900, 1999

Ryan CM: Effects of diabetes mellitus on neuropsychological function: a lifespan perspective. *Semin Clin Neuropsychiatry* 2:4-14, 1997

Ryan C, Longstreet C, Morrow L: The effects of diabetes mellitus on the school attendance and school achievement of adolescents. *Child: Care, Health, & Development* 11:229-240, 1985a

Ryan C, Vega A, Drash A: Cognitive deficits in adolescents who developed diabetes early in life. *Pediatr* 75:921-927, 1985b

Ryan C, Vega A, Longstreet C, Drash A: Neuropsychological changes in adolescents with insulin-independent diabetes. *J Consult Clin Psychol* 52:335-342, 1984

Ryden O, Nevander L, Johnsson P, Hansson K, Kronvall P, Sjoblad S, Westbom L: Family therapy in poorly controlled juvenile IDDM: effects on diabetes control, self-evaluation, and behavioral symptoms. *Acta Paediatr* 83:285-291, 1994

Saha ME, Huuppone T, Mikael K, Juuti M, Komulainen J: Continuous subcutaneous insulin infusion in the treatment of children and adolescents with type 1 diabetes mellitus. *J Pediatr Endocrinol Metab* 15:1005-1010, 2002

Sallis JF: Influences on physical activity of children, adolescents, and adults. In *Toward a Better Understanding of Physical Fitness and Activity.* Corbin CB, Pangrazi RP, Eds. Scottsdale, AZ, Holcomb Hathaway, 1999, p. 27-32

Satin W, La Greca AM, Zigo S, Skyler JS: Diabetes in adolescence: effects of multifamily group intervention and parent simulation of diabetes. *J Pediatr Psychol* 14:259-276, 1989

Schafer LC, Glasgow RE, McCaul KD: Increasing the adherence of diabetic adolescents. *J Behav Med* 5:353-362, 1982

Schilling L, Dixon J, Knafl K, Lynn M, Murphy K, Dumser S, Grey M: A new self-report measure of self-management of type 1 diabetes for adolescents. *Nurs Res* 58:228-236, 2009

Schilling L, Grey M, Knafl K: A review of measures of self management of type 1 diabetes by youth and their parents. *Diabetes Educator* 28:796-808, 2002

Schoenle EJ, Schoenle D, Molinari L, Largo RH: Impaired intellectual development in children with type 1 diabetes: association with HbA1c, age at diagnosis and sex. *Diabetologia* 45:108-114, 2002

Shehadeh N, Battelino T, Galatzer A, Naveh T, Hadash A, de Vries L, Phillip M: Insulin pump therapy for 1-6 year old children with type 1 diabetes. *Isr Med Assoc J* 6:284-286, 2004

Silverman AH, Haines AA, Davies WH, Parton E: A cognitive behavioral adherence intervention for adolescents with type 1 diabetes. *J Clin Psychol Med Settings* 10:119-127, 2003

Silverstein JH, Johnson S: Psychosocial challenge of diabetes and the development of a continuum of care. *Pediatr Ann* 23:300-305, 1994

Snyder J: Behavioral analysis and treatment of poor diabetic self-care and antisocial behavior: a single-subject experimental study. *Behav Ther* 18:251-263, 1987

Soltesz G, Patterson C, Dahlquist G: Global trends in childhood type 1 diabetes. In *Diabetes Atlas.* 3rd ed. Chapter 2.1. Brussels, Belgium, International Diabetes Federation, 2006, p. 153-190

Sperling M, Ize-Ludlow D: The classification of diabetes mellitus: a conceptual framework. *Pediatr Clin N Amer* 52:1533-1552, 2005

Steel JM, Young RJ, Lloyd GG, Clark BF: Clinically apparent eating disorders in young diabetic women: associations with painful neuropathy and other complications. *BMJ* 294:859-862, 1987

Stinson JN, McGrath PJ, Yamada JT: Clinical trials in the Journal of Pediatric Psychology: Applying the CONSORT Statement. *J Pediatr Psychol* 28:59-167, 2003

Sullivan-Bolyai S, Deatrick J, Gruppuso P, Tamborlane W, Grey M: Constant vigilance: mothers' work parenting young children with type 1 diabetes. *J Pediatr Nurs* 18:21-29, 2003

Tan CY, Wilson DM, Buckingham B: Initiation of insulin glargine in children and adolescents with type 1 diabetes. *Pediatr Diabetes* 5:80-86, 2004

Thomas AM, Peterson L, Goldstein D: Problem solving and diabetes regimen adherence by children and adolescents with IDDM in social pressure situations: a reflection of normal development. *J Pediatr Psychol* 22:541-561, 1997

TODAY Study Group, Zeitler P, Hirst K, Pyle L, Linder B, Copeland K, et al.: A clinical trial to maintain glycemic control in youth with type 2 diabetes. *N Engl J Med* 366:2247-2256, 2012

Tubiana-Rufi N, de Lonlay P, Bloch J, Czernichow P: Remission of severe hypoglycemic incidents in young diabetic children treated with subcutaneous infusion. *Arch Pediatr* 3:969-976, 1996

Vehik K, Dabelea D: The changing epidemiology of type 1 diabetes: why is it going through the roof? *Diabetes Metab Res Rev* 27:3-13, 2011

Viner R, McGrath M, Trudinger P: Family stress and metabolic control in diabetes. *Arch Dis Child* 74:418-421, 1996

Waller D, Chipman JJ, Hardy BW, Hightower MS, North AJ, Williams SB, Babick AJ: Measuring diabetes-specific family support and its relation to metabolic control: a preliminary report. *J Am Acad Child Psychol* 25:415-418, 1986

Weibe DJ, Berg CA, Korbel C, Palmer DL, Beveridge RM, Upchurch R, Lindsay R, Swinyard MT, Donaldson DL: Children's appraisals of maternal involvement in coping with diabetes: enhancing our understanding of adherence, metabolic control, and quality of life across adolescence. *J Pediatr Psychol* 30:167-178, 2005

Weissberg-Benchell J, Glasgow AM, Tynan WD, Wirtz P, Turek J, Ward J: Adolescent diabetes management and mismanagement. *Diabetes Care* 18:77-82, 1995

Wolfsdorf JI, Anderson BA, Pasquarello C: Treatment of the child with diabetes. In *Joslin's Diabetes Mellitus.* 13th ed. Kahn CR, Weir G, Eds. Philadelphia, Lea & Febiger, 1994, p. 430-451

Wysocki T, Nansel TR, Holmbeck G, Chen RS, Laffel L, Anderson BJ, Weissberg-Benchell J: Collaborative involvement of primary and secondary caregivers: associations with youths' diabetes outcomes. *J Pediatr Psychol* 34:869-881, 2009

Wysocki T, Harris MA, Buckloh L, Mertlich D, Lochrie A, Taylor A, Sadler M, White NH: Randomized controlled trial of behavioral family systems therapy for diabetes: maintenance and generalization of effects on parent-adolescent communication. *Behav Ther* 39:33-46, 2008a

Wysocki T, Iannotti R, Weissberg-Benchell J, Hood K, Laffel L, Anderson BJ, Chen R: Diabetes problem solving by youths with type 1 diabetes and their caregivers: measurement, validation and longitudinal associations with glycemic control. *J Pediatr Psychol* 33:875-884, 2008b

Wysocki T, Harris MA, Buckloh LM, Mertlich D, Lochrie AS, Mauras N, White NH: Randomized controlled trial of behavioral family systems therapy for diabetes: maintenance of effects on diabetes outcomes in adolescents. *Diabetes Care* 30:555–560, 2007

Wysocki T, Greco P: Social support and diabetes management in childhood and adolescence: influence of parents and friends. *Current Diabetes Reports* 6:117–122, 2006a

Wysocki T, Harris MA, Buckloh LM, Mertlich D, Lochrie AS, Taylor A, Sadler M, Mauras N, White NH: Effects of behavioral family systems therapy for diabetes on adolescents' family relationships, treatment adherence and metabolic control. *J Pediatr Psychol* 31:928–938, 2006b

Wysocki T, Buckloh LM, Lochrie A, Antal H: The psychologic context of pediatric diabetes. *Pediatr Clin N Amer* 52:1755–1778, 2005

Wysocki T: Parents, teens, and diabetes. *Diabetes Spectrum* 15:6–8, 2002

Wysocki T, Meinhold PA, Taylor A, Hough BS, Barnard MU, Clarke WL, Bellando BJ, Bourgeois MJ: Psychometric properties and normative data for the Diabetes Independence Survey - Parent Version. *Diabetes Educ* 22:587–591, 1996a

Wysocki T, Taylor A, Hough BS, Linscheid TR, Yeates KO, Naglieri JA: Deviation for developmentally appropriate self-care autonomy. Association with diabetes outcomes. *Diabetes Care* 19:119–125, 1996b

Wysocki T: Associations among parent-adolescent relationships, metabolic control and adjustment to diabetes in adolescents. *J Pediatr Psychol* 18:443–454, 1993

Wysocki T, Hough BS, Ward KM, Green LB: Diabetes mellitus in the transition to adulthood: adjustment, self-care, and health status. *J Dev Behav Pediatr* 13:194–201, 1992a

Wysocki T, Meinhold P, Abrams K, Barnard M, Clarke WL, Bellando BJ, Bourgeois MJ: Parental and professional estimates of self-care independence of children and adolescents with insulin-dependent diabetes mellitus. *Diabetes Care* 15:43–52, 1992b

Wysocki T, Green LB, Huxtable K: Blood glucose monitoring by diabetic adolescents: compliance and metabolic control. *Health Psychol* 8:267–284, 1989a

Wysocki T, Huxtable K, Linscheid TR, Wayne W: Adjustment to diabetes mellitus in pre-schoolers and their mothers. *Diabetes Care* 2:524–529, 1989b

Young-Hyman D, Davis C: Disordered eating behavior in individuals with diabetes: importance of context, evaluation, and classification. *Diabetes Care* 33:683–689, 2010

Young-Hyman D, Schlundt DG, Herman-Wenderoth L, Bozylinski K: Obesity, appearance, and psychosocial adaptation in young African American children. *J Pediatr Psychol* 28:463–472, 2003

Young-Hyman D, Schlundt DG, Herman L, DeLuca F, Counts D: Evaluation of the insulin resistance syndrome in 5- to 10-year-old overweight/obese African-American children. *Diabetes Care* 24:1359–1364, 2001

第十五章
成人寿命延长问题

发育理论提出成人早期及中年时期的任务可以用四个方面来定义。这四方面包括工作/职业目标和活动、婚姻/伴侣关系、育儿/为人父母和休闲活动。尽管社会和文化因素可能改变时间轨迹和已经选择的工作/家庭方向，但是证据表明工作和个人关系可以预测情绪、生活质量和对健康的掌控感，这也证实了在这些方面的选择对成年过程具有重要的意义。糖尿病对人生的这些方面都有影响，而这些方面的问题对糖尿病也有显著的影响。本章主要论述除休闲活动以外的其他方面。

向成人护理过渡

传统性的发育阶段分类包括儿童、青春期、成人或老年。然而，最近有证据表明另一种类别即"青中年"（YA），可能也是重要的一个类别，尤其是讨论糖尿病患者的时候。Arnett 认为 18～25 岁年龄段定义为"成人初显期"，尤其对于中产或上流社会的白人，他们在利用这段时间来探索在伴侣、为人父母和工作方面的身份、目标和选择。有证据显示患有 1 型糖尿病的青中年更可能在医疗随访中丢失、没有管理依从性及较差的医疗结果、并且容易死亡（通常由于胰岛素缺乏而导致糖尿病酮症酸中毒）和自杀，这使得人们对这一年龄群体的关注不断增加。事实上，对这种常见在管理失效和较差的医疗结果的认知使得美国糖尿病学会起草了儿童向青中年保健过渡的意见书。

随后所有的文献都关注患有 1 型糖尿病的青中年。尽管越来越多的青年人患 2 型糖尿病，但这仍是一个相对较新的现象，而且有关这方面的数据正在收集和传播，因此，本章着重讨论患有 1 型糖尿病的青中年。

过渡是指青春期向成人的发育。这个阶段，患有 1 型糖尿病的青中年必须对自己的健康管理富有更大的责任，而且自行决定自己的管理计划。他们正在建立其成人的身份、伴随新的目标、关系及对生活和糖尿病相关的各方面的需求。

尽管有证据表明患有 1 型糖尿病的青中年在心理成熟度上与其同龄人相似，但是 1 型糖尿病的特殊需求（如强化自我管理、卫生保健系统的广泛参与）使得患有 1 型糖尿病的青中年面临着挑战，而他们在过渡期将一直与这些挑战抗争。研究已经发现 1 型糖尿病的青中年中有一小部分人群存在多种身体和心理方面的合并症，包括血糖控制不佳、微血管并发症进展迅速和精神疾病（如抑郁、进食异常），因此需要持久的多学科的支持来帮助他们克服这些疾病和完成过渡。

过渡还指由儿童卫生保健系统和儿科医生转向成人卫生保健系统及成人医生。一项研究中，超过 50%的 1 型糖尿病的青中年报告其在这种过渡过程中存在困难。当 1 型糖尿病的青中年被问及他们最需要什么来完成平稳过渡时，他们强调需要与卫生保健人员连续接触，同时还需要能够理解他们生活境遇的卫生保健人员。当临床工作者被问及同样的问题时，他们认为需要有特定的患者教育材料和培训，尤其是因为 1 型糖尿病是一种起病于儿童时期的慢性疾病。两项研究介绍了针对 1 型糖尿病青中年的过渡计划。这些过渡计划被认为是可行且可接受的，其中一项研究（非对照研究）报告该计划的参加者临床就诊次数更多且血糖控制更好，糖尿病酮症酸中毒的住院率也更低。

工作/职业目标和活动

当进入成年后，一项关键的任务就是认识到，何种工作对于实现个人人生目标都是有意义、令人满意和有益的。糖尿病对这些选择和活动具有重要的影响。

糖尿病对工作的影响

研究表明糖尿病对与社会和个人相关的工作问题具有重要影响。基于人群的研究评估了糖尿病（1 型和 2 型糖尿病患者）对工作相关领域的影响。糖尿病预示着劳动生产力的下降，包括因为提前退休带来的收入减少、病假天数和残疾、早死亡。雇主为糖尿病工人支付更多的医疗和药品费用，但是生产力却降低，与之相对，工人身体和精神更容易受到伤害，工作不但收入低，而且更容易被解雇。

　　糖尿病自我管理也对工作问题有重要影响。使用胰岛素的 2 型糖尿病患者报告糖尿病会影响他们对工作的选择，包括工作如何影响他们自我管理计划。例如，工作的选择可能基于他们需要一种固定的工作时间而不是倒班、工作对体力的消耗、保险福利情况及是否可以安排时间测定血糖或规律进餐。一旦他们被雇佣，糖尿病可能影响其在工作中的关系，如糖尿病患者可能需要同事或上级领导的支持。

　　患糖尿病的工人之中血糖控制较差的个体更可能出现旷工，患有糖尿病相关并发症的个体更可能被解雇。一项旨在采用活性药物治疗（格列吡嗪）来使 2 型糖尿病患者血糖控制达标的随机对照研究显示，血糖控制改善可以预测积极的工作和功能结果。HbA1C 的改善使就业率更高、旷工率更低、受限活动及住院时间减少。因此很明显，糖尿病管理在与员工和雇主均相关的工作结局中扮演重要的角色。

　　尽管工作场所出现重度低血糖非常罕见也极少引起严重问题，但雇主和工友的一个主要担忧是糖尿病患者在工作时可能出现低血糖，因此他/她或其他人可能存在受伤的风险。低血糖通常发生于 1 型糖尿病的个体或使用胰岛素的 2 型糖尿病个体，但是其通常有预警信号，因此可以预防和治疗，极少引起严重损害。尽管有证据表明重度低血糖发作（定义为需要他人帮助的低血糖发作）很少发生在工作场所，1 型糖尿病个体中的总体发生率约每年每人 0.14 次，但是这种担忧还是持续存在。

　　这种担忧及其他与糖尿病对工作的影响相关的担心可能导致出现就业歧视。一项研究报告糖尿病患者与患其他疾病的患者相比在就业时更容易遭受歧视（如就业领域、停职或解雇）。

　　为了阐述这种担忧，ADA 于 1984 年发布了正式的就业立场声明，指出"任何糖尿病患者，无论胰岛素依赖或非胰岛素依赖都能胜任其本人能胜任的任何职业"。美国残疾人法案规定，应向糖尿病患者提供"合理的膳宿"便于其工作时管理糖尿病。这些膳宿条件可能是：可以频繁休息和进餐、有冰箱用于药物储存。患有糖尿病并发症的个体还需要一些场所（如对于视力受损患者的阅读辅助设施）（www.eeoc.gov /facts/diabetes.html）。美国糖尿病学会已经制定了一系列指南来评估糖尿病患者的就业情况及他们需要的工作场所。尽管对这些膳宿条件的需求频率，以及是否应该给予提供还不清楚，但是糖尿病患者与其他疾病患者相比，在雇佣过程中及合理膳宿的诉求方面报告的歧视更少。

工作对糖尿病的影响

成功就业可以直接及间接影响健康。未就业的个体通常收入较低。低收入又使得患者无法获得重要的医疗保健，例如，就诊于内分泌专科医生，或每年进行糖化血红蛋白监测及每两年行眼部检查。工资较低的工作其工作环境不利于健康（如快速、重复、强体力），这也部分解释了为什么工资较低的工人其疾病发生率更高。研究还显示"工作紧张"（劳动需求大但控制性较低）及"付出-回报失衡"（低保障、劳动需求大及职业机会有限）都将导致心血管疾病，尽管这一领域还没有对糖尿病患者进行特别的关注，但是糖尿病和心血管疾病之间密切的关系指向了一个潜在的重要领域。

把工作和糖尿病合为一体——工作场所的干预

已经有人建议在工作场所进行饮食和运动干预来帮助患者改善健康并减少雇主的长期花费。针对肥胖的工作场所资助项目的数量越来越多，其中大多数都是由大型的私人雇主所执行的。然而，工作场所项目的结果发表很少，而且在少数发表的结果中，其效应微弱且多为短期，而且其方法学较差。近期对工作场所进行饮食和运动干预来减轻体重的效果进行 Meta 分析后发现其可以使体重略减轻（约 1.27kg），但是值得注意的是，即使微小的体重下降也能使全身健康状况获益。

婚姻/伴侣

发展一段健康的婚姻/伴侣关系是成人时期的重要任务之一。研究显示患者从其他人那里可以获得社会和感情的帮助，尤其是从家庭和配偶，表现为免疫功能、心血管内内分泌功能更强，疾病和创伤恢复更快、而且对于疾病的心理适应力更强、更多地参与管理行为且对医疗保健方案的依从性更好。

相反，这种关系对健康结果也可以有负面影响。婚姻关系中的相互作用（如支持是如何给予和接受的）也影响到婚姻质量和健康功能状况。一项有关婚姻关系中相互作用的综述表明负面的相互作用可以导致负面的健康习惯和抑郁，从而间接影响健康。对于 1 型糖尿病患者，家庭成员的过度责备与血糖控制不佳密切相关。

家庭支持/婚姻质量对糖尿病的影响

对于糖尿病患者，关系变量可能尤其重要，因为糖尿病治疗方案（如食物的购买和准备、运动、给药、低血糖的处置）通常需要配偶的参与。对于 1 型糖尿病和 2 型糖尿病患者来说，更大的社会支持可以带来更好的疾病适应、治疗依从性更好且血糖控制更佳。而且，婚姻满意度越高，出现代谢综合征的风险越低，其次降低与体重相关的糖尿病的前期表现。更好的婚姻质量（亲密、调整）也与 2 型糖尿病患者更高的生活质量和治疗依从性密切相关。

这些资料使得有人建议对于成人也采用一种家庭式的糖尿病管理，这种方式一直被鼓励用于 1 型糖尿病的青少年。这种方式把家庭关系和环境作为干预的目标，因为家庭关系可以影响患者生理状态，而家庭互动又可以影响自我管理。

然而，这些少量的针对家庭或婚姻中的相互作用与健康关系的研究就夫妻干预对健康结果的影响这一命题仅仅提供了一些数量有限且结果令人失望的数据。一项随机对照研究的 Meta 分析评价了对患有慢性疾病的成人其家庭成员进行干预的益处，结果发现当配偶参与其中时，对抑郁有积极的影响，但对于焦虑、身体残疾或夫妻关系的满意度没有影响。该分析还发现家庭干预的结果之一是死亡率下降，但是这仅发生在干预不局限于配偶也不涉及婚姻关系问题时。最近对以夫妻而不是单个患者为目标的 25 项随机干预试验进行的跨疾病 Meta 分析发现当伴侣参与其中时，疼痛、抑郁和婚姻功能都得到明显改善，虽然这种效应比较微弱。一项体重干预的 Meta 分析发现伴侣参与是有意义的，但是益处比较微弱且时间较短。然而，配偶参与的戒烟干预并没有带来更好的结果。

有一些证据表明配偶参与糖尿病教育和肥胖计划可以带来更好的结果。一项糖尿病教育计划中（非随机试验），老年 2 型糖尿病患者与其配偶共同参与可以学到更多，压力更小，且血糖控制改善更明显。一项减重的随机试验中，既有糖尿病患者也有非糖尿病患者，如果与肥胖的配偶共同参与而不是自己一个人，肥胖的女性而不是男性，其体重减轻更多。一项对家庭参与的体重控制干预试验的系统综述表明配偶的参与作用有限，关键是要仔细挑选家庭成员并使他/她积极参与到目标设定和行为改变中来。由于许多研究尚存在设计缺陷，因此对于是否及如何让家庭成员或伴侣参与的问题还没有很好的答案。

这些研究中使用的模式是配偶参与。然而，更广泛的文献回顾表明该模型过于简单，一种"双向水平"的模式可能更合适。这种方法强调伴侣的相互依赖性，因为伴侣间的相互作用也可以影响到双方。两项研究正在采用这种方式所倡导的协作性解决问题的方法在 2 型糖尿病患者中进行验证。初步数据能够令人看到希望，但是还没有得到最终结果。

糖尿病对婚姻关系的影响

配偶在处理伴侣的糖尿病过程中会感受到明显的负担。这包括责任（如食物制备、药物注射）、角色和作用（尤其是当伴侣患有 2 型糖尿病并发症或出现功能受限时）的改变。配偶通常是患者的主要支持，但同时又需要自己得到支持。针对患有其他慢性疾病的患者配偶的研究显示他们通常也更容易出现焦虑和抑郁、压力相关的症状及工作表现降低。这些问题又影响到伴侣的精神健康及结成对子来解决疾病的能力。家庭干预随机对照研究的 Meta 分析显示对家庭成员有正面影响，尤其是当干预措施仅以家庭成员为目标且仅涉及关系问题。

虽然关于糖尿病伴侣压力的研究有限，但有证据显示 2 型糖尿病患者的伴侣感到的痛苦与患者本人相当甚至更多，即使糖尿病患者本人并没有感到痛苦。同时，他们的痛苦不仅限于糖尿病，还与其他生活的压力源有关（如经济、家庭关系）。在没有被打扰或批评的情况下，伴侣努力想提供帮助及合适且适时的支持。

性别之间有差异吗?

性别角色(如谁做什么)也影响到糖尿病夫妻如何有效应对糖尿病。女性仍然倾向认为在维持家庭功能、疾病管理和提供情感支持方面负有更大的责任,因此她们最终承受更多的负担。一项有关肥胖夫妻的研究中,夫妻双方至少一人患有 2 型糖尿病,结果显示与其配偶共同治疗后,女性结局更好,而当单独治疗时男性结局更好。还有证据表明丈夫和妻子应对疾病存在差异,如果他们处理的方式存在一致则会最有效。例如,当进行更多的"关系探讨"(谈论关系的状态)时,那么女性比男性更满意他们之间的关系,尤其是夫妻一方有疾病时。

生儿育女/为人父母

对于成人来说作出生儿育女的决定是一个里程碑,但是当女性患有糖尿病时又带来额外的刺激和负担。如果有很好的自我管理及出生前的保健,糖尿病妇女可以安全的妊娠并孕育健康的孩子。然而对于母亲和孩子来说仍然存在额外的风险。妊娠前糖尿病相关的并发症通常在妊娠期间会加重。高血糖增加流产和早产的风险,而且可能引起先天畸形(如神经管缺陷)、肺不成熟和巨大儿(www.cdc.gov/NCBDDD/ pregnacy_gateway/diabetes.htm)。尽管既往关注的重点一直是 1 型糖尿病妇女,但是目前认识到 2 型糖尿病妇女也存在风险,而且可能在妊娠期间接受胰岛素治疗。因此,基于治疗方案的压力同样会发生。

患者有自己的恐惧。一项研究中,1 型糖尿病青中年报告明显担心糖尿病对未来为人父母和婚姻的影响。这些恐惧包括害怕遗传给孩子,害怕未来的并发症影响其养育子代,而且明显害怕糖尿病会导致自己提前死亡,从而缩短与孩子的相处时间。

妊娠糖尿病妇女也代表着一群需要特殊医疗和情绪关心的群体。3%～5%的健康妇女会有妊娠糖尿病,除了带来额外的负担外,超过半数在分娩后的 5～10 年会患 2 型糖尿病。妊娠糖尿病会引起巨大儿从而导致早产和(或)剖宫产,这都会给母亲和孩子带来风险。当母亲患有妊娠糖尿病时,其他新生儿状况(如喂养差、低血糖)也更可能发生。

妊娠糖尿病的治疗包括营养治疗和每日自我监测血糖及必要时的胰岛素治疗。两项随机试验中，以上干预使新生儿死亡率相对于常规保健的死亡率明显降低。治疗的强度会随胎儿的生长监测进行调整，对胎儿的监测应定期进行。对于正常生长的胎儿，不太强化的管理可能就足够，但对于大于实际胎龄的胎儿应给予更强化的管理。正如先前所述，妊娠糖尿病的妇女发生 2 型糖尿病的风险明显增加。妊娠糖尿病的诊断意味着这是唯一的机会去干预阻止。

　　应鼓励糖尿病的妇女（1 型糖尿病，2 型糖尿病或妊娠糖尿病）在妊娠前和妊娠期间严格控制血糖。然而，这可能是一项令人畏缩的任务。我们可以参考一下 DCCT 研究中强化治疗组中的 1 型糖尿病患者。这些患者每周接受辅助性电话随访，每月进行健康小组教育和免费的医疗支持，然而低于 5% 的患者能够维持在正常 HbA1C 范围。妊娠糖尿病期间血糖的控制需要密切监测血糖水平、经常与健康管理团队接触、对母亲和胎儿进行多次的检测、胰岛素治疗的开启及调整，以及与这些步骤相关的额外情感和经济上的负担。

　　由于肥胖的妇女患妊娠糖尿病的风险增加，因此无论其是否有糖尿病，都应该更广泛的关注肥胖对妊娠的影响。医学研究所回顾了妊娠体重增加的相关文献，结果发现肥胖妇女在妊娠和分娩期间出现并发症的风险明显增高，包括死亡，其孩子比正常体重妇女的孩子出现先天性缺陷的风险更高。尽管大多数证据强度并不太强，且这些研究均为观察性研究，但是 IOM 还是修改了妊娠期间体重增加的指南。有一些小型的通过行为干预来减少妊娠期间体重增加的随机对照试验研究显示出一定的效果，其中一项研究发现限制体重对妊娠引起的糖代谢改变有益，这表明干预可能对糖尿病的妇女有益。帮助妇女管理妊娠期间体重及增加其活动量的生活方式干预计划应该是有益的。

　　考虑到妊娠期间体重和糖尿病的管理需要行为改变（如计算糖类、食物限制、增加活动量、胰岛素治疗），也应该评估那些可能影响妇女自我管理方案依从性的心理因素。这些包括抑郁、压力、和（或）饮食障碍，以上都显示与治疗依从性差有关而且对妊娠妇女依从性的影响程度相似。

　　新技术可以改善结果。每日注射（MDI）和胰岛素泵（连续皮下胰岛素输注，或 CSII）可以使 1 型糖尿病的妊娠妇女血糖控制良好。而且，无论采用何种治疗方式，计划妊娠的妇女比非计划妊娠的妇女血糖控制得好。

普遍认为对于 1 型糖尿病妇女进行孕前咨询和妊娠计划是标准的保健，因为这对于降低妊娠相关的风险非常重要。接受孕前咨询的妇女其 HbA1C 更低且母亲和胎儿的不良结局更少。然而，一项健康教育者的调查发现，仅 68% 的人强烈同意提供孕前咨询是非常重要的，大多数未接受过孕前咨询的培训，而且 30%～40% 的人未向其成人或青少年患者提供孕前咨询。

尽管孕前咨询和妊娠计划的价值得到认可，极少的研究对糖尿病如何影响妊娠的决定或妊娠期间生活质量进行探讨。而且，尽管为人父母是成年时期最重要的发展任务，但糖尿病如何影响孩子出生后的为人父母或心理结局方面的文献尚未见报道。因此糖尿病和为人父母之间关系的研究必须进行。

生命的评估

还有两个问题必须澄清才能理解本文的内容及建议。

第一，报道的理论和研究均来源于患者，大多数为白种人，生活在发达的西方国家。因此结论及建议并非适用于其他人种或民族或生活在发展中国家的个体。

第二，当选择治疗、目标和干预时，我们应该考虑到包含生命中很长的一段时间和一个阶段的"成人时期"。我们引用的文献建议将成人早期定义为显著不同的"青中年"阶段，这个阶段的个体开始逐渐过渡到具有责任和需求的成年期。同样，发展理论通常还根据一生中的得与失定义了其他人生阶段。成年早期被认为是得大于失，而中年则相对平衡，晚年可能是失大于得。中年时期（35～50 岁）通常被定义为发展个人的工作和生活，建立稳定的职业和伴侣从而为未来打下基础。一些人还认为晚年应定义为三个不同的阶段，即中年后期（50～64 岁）、早老年（65～74 岁）及长寿老年（≥75 岁）。每一阶段有正常的发展调整。中年后期通常表现为经济稳定而且可能是事业的高峰期，这个阶段的个体感到自信和有自控力。个体通常开始改变角色，从生理性任务（如养育子女）和社会性需要（如寻找工作、寻找伴侣）过渡到减少预期和需要。早老年个体着重于为人生的下一个阶段寻找新目标，他们开始面临死亡。退休通常在这个阶段出现，而且可能引起自由和自我表达和（或）迷茫和孤独。最后，长寿老年面临的特殊挑战与生理和认知的能力下降、社会接触的减少及依赖性增加有关。

　　虽然目前认识到这些具有广泛的普遍性，但是近来的数据显示这些过程也正在改变，其包括现代生活的各种影响（如早老年时期的养老保健）和越来越不典型的发展过程（如没有工作的父母、一直工作的单身）。然而，这种发展的观点强调了理解每一个人的挑战和压力，以及他/她满意和支持的来源的重要性。

临床保健的建议

　　卫生保健工作者应该通过他/她人生阶段中的典型特征来评估患者面对的生理、社会和情感阶段。通过理解糖尿病对于每一个人的全面含义，卫生保健工作者将站在更好的角度来制订和实施最合适的干预，从而激励患者成长并成功适应糖尿病。另外，每个人的人生阶段并不是实施自我管理计划或具备优化疾病结局能力的标志或禁忌。相反，卫生保健工作者应与患者一起根据不同的人生阶段，体力、资源的限制，以及对疾病管理和结局的预期共同来优化治疗方案。

过渡到成人护理

　　1. 1型糖尿病中青年的评估应包括精神健康及可能影响自我管理的依从性和医疗接触的药品使用问题。

　　2. 卫生保健工作者应监测中青年时期的特殊挑战，使得他/她能够注意到青中年时期的所有可能影响其参与卫生保健和进行良好自我管理的因素。

　　3. 应制订过渡时期保健的新模型并评估其效力。包括辅助中青年患者预约、保险和接受其他服务的导诊系统。

工作/就业目标和活动

　　1. 应该在工作场所实施有助于患者获得更好血糖控制的干预措施。帮助患者改善血糖控制和减轻体重可以降低糖尿病对旷工、生产力和残疾的负面影响。

2. 应评估低血糖的风险并积极评价每个患者和特殊的工作环境。应该摒弃所有糖尿病患者都有低血糖的风险，以及无法成功处理低血糖的误区。这种观点可能导致工作歧视。风险评估也能增强工人的安全感。患者的医生可以通过讲述患者的风险、这些风险在特殊工作环境下如何影响患者，以及何种合理的场所能降低风险来指导雇主。ADA 立场声明指出了一系列建议：四条建议与全面的个体评估及卫生保健工作者采用最新的糖尿病专业知识进行评估的重要性有关，四条建议与适当和不适当的安全性评估有关，一条建议与合理的工作场所有关。

3. 应该鼓励雇主对患有糖尿病的雇员提供情感和设备上的支持。老板和工友的支持可以使糖尿病患者更加开放而且更可能在工作场所获得良好的血糖自我管理。

4. 应该鼓励在工作时努力进行糖尿病管理的患者要求合理的工作场所。改变工作时间表、工作任务、和（或）环境可以使工人更能胜任工作和更好地进行自我管理。应根据美国残疾人法指导雇主。不能保证其有合理工作场所的雇员应交由平等就业委员会指导并给予法律支持。

婚姻/伴侣

1. 健康保健提供者应选择性地将家庭成员纳入糖尿病教育及其他干预计划中以改善糖尿病结局。伴侣可能是最适合参与的人选，但是其他家庭成员可能具有更好的支持性，因此可能更适合这个角色。健康保健工作者应该认识并支持这个人（或这些人），因为他/她可以帮助糖尿病患者。另外，健康保健工作者还应该意识到仅仅是参与还不能影响结局，可能还需要积极地融入目标设定和行为改变过程中，并努力协助。这些干预措施也可能对伴侣有益。

2. 当与患者及其伴侣共同工作时，健康保健工作者应注意到他们之间的关系。应意识到患者可能处于有矛盾的关系之中而需要特别给予关注，尤其是当伴侣给予过多的指责及婚姻质量不高时。夫妻可能需要进行夫妻咨询以改变其负面关系模式。

3. 糖尿病对于伴侣来说也是一种压力性疾病，而且正面的支持对于其生理和精神健康非常重要。健康保健工作者应指导伴侣让合适的支持小组帮助其解决夫妻在处理糖尿病过程中面临的情感上的困难。

生儿育女/为人父母

1. 健康保健工作者应评估糖尿病孕妇整个孕期的精神状态。包括潜在的抑郁、焦虑及其他可能影响糖尿病孕妇在孕期坚持治疗方案的精神问题的评估。当确实有担忧时，健康保健工作者应该提供必要的支持并进行必要的精神卫生治疗。这些建议是基于对糖尿病的人群而不是糖尿病孕妇的研究，但是专家的观点表明应将这些建议应用于糖尿病孕妇。

2. 健康保健工作者应向所有患有糖尿病的育龄期妇女强调并提供妊娠计划和咨询。

3. 应指导肥胖妇女及患有妊娠糖尿病的妇女在孕期管理体重以避免肥胖和妊娠糖尿病所带来的负面结果，并减少其以后出现 2 型糖尿病的风险。

参 考 文 献

American Diabetes Association: Diabetes and employment. *Diabetes Care* 34 (Suppl. 1):S82–S86, 2011a

American Diabetes Association: Standards of Medical Care in Diabetes-2011. *Diabetes Care* 34 (Suppl. 1), S11–S61, 2011b

American Diabetes Association: Recommendations for transition from pediatric to adult diabetes care systems. *Diabetes Care* 34:2477–2485, 2011c

American Diabetes Association: Gestational diabetes mellitus. *Diabetes Care* 27 (Suppl. 1):S88–S90, 2004a

American Diabetes Association: Preconception care of women with diabetes. *Diabetes Care* 27 (Suppl. 1):S76–S78, 2004b

Anderson BJ, Wolpert HA: A developmental perspective on the challenges of diabetes education and care during the young adult period. *Patient Education and Counseling* 53:347–352, 2004

Anderson LM, Quinn TA, Glanz K, Ramirez G, Kahwati LC, Johnson DB, et al.: The effectiveness of worksite nutrition and physical activity interventions for controlling employee overweight and obesity: a systematic review. *American Journal of Preventive Medicine* 37:340–357, 2009

Arnett JJ: *Emerging Adulthood: The Winding Road from the Late Teens through the Twenties.* New York, Oxford University Press, 2004

Badr H, Acitelli LK: Dyadic adjustment in chronic illness: does relationship talk matter? *Journal of Family Psychology* 19:465–469, 2005

Bailey BJ, Kahn A: Apportioning illness management authority: how diabetic individuals evaluate and respond to spousal help. *Qualitative Health Research* 3:55–73, 1993

Baltes PB, Smith J: New frontiers in the future of aging: from successful aging of the young old to the dilemmas of the fourth age. *Gerontology* 49:123–135, 2003

Baltes PB: Theoretical propositions of life-span developmental psychology: on dynamics between growth and decline. *Developmental Psychology* 23:611–626, 1987

Baltrusch HJ, Seidel J, Stangel W, Waltz ME: Psychosocial stress, aging and cancer. *Annals of the New York Academy of Sciences* 521:1–15, 1988

Barham K, West S, Trief P, Morrow C, Wade M, Weinstock RS: Diabetes prevention and control in the workplace: a pilot project for county employees. *J Public Health Management Practice* 17:233–241, 2011

Bastida E, Pagan JA: The impact of diabetes on adult employment and earnings of Mexican Americans: findings from a community based effort. *Health Economics* 11:403–413, 2002

Benedict MA, Arterburn D: Worksite-based weight loss programs: a systematic review of recent literature. *American Journal of Health Promotion* 22:408–416, 2008

Black DR, Gleser LJ, Kooyers KJ: A meta-analytic evaluation of couples weight-loss programs. *Health Psychology* 9:330–347, 1990

Brim OG, Ryff CD, Kessler RC, Eds.: *How Healthy Are We? A National Study of Well-Being at Midlife.* Chicago, University of Chicago Press, 2003

Brummett BH, Babyak MA, Barefoot JC, Bosworth HB, Clapp-Channing NE, Siegler IC, et al.: Social support and hostility as predictors of depressive symptoms in cardiac patients one month after hospitalization: a prospective study. *Psychosom Med* 60:707–713, 1998

Bryden KS, Dunger DB, Mayou RA, Peveler RC, Neil HA: Poor prognosis of young adults with type 1 diabetes: a longitudinal study. *Diabetes Care* 26:1052–1057, 2003

Bryden KS, Peveler RC, Stein A, Neil A, Mayou RA, Dunger DB: Clinical and psychological course of diabetes from adolescence to young adulthood: a longitudinal cohort study. *Diabetes Care* 24:1536–1540, 2001

Bryden KS, Neil A, Mayou RA, Peveler RC, Fairburn CG, Dunger DB: Eating habits, body weight, and insulin misuse. A longitudinal study of teenagers and young adults with type 1 diabetes. *Diabetes Care* 22:1956–1960, 1999

Campbell TA: Physical disorder and effectiveness research in marriage and family therapy. In *Effectiveness Research in Marriage and Family Therapy.* Sprenkle D, Ed. Alexandria, VA, American Association for Marriage and Family Therapy, 2002, p. 311–337

Cardenas L, Vallbona C, Baker S, Yusim S: Adult onset DM: glycemic control and family function. *American Journal of the Medical Sciences* 293:28–33, 1987

Centers for Disease Control and Prevention: Pregnancy: diabetes and pregnancy. Available at www.cdc.gov/NCBDDD/pregnancy_gateway/diabetes.html. Accessed 26 July 2010

Charron-Prochownik D, Hannan MF, Fischl AR, Slocum JM: Preconception planning: are we making progress? *Current Diabetes Reports* 8:294–298, 2008

Claesson IM, Sydsjo G, Brynhildsen J, Cedergren M, Jeppsson A, Nystrom F, Sydsjo A, Joseffsson A: Weight gain restriction for obese pregnant women: a case-control intervention study. *BJOG* 115:44–50, 2008

Coyne JC, Fiske V: Couples coping with chronic and catastrophic illness. In *Family Health Psychology.* Nakamatsu TJ, Stephs MAP, Hobfoll SS, Crowther J, Eds. Washington, DC, Hemisphere, 1992, p. 129–149

Crowther CA, Hiller JE, Moss JR, McPhee AJ, Jeffries WS, Robinson JS, et al.: Effect of treatment of gestational diabetes mellitus on pregnancy outcomes. *N Engl J Med* 352:2477–2486, 2005

Cyganek K, Hebda-Szydlo A, Katra B, Skupien J, Klupa T, Janas I, et al.: Glycemic control and selected pregnancy outcomes in type 1 diabetes women on continuous subcutaneous insulin infusion and multiple daily injections: the significance of pregnancy planning. *Diabetes Technology & Therapeutics* 12:41–47, 2010

De Bacquer D, Pelfrene E, Clays E, Mak R, Moreau M, de Smet P, et al.: Perceived job stress and incidence of coronary events: 3-year follow-up of the Belgian Job Stress Project cohort. *American Journal of Epidemiology* 161:434–441, 2005

Diabetes Control and Complications Research Group: The effect of intensive treatment of diabetes on the development and progression of long-term complications in insulin-dependent diabetes mellitus. *N Engl J Med* 329:977–986, 1993

DiMatteo MR: Social support and patient adherence to medical treatment: a meta-analysis. *Health Psychology* 23:207–218, 2004

Dovey-Pearce G, Hurrell R, May C, Walker C, Doherty Y: Young adults' (16-25 years) suggestions for providing developmentally appropriate diabetes services: a qualitative study. *Health & Social Care in the Community* 13:409–419, 2005

Duke DJ: Diabetes in the workplace. *Diabetes Self-Management* 21:62, 64–66, 2004

Eaton WW, Mengel M, Mengel L, Larson D, Campbell R, Montague RB: Psychosocial and psychopathologic influences on management and control of insulin-dependent diabetes. *International Journal of Psychiatry in Medicine* 22:105–117, 1992

Equal Employment Opportunity Commission: Questions and answers about diabetes in the workplace and the Americans with Disabilities Act. Available at www.eeoc.gov/facts/diabetes.html. Accessed 16 July 2010

Eyetsemitan FE, Gire JT: *Aging and Adult Development in the Developing World*. Westport, CT, Praeger, 2003

Fisher L, Chesla CA, Skaff MA, Mullan J, Kanter R: Depression and anxiety among partners of European-American and Latino patients with type 2 diabetes. *Diabetes Care* 25:1564–1570, 2002

Fisher L, Wiehs KL: Can addressing family relationships improve outcomes in chronic disease? Report of the National Working Group on Family-Based Interventions in Chronic Disease. *Journal of Family Practice* 49:561–566, 2000

Fisher L, Chesla CA, Bartz RJ, Gilliss C, Skaff MA, Sabogal F, et al.: The family and type 2 diabetes: a framework for intervention. *Diabetes Educ* 24:599–607, 1998

Fisher L, Ransom DC, Terry HE: The California Family Health Project: VII. Summary and integration of findings. *Family Process* 32:69–86, 1993

Galindo A, Burguillo AG, Azriel S, Fuente Pde L: Outcome of fetuses in women with pregestational diabetes mellitus. *Journal of Perinatal Medicine* 34:323–331, 2006

Gilden JL, Hendryx M, Casia C, Singh SP: The effectiveness of diabetes education programs for older patients and their spouses. *Journal of the American Geriatric Society* 37:1023–1030, 1989

Gonzalez JS, Safren SA, Delahanty LM, Cagliero E, Wexler DJ, Meigs JB, et al.: Symptoms of depression prospectively predict poorer self-care in patients with type 2 diabetes. *Diabet Med* 25:1102–1107, 2008

Gottlieb BH, Wager F: Stress and support processes in close relationships. In *The Social Context of Coping*. Eckenrode J, Ed. New York, Plenum, 1991, p. 165–188

Guralnik JM, Land KC, Blazer D, Fillenbaum GG, Branch LG: Educational status and active life expectancy among older blacks and whites. *N Engl J Med* 329:110–116, 1993

Harden J: Developmental life stage and couples' experiences with prostate cancer: a review of the literature. *Cancer Nursing* 28:85–98, 2005

Health Canada: *Responding to the Challenge of Diabetes in Canada: First Report of the National Diabetes Surveillance System* (Pub H39-4/21-2003E ed.). Ottawa, ON, Ministry of Health, 2003

Heinen L, Darling H: Addressing obesity in the workplace: the role of employers. *Milbank Quarterly* 87:101–122, 2009

Helgeson VS, Cohen S: Social support and adjustment to cancer: reconciling descriptive, correlational, and intervention research. *Health Psychology* 15:135–148, 1996

Herquelot E, Gueguen A, Bonenfant S, Dray-Spira R: Impact of diabetes on work cessation: data from the GAZEL cohort study. *Diabetes Care* 34:1344–1349, 2011

Holmes J, Gear E, Bottomley J, Gibbons S, Murphy M, Williams R: Do people with type 2 diabetes and their careers lose income? (T2ARDIS-4). *Health Policy* 64:291–296, 2003

Holmes-Walker DJ, Llewellyn AC, Farrell K: A transition care programme which improves diabetes control and reduces hospital admission rates in young adults with type 1 diabetes aged 15-25 years. *Diabet Med* 24:764–769, 2007

Jaser SS: Psychological problems in adolescents with diabetes. *Adolescent Medicine: State of the Art Reviews* 21:138–151, x–xi, 2010

Kaplan G: *Reflections on Present and Future Research on Bio-behavioral Risk Factors: New Research Frontiers in Behavioral Medicine, Proceedings of the National Conference*. Washington, DC, NIH, US Government Printing Office, 1994, p. 119–134

Katon W, Russo J, Lin EH, Heckbert SR, Karter AJ, Williams LH, et al.: Diabetes and poor disease control: is comorbid depression associated with poor medica-

tion adherence or lack of treatment intensification? *Psychosom Med* 71:965–972, 2009

Katz DL, O'Connell M, Yeh MC, Nawaz H, Njike V, Anderson LM, et al.: Public health strategies for preventing and controlling overweight and obesity in school and worksite settings: a report on recommendations of the Task Force on Community Preventive Services. *MMWR* 54:1–12, 2005

Keogh KM, White P, Smith SM, McGilloway S, O'Dowd T, Gibney J: Changing illness perceptions in patients with poorly controlled type 2 diabetes: a randomized controlled trial of a family-based intervention: protocol and pilot study. *BMC Family Practice* 8:36, 2007

Kiecolt-Glaser JK, Newton TL: Marriage and health: his and hers. *Psychological Bulletin* 127:472–503, 2001

Kinnunen TI, Pasanen M, Aittasalo M, Fogelholm M, Weiderpass E, Luoto R: Reducing postpartum weight retention—a pilot trial in primary health care. *Nutrition Journal* 6:21, 2007

Kitzmiller JL, Block JM, Brown FM, Catalano PM, Conway DL, Coustan DR, et al.: Managing preexisting diabetes for pregnancy: summary of evidence and consensus recommendations for care. *Diabetes Care* 31:1060–1079, 2008

Kitzmiller JL, Buchanan TA, Kjos S, Combs CA, Ratner RE: Pre-conception care of diabetes, congenital malformations, and spontaneous abortions. *Diabetes Care* 19:514–541, 1996

Kivimaki M, Leino-Arjas P, Luukkonen R, Riihimaki H, Vahtera J, Kirjonen J: Work stress and risk of cardiovascular mortality: prospective cohort study of industrial employees. *BMJ* 325:857, 2002

Klausner EJ, Koenigsberg HW, Skolnick N, Chung H, Rosnick P, Pelino D, et al.: Perceived familial criticism and glucose control in IDDM. *International Journal of Mental Health* 24:64–75, 1995

Kulik JA, Mahler A, Hcika I: Emotional support as a moderator of adjustment and compliance after coronary artery bypass surgery: a longitudinal study. *Journal of Behavioral Medicine* 16:45–63, 1993

Kulik JA, Mahler HI: Social support and recovery from surgery. *Health Psychology* 8:221–238, 1989

Lackman MF: *Psychology of Adult Development*. Miamisburg, OH, Science Direct, 2001

Landon MB, Spong CY, Thom E, Carpenter MW, Ramin SM, Casey B, Wapner RJ, Varner MW, Rouse DJ, Thorp JM Jr, Sciscione A, Catalano P, Harper M, Saade G, Lain KY, Sorokin Y, Peaceman AM, Tolosa JE, Anderson GB: A multicenter, randomized trial of treatment for mild gestational diabetes. *N Engl J Med* 361:1339–1348, 2009

Leckie AM, Graham MK, Grant JB, Ritchie PJ, Frier BM: Frequency, severity, and morbidity of hypoglycemia occurring in the workplace in people with insulin-treated diabetes. *Diabetes Care* 28:1333–1338, 2005

Lewis FM, Woods NF, Hough EE, Bensley LS: The family's functioning with chronic illness in the mother: the spouse's perspective. *Social Science & Medicine* 29:1261–1269, 1989

Lewis MA, McBride CM, Pollak KI, Puleo E, Butterfield RM, Emmons KM: Understanding health behavior change among couples: an interdependence and communal coping approach. *Social Science & Medicine* 62:1369–1380, 2006

Lin FH, Katon W, Von Korff M, Rutter C, Simon GE, Oliver M, et al.: Relationship of depression and diabetes self-care, medication adherence, and preventive care. *Diabetes Care* 27:2154–2160, 2004

Lloyd CE, Robinson N, Andrews B, Elston MA, Fuller JH: Are the social relationships of young insulin-dependent diabetic patients affected by their condition? *Diabet Med* 10:481–485, 1993

Lyons RF, Sullivan MJL, Rivo PG: *Relationships in Chronic Illness and Disability*. Thousand Oaks, CA, Sage Publications, 1995

Martire LM, Schulz R, Helgeson VS, Small BJ, Saghafi EM: Review and meta-analysis of couple-oriented interventions for chronic illness. *Annals of Behavioral Medicine* 40:325–342, 2010

Martire LM, Lustig AP, Schulz R, Miller GE, Helgeson VS: Is it beneficial to involve a family member? A meta-analysis of psychosocial interventions for chronic illness. *Health Psychology* 23:599–611, 2004

Mayfield JA, Deb P, Whitecotton L: Work disability and diabetes. *Diabetes Care* 22:1105–1109, 1999

McBride CM, Baucom DH, Peterson BL, Pollak KI, Palmer C, Westman E, et al.: Prenatal and postpartum smoking abstinence a partner-assisted approach. *Am J Prev Med* 27:232–238, 2004

McBroom LA, Enriquez M: Review of family-centered interventions to enhance the health outcomes of children with type 1 diabetes. *Diabetes Educ* 35:428–438, 2009

McCall DT, Sauaia A, Hamman RF, Reusch JE, Barton P: Are low-income elderly patients at risk for poor diabetes care? *Diabetes Care* 27:1060–1065, 2004

McDonagh JE, Minnaar G, Kelly K, O'Connor D, Shaw KL: Unmet education and training needs in adolescent health of health professionals in a UK children's hospital. *Acta Paediatrica* 95:715–719, 2006

McDonagh JE, Southwood TR, Shaw KL, British Paediatric Rheumatology Group: Unmet education and training needs of rheumatology health professionals in adolescent health and transitional care. *Rheumatology* 43:737–743, 2004

McLean N, Griffin S, Toney K, Hardeman W: Family involvement in weight control, weight maintenance and weight-loss interventions: a systematic review of randomised trials. *International Journal of Obesity and Related Metabolic Disorders* 27:987–1005, 2003

McMahon BT, West SL, Mansouri M, Belongia L: Workplace discrimination and diabetes: the EEOC Americans with Disabilities Act research project. *Work* 25:9–18, 2005

Michel B, Charron-Prochownik D: Diabetes nurse educators and preconception counseling. *Diabetes Educ* 32:108–116, 2006

Mollenkopf J, Waters MC, Holdaway J, Kasinitz P: The ever-winding path: ethnic and racial diversity in the transition to adulthood. In *On the Frontier of Adulthood: Theory, Research, and Public Policy*. Settersten RA Jr, Furstenberg FF Jr, Rumbaut RG, Eds. Chicago, University of Chicago Press, 2005, p. 454–497

Munir F, Leka S, Griffiths A: Dealing with self-management of chronic illness at work: predictors for self-disclosure. *Social Science & Medicine* 60:1397–1407, 2005

Newman B, Newman P: *Development Through Life: A Psychosocial Approach*. Belmont, CA, Wadsworth Publishing, 1999

Osgood DW, Ruth G, Eccles JS, Jacobs JE, Barber BL: Six paths to adulthood: fast starters, parents without careers, educated partners, educated singles, working singles, and slow starters. In *On the Frontier of Adulthood: Theory, Research and Public Policy*. Settersten RA Jr, Furstenberg FF Jr, Rumbaut RG, Eds. Chicago, University of Chicago Press, 2005, p. 320–355

Pacaud D, Crawford S, Stephure DK, Dean HJ, Couch R, Dewey D: Effect of type 1 diabetes on psychosocial maturation in young adults. *Journal of Adolescent Health* 40:29–35, 2007

Palmer CA, Baucom DH, McBride CM: Couple approaches to smoking cessation. In *The Psychology of Couples and Illness*. Schmaling T, Sher TG, Eds. Washington, DC, American Psychological Association, 2000, p. 311–336

Peveler RC, Bryden KS, Neil HA, Fairburn CG, Mayou RA, Dunger DB, et al.: The relationship of disordered eating habits and attitudes to clinical outcomes in young adult females with type 1 diabetes. *Diabetes Care* 28:84–88, 2005

Peyrot M, McMurry JF, Hedges R: Marital adjustment to adult diabetes: interpersonal congruence and spouse satisfaction. *Journal of Marriage & the Family* 50:363–376, 1988

Polonsky WH, Anderson BJ, Lohrer PA, Aponte JE, Jacobson AM, Cole CF: Insulin omission in women with IDDM. *Diabetes Care* 17:1178–1185, 1994

Poston L, Harthoorn LF, Van Der Beek EM: Obesity in pregnancy: implications for the mother and lifelong health of the child. A consensus statement. *Pediatric Research* 69:175–180, 2011

Ramsey S, Summers KH, Leong SA, Birnbaum HG, Kemner JE, Greenberg P: Productivity and medical costs of diabetes in a large employer population. *Diabetes Care* 25:23–29, 2002

Rasmussen K, Yaktine A: *Weight Gain During Pregnancy: Reexamining the Guidelines*. Washington, DC, National Academies Press, 2008

Revenson RA: Social support and marital coping with chronic illness. *Annals of Behavioral Medicine* 16:122–130, 1994

Revenson TA, Majerovitz SD: The effects of chronic illness on the spouse. Social resources as stress buffers. *Arthritis Care Res* 4:63–72, 1991

Roberts SE, Goldacre MJ, Neil HA: Mortality in young people admitted to hospital for diabetes: database study. *BMJ* 328:741–742, 2004

Rydall AC, Rodin GM, Olmsted MP, Devenyi RG, Daneman D: Disordered eating behavior and microvascular complications in young women with insulin-dependent diabetes mellitus. *N Engl J Med* 336:1849–1854, 1997

Saarni C, Crowley M: The development of emotion regulation: effects on emotional state and expression. In *Emotions and the Family: For Better or For Worse*. Blechman E, Ed. Hillsdale, NJ, Lawrence Erlbaum Associates, 1990, p. 53–74

Schafer LC, McKaul KD, Glasgow RE: Supportive and non-supportive family behaviors: relationship to adherence and metabolic control in persons with type 1 diabetes. *Diabetes Care* 9:179–185, 1986

Schmaling KB, Sher TB: *The Psychology of Couples and Illness: Theory, Research, and Practice*. Washington, DC, American Psychological Association, 2000

Temple RC, Aldridge VJ, Murphy HR: Prepregnancy care and pregnancy outcomes in women with type 1 diabetes. *Diabetes Care* 29:1744–1749, 2006

Testa MA, Simonson DC: Health economic benefits and quality of life during improved glycemic control in patients with type 2 diabetes mellitus: a randomized, controlled, double-blind trial. *JAMA* 280:1490–1496, 1998

TODAY Study Group, Zeitler P, Epstein L, Grey M, Hirst K, Kaufman F, Tamborlane W, Wilfley D: Treatment options for type 2 diabetes in adolescents and youth: a study of the comparative efficacy of metformin alone or in combination with rosiglitazone or lifestyle intervention in adolescents with type 2 diabetes. *Pediatric Diabetes* 8:74–87, 2007

Trief PM, Sandberg JG, Fisher L, Dimmock JA, Scales K, Hessler D, Weinstock RS: Challenges and lessons learned in the development and implementation of a couples-focused telephone intervention for adults with type 2 diabetes: the Diabetes Support Project. *Translational Behavioral Medicine* 2011a, doi: 10.1007/s13142-011-0057-8.

Trief PM, Sandberg JG, Ploutz-Snyder R, Brittain R, Cibula D, Scales K, Weinstock RS: Promoting couples collaboration in type 2 diabetes: the diabetes support project pilot data. *Families, Systems & Health* 29:253–261, 2011b, doi: 10.1037/a0024564.

Trief PM, Morin PC, Izquierdo R, Teresi J, Starren J, Shea S, et al.: Marital quality and diabetes outcomes: the IDEATel project. *Families, Systems & Health* 24:318–331, 2006

Trief PM, Wade MJ, Brittain KD, Weinstock RS: A prospective analysis of marital relationship factors and quality of life in diabetes. *Diabetes Care* 25:1154–1158, 2005

Trief PM, Ploutz-Snyder R, Brittain KD, Weinstock RS: The relationship between marital quality and adherence to the diabetes care regimen. *Annals of Behavioral Medicine* 27:148–154, 2004

Trief PM, Sandberg J, Greenberg RP, Graff K, Castranova N, Yoon M, et al.: Describing support: a qualitative study of couples living with diabetes. *Families, Systems & Health* 21:57–67, 2003

Trief PM, Himes CL, Orendorff R, Weinstock RS: The marital relationship and psychosocial adaptation and glycemic control of individuals with diabetes. *Diabetes Care* 24:1384–1389, 2001

Trief PM, Aquilino C, Paradies K, Weinstock RS: Impact of the work environment on glycemic control and adaptation to diabetes. *Diabetes Care* 22:569–574, 1999

Trief PM, Grant W, Elbert K, Weinstock RS: Family environment, glycemic control and the psychosocial adaptation of adults with diabetes. *Diabetes Care* 11:241–245, 1998

Troxel WM, Matthews KA, Gallo LC, Kuller LH: Marital quality and occurrence of the metabolic syndrome in women. *Archives of Internal Medicine* 165:1022–1027, 2005

Tunceli K, Bradley CJ, Lafata JE, Pladevall M, Divine GW, Goodman AC, et al.: Glycemic control and absenteeism among individuals with diabetes. *Diabetes Care* 30:1283–1285, 2007

Uchino BN, Cacioppo JT, Kiecolt-Glaser JK: The relationship between social support and psychological processes: a review with emphasis on underlying mechanisms and implications for health. *Psychological Bulletin* 119:488–531, 1996

Valdmanis V, Smith DW, Page MR: Productivity and economic burden associated with diabetes. *American Journal of Public Health* 91:129–130, 2001

Van Walleghem N, MacDonald CA, Dean HJ: Building connections for young adults with type 1 diabetes mellitus in Manitoba: feasibility and acceptability of a transition initiative. *Chronic Diseases in Canada* 27:130–134, 2006

Vijan S, Hayward RA, Langa KM: The impact of diabetes on workforce participation: results from a national household sample. *Health Services Research* 39 (6 Pt 1):1653–1669, 2004

Von Korff M, Katon W, Lin EH, Simon G, Ciechanowski P, Ludman E, et al.: Work disability among individuals with diabetes. *Diabetes Care* 28:1326–1332, 2005

Weissberg-Benchell J, Wolpert H, Anderson BJ: Transitioning from pediatric to adult care: a new approach to the post-adolescent young persons with type 1 diabetes. *Diabetes Care* 30:2441–2446, 2007

Whittaker C: Transfer of young adults with type 1 diabetes from pediatric to adult diabetes care. *Diabetes Quarterly* (Spring):10–14, 2004

Wing RR, Marcus MD, Epstein LH, Jawad A: A family based approach to the treatment of obese type II diabetic patients. *Journal of Consulting & Clinical Psychology* 59:156–162, 1991

Wolff S, Legarth J, Vansgaard K, Toubro S, Astrup A: A randomized trial of the effects of dietary counseling on gestational weight gain and glucose metabolism in obese pregnant women. *International Journal of Obesity* 32:495–501, 2008

Wrightsman LS: *Adult Personality Development: Theories and Concepts*. Thousand Oaks, CA, Sage Publications, 1994

Wysocki T, Nansel TR, Holmbeck GN, Chen R, Laffel L, Anderson BJ, et al.: Collaborative involvement of primary and secondary caregivers: associations with youths' diabetes outcomes. *Journal of Pediatric Psychology* 34:869–881, 2009

第十六章

糖尿病相关功能损害和残疾

功能和残疾的评估和诊断

世界卫生组织的功能、残疾和健康国际分类（ICF）作为健康和残疾的诊断及分类框架可以用于临床、社会、政策、经济和研究。ICF 将健康和功能分为三个水平：身体或部分身体，整个人和社会背景中的整个人。残疾被定义为以下一个或多个区域出现功能障碍。

受损（身体功能或结构的问题如明显移位或丧失）

■ 身体功能——身体系统的生理功能（包括心理和认知功能）。

■ 身体结构——身体的解剖部位如器官、肢体，以及其组成部分。

活动和参与（一项任务或动作的执行和生活情况）

■ 活动受限——个体在执行活动时可能存在的困难。

■ 参与限制——个体在生活状况中可能经历的困难。

包含活动受限和参与受限的生命活动都与社会心理的功能有关，包括：学习和应用知识、进行日常活动、交流、运动、自我保健（包括照顾和保持自我健康）、家务劳动、人际交流和关系、主要的生活领域（包括教育、工作、经济生活），以及社区、社会和公民生活。另外，ICF 残疾框架还指出环境因素的作用，并鼓励考虑产品和科技、自然环境支持、关系、态度，以及服务、系统和政策对损伤、活动和参与的影响。

糖尿病作为一种致残疾病

ICF 框架内，残疾是影响大多数糖尿病患者的事情。如果扩大到所有人在生活的一个或多个领域都可能受到疾病的影响，每一个糖尿病患者都经历某种程度的残疾。糖尿病是一种受美国残疾法修正案保护的慢性疾病（http://www.diabetes.org/living-with-diabetes/know–your-rights/discrimination/employment-discrimination/Americans-with-diabilities-act-amendments-act）。糖尿病患者身体残疾的患病率及新发残疾的发病率为无糖尿病个体的两倍。这额外的残疾负担独立于糖尿病的并发症和合并症。关心糖尿病患者可以影响其生活的多个方面包括自我管理、主要生命活动如工作或休闲及人际关系。ICF 框架内，环境因素如态度、科技和其他人的支持被认为可以潜在减少或增加疾病的影响，如糖尿病对患者生命活动的影响。

除了糖尿病作为一种致残疾病本身的影响，糖尿病并发症也会带来很多的限制、活动损害及参与受限。患有糖尿病并发症的患者由于糖尿病相关残疾可能影响情绪、生活质量、心理和人际关系及糖尿病自我管理，因此可能被认为是一个特殊群体。

糖尿病足溃疡和截肢

在美国，糖尿病引起 60%以上的非创伤性截肢，而且每年糖尿病患者的截肢＞65 000 例。周围神经病变在成人糖尿病患者中的患病率为 30%，是导致足部伤口和下肢截肢的主要原因之一。出现任何足部并发症（如足溃疡、未截肢的愈合伤口或截肢）的 1 型和 2 型糖尿病患者其生活质量低于无足部问题的糖尿病患者。足部溃疡或截肢患者的心理症状和不适包括轻至中度的抑郁症状、因担心伤口和足部产生的焦虑症状、对其足部的负面感受、态度和自我意识、对症状和治疗感到不可预知及疼痛或幻痛。因为害怕感染或溃疡复发及在溃疡期间比截肢后出现更多的制动，足溃疡引起的情感障碍可能比截肢要多。足溃疡或截肢的患者身体功能下降、日常活动能力降低、自我保健能力减弱、药物依从性变差、社会和家庭角色受到影响。关于截肢，术前患者就已经对截肢后的生活存在心理担忧，包括害怕和担心未来的经济状况及截肢后不能参加社会活动和功能行为（如行走、驾车）。某些糖尿病患者在面对即将来临的截肢时，可能出现严重的抑郁甚至自杀。糖尿病足患者的护理人员及配偶也会经历心理的不适。可能存在的担忧包括糖尿病足患者的日常功能和活动受损，护理人员所面对的责任和任务，以及足溃疡对失业和家庭生活的影响。

周围神经病变不仅是导致糖尿病足溃疡和下肢截肢的主要原因，还可以引起功能损害和活动及参与受限。周围神经病变引起的身体损害会导致不能工作。慢性神经性疼痛，其在神经病变的患者中为11%～32%，是引起心理不适、抑郁、睡眠障碍及生活质量降低的另一原因。

对于治疗，有糖尿病患者截肢后的康复指南，内容包括情绪、功能损害和导致生活质量下降的活动和参与问题。对于慢性疼痛引起的限制，有证据表明认知行为治疗对于成人慢性、非头痛性疼痛的疗效有限。然而，还需要进一步研究来判断心理干预对糖尿病足溃疡及肢体丧失的患者其慢性疼痛、疼痛的处理、自我保健和生活质量的影响。

一项随机对照研究表明固定的同伴自我管理干预，但并非是一个同伴支持小组的干预，对肢体丧失的患者多个心理结局改善是有效的。提高残疾人生活技能（PALS）的研究，其中共纳入500名截肢者，约37%是由于糖尿病所导致的，结果发现有经过培训的截肢同伴进行的九次（每次90分钟）结构化自我管理干预可以降低抑郁和功能受损的可能性并提高自我效能。

糖尿病相关视力受损和失明

糖尿病视网膜病变在美国每年导致 12 000～24 000 的新发失明病例，糖尿病是20～74岁人群中新发失明的主要原因。出现糖尿病相关视力受损或失明的糖尿病患者有发生社会心理痛苦的风险，包括焦虑、恐惧、抑郁症状、躯体化、容易受伤害、生活质量差及家庭危机的风险。即使在失明之前，糖尿病视网膜病变的患者也可能报告对目前或未来失明的焦虑。导致生活质量降低的因素包括独立性降低、控制感/能力丢失、休闲和社会活动参与受限及由于活动受限导致的日常活动能力下降。家庭中，糖尿病导致的视力损害是婚姻关系的重要压力源，与较高的夫妻分居比率相关。

视力受损和失明的患者在糖尿病自我管理的参与也受到限制。参与自我管理的障碍包括：对卫生保健专业知识不能理解、行动及出行不便导致不能及时就诊、参加教育活动或互助小组、缺少可获得的糖尿病相关健康信息，以及缺乏便携式的糖尿病设备。这些障碍都导致患者在卫生保健过程中的控制感和参与感下降。

糖尿病患者初发视力受损或失明后的心理适应性治疗领域仍被忽视。还需要研究情绪或调节障碍的患病率及个体和婚姻/家庭干预措施。有研究已经探讨了糖尿病伴视力受损患者的教育诉求，而且发现专门针对视力受损患者的糖尿病设计的自我管理计划在改善生活质量、自我依赖和糖尿病自我管理技能方面具有一定作用。

卒中和心肌梗死带来的心理后遗症

糖尿病患者中心血管疾病的患病率约为 30%（http://www.cdc.gov/diabetes/pubs/estimates11.htm#12），糖尿病患者卒中的风险高出 200%～400%。卒中或心肌梗死后常见的心理并发症包括抑郁、认知障碍、生活质量下降及影响日常生活能力的功能受损。卒中或心肌梗死后的抑郁死亡率更高。

家庭成员和保健工作者也经历与管理负担及受损和残疾对角色功能、人际关系和生活质量带来的影响相关的恐惧、担忧和抑郁症状。保健工作者的痛苦主要来自于心肌梗死后患者恢复不佳。对保健工作者进行压力、幸福感、角色转换、关系担忧，以及经济问题方面的心理干预可以改善卒中或心肌梗死后保健工作者的生活质量。

越来越多的证据表明卒中后的康复可以使糖尿病患者和非糖尿病患者都获得相似的整体功能改善（包括活动、认知、交流和个人日常生活照料）。然而，尚需要研究来判断语言、视力、认知、行动方面的损害对自我管理行为和参加糖尿病保健的影响。

卒中后出现轻瘫（乏力）和瘫痪并影响到手的使用的患者中，自我注射胰岛素和自我血糖监测也受到负面影响，从而导致自我管理的独立性丧失，并明显影响生活质量和功能健康状态。病例研究已经关注了卒中后偏瘫的患者自我管理活动受限的问题。这些病例表明通过设计能够弥补功能损害并能够利用保留的功能来完成任务的装置，可以恢复自我管理能力或胰岛素注射。

糖尿病患者的认知障碍和痴呆

认知障碍和失忆会导致糖尿病患者额外的残疾负担。老年糖尿病患者阿尔茨海默病的风险增加 50%～100%，血管性痴呆的风险增加100%～150%。糖尿病还与轻度认知受损和神经影像表现为结构功能性异常有关。执行功能、处理速度和记忆容易出现减退，也是非糖尿病对照组中最常研究的领域。

出现认知障碍的症状及进行性痴呆对家庭和保健工作者的情感和心理具有毁灭性影响。糖尿病对其影响程度还不清楚。同样，还需要研究糖尿病及其管理对保健工作者压力、负担和行为的相互影响。

非痴呆的糖尿病患者出现认知障碍，则日常生活中的器械性活动（如使用电话、外出长途旅行、购物、做饭、做家务、操作性工作、洗衣、服药和管理钱财）需要一定的辅助，同时对这种功能损害意识较差。然而，尚需要研究来判断轻度、中度和重度认知障碍对糖尿病自我管理如服药、自我血糖监测、健康饮食、体育锻炼和处理急性高和低血糖的影响。

一项研究表明存在轻度和中度认知障碍的成年 2 型糖尿病患者在接受方便而实用的打印和口头表述方法的糖尿病自我管理教育后展现出一定的学习能力。另外，随访性随机对照试验在认知受损的人群中检验了基于问题解决的糖尿病自我管理训练，结果显示一种采用方便可行材料进行的九次结构化计划可以提高糖尿病知识、问题解决能力、自我管理和糖尿病控制。

认知障碍对糖尿病患者的情绪、处理、生活质量的影响还需进一步研究。而且，还需要研究认知干预（如认知康复、药物）的时间及其对糖尿病认知障碍患者实施自我管理活动的影响效果。最后，还需要进行糖尿病认知障碍或痴呆患者进行糖尿病自我管理辅助培训方法及如何有效进行糖尿病管理辅助的研究。

智力残疾

智力残疾（ID）的患者智力功能（通常 IQ＜70～75 分）和适应性行为方面明显受损，而且在 18 岁之前就出现残疾（http://www.aamr.org/cntent_100.cfm?navID=21）。研究已经显示 ID 患者中糖尿病的患病率为 11%～24%，部分是来源于 ID 人群中超重和肥胖的患病率。尽管糖尿病的患病率较高，但仍缺乏 ID 人群中糖尿病状况的研究。定性研究发现 ID 伴糖尿病的患者可能体验丧失感、缺乏控制，以及不能获得可理解的糖尿病自我管理的信息，然而专业的保健工作者也可能苦于缺乏糖尿病知识，且在自我管理过程中是自主还是辅助的两难境地中挣扎。未来还需要研究来明确这一群体的心理需求，并设计和验证以 ID 伴糖尿病患者及它们的保健工作者共同需求为目标的干预措施的有效性。

临床保健的建议

足溃疡和截肢

1. 康复心理师、咨询师，以及经过培训能对功能损害和残疾的适应进行评估和干预的健康心理师，可能适合对足溃疡和伤口、慢性疼痛，以及下肢截肢相关的心理痛苦和适应来进行评估和治疗安排。

2. 作为保健的一部分，采用标准的问卷或访视表来评估功能或损害、认知能力包括精神健康状况。

3. 对于如何处理慢性疼痛，建议使用认知-行为治疗。这种方法可以改善情绪并且减轻痛苦。

4. 应筛查具有足溃疡风险的糖尿病患者是否存在抑郁，因为会使患病时抑郁风险增加，而且足部护理恶化的可能性增加。

5. 建议参加能够提供社区融入（平衡感情和处理健康、恢复家庭角色和社区活动、休闲活动的措施）的康复计划及职业康复（评估和计划职业能力和机会、教育需求）。

6. 下肢截肢后，除了继续康复训练以恢复活动和参与日常生活及糖尿病自我管理以外，还应该进行心理需求及精神健康的评估。另外，结构化同伴自我管理干预对于改善截肢后的心理结局也有帮助。

视力受损和失明

1. 建议开展糖尿病自我管理教育计划及专门为视力受损或失明患者设计的康复计划。重点以处理、更新糖尿病知识、辅助选择适当的自我管理设备、训练患者使用适应性器械（如注射器放大镜、注射器装药装置和有语言功能及可触摸辅助功能的血糖监测设备）和低视力措施等方面干预为主。

2. 提高视力受损和失明患者参与糖尿病自我管理，包括以下几点

（1）建议采用具有特殊功能的试纸和血糖监测仪，如语言输出、适当尺寸、建议模版、操作方法、试纸使用方法和可触摸。

（2）提供对视力无要求或仅语音格式和包括字体、背景颜色和纸张等符合低视力指南要求的糖尿病教育纸质材料。

（3）使用剂量调整更方便、更耐用、且有使用说明和错误操作说明的胰岛素注射工具。

（4）使用胰岛素泵，包括使用具备语音输出功能的胰岛素泵时，应保证对比清晰，且字体较大。

（5）保证纸张材料、血糖监测仪和胰岛素泵，适合失明和视力受损患者，但目前，糖尿病自我管理工具仅具备部分特征而并非全部特征。

3. 向有循证医学证据的心理治疗转诊，当确定抑郁、焦虑、难以适应受损或残疾、糖尿病相关视力受损或失明而导致的家庭配偶压力时建议行认知行为治疗和人际关系治疗。

4 建议确认视力受损的患者依靠人际支持来监测或辅助治疗方案的执行。

卒中和心梗

1. 因为残疾并不意味着不能进行糖尿病自我管理，建议对所有卒中后或心肌梗死后残疾的患者进行糖尿病自我管理相关的功能限制和能力

评估（如手灵活性、视力和认知功能），并为其提供合理的场所，包括教育工具和糖尿病设备。重点在于患者是否能独立进行糖尿病自我管理行为或是否需要帮助或监督。

2. 建议对卒中后认知受损的患者进行认知康复，采用纠正措施和代偿训练。根据指南应采用目前基于循证且证明有效的措施。另外，卒中后患者增加活动和个人保健、适应日常器械性活动和维持交流方面的治疗应遵循指南。保持个人保健和交流是糖尿病卒中后患者健康的关键。

3. 对于卒中后由于瘫痪而不能自我注射胰岛素或自我血糖监测的糖尿病患者可以使用辅助装置以帮助其单手独立进行糖尿病自我管理。

4. 建议卒中或心肌梗死后筛查抑郁和其他不能适应疾病的心理表现。功能恢复差及死亡率高与抑郁/明显心理疾病相关。健康管理保健专业人员应根据操作标准和指南进行心理和认知筛查或神经心理评估，包括试验选择、使用和修改。

5. 基于循证的心理治疗包括用于治疗糖尿病患者卒中后的抑郁、焦虑、受损或残疾适应困难及心理应激的认知行为治疗和人际关系治疗。当向功能或认知障碍的患者如卒中后的患者进行心理治疗或咨询时，应特别注意感觉缺陷和信息加工困难对完全投入治疗的影响。

6. 仔细评估卒中或心肌梗死后的身体系统、功能状态和心理状态后如果发现受损明显，则可能是适应较差及出现严重的后遗症，这时应考虑给予药物治疗。抗抑郁药一直被用于卒中后抑郁的治疗。尽管不能加速认知或功能恢复，但氟西汀的耐受性好且可以缓解卒中后抑郁症状。去甲替林可以缓解卒中后抑郁而且可以改善焦虑症状并提高日常活动的功能恢复。去甲替林和氟西汀减少卒中后数年的死亡率。

7. 建议对糖尿病相关残疾患者的家庭成员和保健人员提供卒中或心肌梗死后应激/危象的处理和咨询以明确受损或残疾的影响并提高保健人员的生活质量。

认知受损

1. 采用方便易行且清晰简单的糖尿病自我管理教育以促进轻度至中度的认知受损患者学习。

2. 如果怀疑存在认知受损，应该采用标准的神经心理测量方法和程序来明确认知受损的程度和类型。对糖尿病可疑合并或明确合并认知功能障碍的患者应遵循现有推荐的认知受损和痴呆的评估和干预指南。

3. 评估和治疗认知障碍范畴内的情绪状态应遵循标准的和普遍接受的准则并采用标准的诊断工具或正规精神访视工具，如 SCID。

4. 糖尿病管理团队应该对帮助认知障碍、痴呆或智力受损患者进行糖尿病自我管理的保健人员教育和训练。

参 考 文 献

American Association of Diabetes Educators (AADE): Diabetes education for people with disabilities. *Diabetes Educ* 28:916–921, 2002

American Association on Intellectual and Developmental Disabilities: Definition of Intellectual Disability. Available at http://www.aamr.org/content_100.cfm?navID=21. Accessed 20 July 2012

American Diabetes Association: Americans with Disabilities Act Amendments Act. Available at http://www.diabetes.org/living-with-diabetes/know-your-rights/discrimination/employment-discrimination/americans-with-disabilities-act-amendments-act/. Accessed 2 July 2012

American Educational Research Association, American Psychological Association, National Council on Measurement in Education: Testing individuals with disabilities. In *Standards for Educational and Psychological Testing*. Washington, DC, American Educational Research Association, 1999, p. 101–108

American Geriatrics Society Clinical Practice Committee: Guidelines Abstracted from the American Academy of Neurology's Dementia Guidelines for Early Detection, Diagnosis. and Management of Dementia. *J Am Geriatr Soc* 51:869–873, 2003

Antman EM, Anbe DT, Armstrong PW, Bates ER, Green LA, et al.: ACC/AHA guidelines for the management of patients with ST-elevation myocardial infarction: a report of the American College of Cardiology/American Heart Association Task Force on Practice Guidelines (Committee to Revise the 1999 Guidelines for the Management of Patients with Acute Myocardial Infarction). *Circulation* 110:e82–e292, 2004

Argoff CE, Cole BE, Fishbain DA, Irving GA: Diabetic peripheral neuropathic pain: clinical and quality-of-life issues. *Mayo Clin Proc* 81 (4 Suppl.):S3–S11, 2006

Bernbaum M, Wittry S, Stich T, Brusca S, Albert SG: Effectiveness of a diabetes education program adapted for people with vision impairment. *Diabetes Care* 23:1430–1432, 2000

Bernbaum M, Albert SG, Duckro PN, Merkel W: Personal and family stress in individuals with diabetes and vision loss. *J Clin Psychol* 49:670–677, 1993

Bernbaum M, Albert SG, Brusca SR, Drimmer A, Duckro PN, et al.: A model clinical program for patients with diabetes and vision impairment. *Diabetes Educ* 15:325–330, 1989

Bernbaum M, Albert SG, Brusca SR, Drimmer A, Duckro PN: Promoting diabetes self-management and independence in the visually impaired: a model clinical program. *Diabetes Educ* 14:51–54, 1988a

Bernbaum M, Albert SG, Duckro PN: Psychosocial profiles in patients with visual impairment due to diabetic retinopathy. *Diabetes Care* 11:551–557, 1988b

Biessels GJ, Staekenborg S, Brunner E, Brayne C, Scheltens P: Risk of dementia in diabetes mellitus: a systematic review. *Lancet Neurology* 5:64–74, 2006

Bogey RA, Geis CC, Bryant PR, Moroz A, O'Neill BJ: Stroke and neurodegenerative disorders. 3. stroke: rehabilitation management. *Archives of Physical Medicine and Rehabilitation* 85 (3 Suppl.):S15–S20, 2004

Bowen A, Lincoln NB, Dewey M: Cognitive rehabilitation for spatial neglect following stroke. *Cochrane Database Syst Rev* CD003586, 2007

Brod M: Quality of life issues in patients with diabetes and lower extremity ulcers: patients and care givers. *Qual Life Res* 7:365–372, 1998

Butler JV, Whittington JE, Holland AJ, Boer H, Clarke D, Webb T: Prevalence of, and risk factors for, physical ill-health in people with Prader-Willi syndrome: a population based study. *Developmental Medicine and Child Neurology* 44:248–255, 2002

Cameron JI, Cheung AM, Streiner DL, Coyte PC, Stewart DE: Stroke survivors' behavioral and psychologic symptoms are associated with informal caregivers' experiences of depression. *Archives of Physical Medicine and Rehabilitation* 87:177–183, 2006

Candrilli SD, Davis KL, Kan HJ, Lucero MA, Rousculp MD: Prevalence and the associated burden of illness of symptoms of diabetic peripheral neuropathy and diabetic retinopathy. *J Diabetes Complications* 21:306–314, 2007

Cardol M, Rijken M, van Schrojenstein Lantman-de Valk H: People with mild to moderate intellectual disability talking about their diabetes and how they manage. *Journal of Intellectual Disability Research* 56:351–360, 2012

Cardol M, Rijken M, van Schrojenstein Lantman-de Valk H: Attitudes and dilemmas of caregivers supporting people with intellectual disabilities who have diabetes. *Patient Educ Couns* 87:383–388, 2011, doi:10.1016/j.pec.2011.11.010

Carrington AL, Mawdsley SK, Morley J, Kincey J, Boulton AJ: Psychological status of diabetic people with or without lower limb disability. *Diabetes Res Clin Pract* 32:19–25, 1996

Cate Y, Baker SS, Gilbert MP: Occupational therapy and the person with diabetes and vision impairment. *Am J Occup Ther* 49:905–911, 1995

Centers for Disease Control and Prevention. National diabetes fact sheet: national estimates and general information on diabetes and prediabetes in the United States, 2011. Atlanta, U.S. Department of Health and Human Services, Centers for Disease Control and Prevention, 2011. Available from http://www.cdc.gov/diabetes/pubs/factsheet11.htm. Accessed 19 September 2012

Centers for Disease Control and Prevention: *Scientific and Technical Information Simply Put*. 2nd ed. Atlanta, Centers for Disease Control and Prevention, 1999

Chambless DL: Compendium of empirically supported therapies. In *Psychologists' Desk Reference*. 2nd ed. Koocher GP, Norcross JC, Hill SS, Eds. Oxford, Oxford University Press, 2005

Christman A, Vannorsdall T, Hill-Briggs F, Schretlen D: Cranial volume, mild cognitive deficits and functional limitations associated with diabetes in a community sample. *Arch Clin Neuropsychol* 25:49–59, 2010

Cicerone KD, Dahlberg C, Malec JF, Langenbahn DM, Felicetti T, et al.: Evidence-based cognitive rehabilitation: updated review of the literature from 1998 through 2002. *Archives of Physical Medicine and Rehabilitation* 86:1681–1692, 2005

Clare L, Woods RT, Moniz Cook ED, Orrell M, Spector A: Cognitive rehabilitation and cognitive training for early-stage Alzheimer's disease and vascular dementia. *Cochrane Database Syst Rev* CD003260, 2003

Cox DJ, Kiernan BD, Schroeder DB, Cowley M: Psychosocial sequelae of visual loss in diabetes. *Diabetes Educ* 24:481–484, 1998

Coyne KS, Margolis MK, Kennedy-Martin T, Baker TM, Klein R, Paul MD, Revicki DA: The impact of diabetic retinopathy: perspectives from patient focus groups. *Fam Pract* 21:447–453, 2004

Duncan PW, Zorowitz R, Bates B, Choi JY, Glasberg JJ, et al.: Management of adult stroke rehabilitation care: a clinical practice guideline. *Stroke* 36:e100–e143, 2005

Eccleston C, Williams AC, Morley S: Psychological therapies for the management of chronic pain (excluding headache) in adults. *Cochrane Database Syst Rev* CD007407, 2009. doi: 10.1002/14651858.CD007407.pub2

Engelgau MM, Geiss LS, Saaddine JB, Boyle JP, Benjamin SM, et al.: The evolving diabetes burden in the United States. *Ann Intern Med* 140:945–950, 2004

Esquenazi A, Meier RH 3rd: Rehabilitation in limb deficiency. 4. Limb amputation. *Archives of Physical Medicine and Rehabilitation* 77 (3 Suppl.):S18–S28, 1996

Etters L, Goodall D, Harrison BE: Caregiver burden among dementia patient caregivers: a review of the literature. *J Am Acad Nurse Pract* 20:423–428, 2008

First MB, Spitzer RL, Gibbon M, Williams JBW: *Structured Clinical Interview for DSM-IV Axis I Disorders, Clinician Version (SCID-CV)*. Washington, DC,

American Psychiatric Press, 1996

Frasure-Smith N, Lesperance F, Talajic M: Depression and 18-month prognosis after myocardial infarction. *Circulation* 91:999–1005, 1995

Fruehwald S, Gatterbauer E, Rehak P, Baumhackl U: Early fluoxetine treatment of post-stroke depression. *Journal of Neurology* 250:347–351, 2003

Golden SH, Hill-Briggs F, Williams K, Stolka K, Mayer RS: Management of diabetes during acute stroke and inpatient stroke rehabilitation. *Archives of Physical Medicine and Rehabilitation* 86:2377–2384, 2005

Goodrige D, Trepman E, Sloan J, Guse L, Strain LA, McIntyre J, Embil JM: Quality of life of adults with unhealed and healed diabetic foot ulcers. *Foot Ankle Int* 27:274–280, 2006

Gore M, Brandenburg NA, Hoffman DL, Tai KS, Stacey B: Burden of illness in painful diabetic peripheral neuropathy: the patients' perspectives. *J Pain* 7:892–900, 2006

Gregg EW, Mangione CM, Cauley JA, Thompson TJ, Schwartz AV, et al.: Diabetes and incidence of functional disability in older women. *Diabetes Care* 25:61–67, 2002

Hackett ML, Anderson CS: Predictors of depression after stroke: a systematic review of observational studies. *Stroke* 36:2296–2301, 2005

Harvey RL, Stachowski KM, Dewulf SK: Independent insulin administration by the hemiplegic patient: stabilization of an insulin pen with a new device. *Arch Phys Med Rehabil* 73:779–781, 1992

Hill-Briggs F, Lazo M, Peyrot M, Chang Y, Doswell A, Hill M, Levine D, Wang N, Brancati F: Effect of problem-solving-based diabetes self-management training on diabetes control in a low income patient sample. *J Gen Intern Med* 26:972–978, 2011

Hill-Briggs F, Lazo M, Renosky R, Ewing C: Usability of a diabetes and cardiovascular disease education module in an African-American, diabetic sample with physical, visual, and cognitive impairment. *Rehabilitation Psychology* 53:1–8, 2008

Hill-Briggs F, Dial J, Morere D: Neuropsychological assessment of persons with physical disability, visual impairment or blindness, and hearing impairment or deafness. *Arch Clin Neuropsychol* 22:389–404, 2007

House A, Knapp P, Bamford J, Vail A: Mortality at 12 and 24 months after stroke may be associated with depressive symptoms at 1 month. *Stroke* 32:696–701, 2001

Jorge RE, Robinson RG, Arndt S, Starkstein S: Mortality and poststroke depression: a placebo-controlled trial of antidepressants. *Am J Psychiatry* 160:1823–1829, 2003

Kendall PC, Chambless DL: Empirically supported psychological therapies. *J Consult Clin Psychol* 66:3–6, 1998

Keon HM, Hanna AK: Self-administration of insulin by a hemiplegic individual. *Diabetes Care* 3:705, 1980

Kleinbeck C, Williams AS: Disabilities, diabetes, and devices. *Home Healthc Nurse* 22:469–475, 2004

Knopman DS, DeKosky ST, Cummings JL, Chui H, Corey-Bloom J, et al.: Practice parameter: diagnosis of dementia (an evidence-based review). Report of the Quality Standards Subcommittee of the American Academy of Neurology. *Neurology* 56:1143–1153, 2001

Kortte KB, Hill-Briggs F: Psychotherapy with cognitively impaired adults. In *Psychologists' Desk Reference*. 2nd ed. Koocher GP, Norcross JC, Hill SS, Eds. Oxford, Oxford University Press, 2005, p. 342–349

Leksell JK, Sandberg GE, Wikblad KF. Self-perceived health and self-care among diabetic subjects with defective vision: a comparison between subjects with threat of blindness and blind individuals. *J Diabetes Complications* 19:54–59, 2005a

Leksell JK, Wikblad KF, Sandberg GE: Sense of coherence and power among people with blindness caused by diabetes. *Diabetes Res Clin Pract* 67:124–129, 2005b

Limb Loss Task Force/Amputee Coalition: *Roadmap for Limb Loss Prevention and Amputee Care Improvement*. Knoxville, TN, Amputee Coalition, 2011. Available from http://www.amputee-coalition.org/WhitePapers/Roadmap-for-Limb-Loss-Prevention-and-Amputee-Care-Improvement.pdf. Accessed 20 July 2012

Lincoln NB, Majid MJ, Weyman N: Cognitive rehabilitation for attention deficits following stroke. *Cochrane Database Syst Rev* CD002842, 2000

Luchsinger JA, Reitz C, Patel B, Tang MX, Manly JJ, Mayeux R: Relation of diabetes to mild cognitive impairment. *Archives of Neurology* 64:570–575, 2007

Mant J, Carter J, Wade DT, Winner S: Family support for stroke: a randomised controlled trial. *Lancet* 356:808–813, 2000

Maty SC, Fried LP, Volpato S, Williamson J, Brancati FL, Blaum CS: Patterns of disability related to diabetes mellitus in older women. *Journal of Gerontology: Medical Sciences* 59:148–153, 2004

McCullagh E, Brigstocke G, Donaldson N, Kalra L: Determinants of caregiving burden and quality of life in caregivers of stroke patients. *Stroke* 36:2181–2186, 2005

Mizrahi EH, Fleissig Y, Arad M, Kaplan A, Adunsky A: Functional outcome of ischemic stroke: a comparative study of diabetic and non-diabetic patients. *Disabil Rehabil* 29:1091–1095, 2007

Moser DK, Dracup K: Role of spousal anxiety and depression in patients' psychosocial recovery after a cardiac event. *Psychosom Med* 66:527–532, 2004

Nair RD, Lincoln NB: Cognitive rehabilitation for memory deficits following stroke. *Cochrane Database Syst Rev* CD002293, 2007

National Academy of Neuropsychology (NAN): Cognitive rehabilitation: official statement of the National Academy of Neuropsychology: NAN position papers. Denver, CO, NAN, May 2002. Available at https://www.nanonline.org/docs/PAIC/PDFs/NANPositionCogRehab.pdf. Accessed 20 July 2012

Nelson DV, Baer PE, Cleveland SE: Family stress management following acute myocardial infarction: an educational and skills training intervention program. *Patient Education and Counseling* 34:135–145, 1998

Petersen RC, Stevens JC, Ganguli M, Tangalos EG, Cummings JL, DeKosky ST: Practice parameter: early detection of dementia: mild cognitive impairment (an evidence-based review). Report of the Quality Standards Subcommittee of the American Academy of Neurology. *Neurology* 56:1133–1142, 2001

Price P: The diabetic foot: quality of life. *Clin Infect Dis* 39 (Suppl. 2):S129–S131, 2004

Price P, Harding K: The impact of foot complications on health-related quality of life in patients with diabetes. *J Cutan Med Surg* 4:45–50, 2000

Ragnarson Tennvall G, Apelqvist J: Health-related quality of life in patients with diabetes mellitus and foot ulcers. *J Diabetes Complications* 14:235–241, 2000

Reichard A, Stolzle H: Diabetes among adults with cognitive limitations compared to individuals with no cognitive disabilities. *Intellect Dev Disabil* 49:141–154, 2011

Renosky R, Hunt B, Hill-Briggs F, Wray L, Ulbrecht JS: Counseling people living with diabetes. *Journal of Rehabilitation* 74:31–40, 2008

Reyerson B, Tieney EF, Thompson TJ, Engelgau MM, Wang J, Gregg EW, et al.: Excess physical limitations among adults with diabetes in the U.S. population, 1997–1999. *Diabetes Care* 26:206–210, 2003

Ripley DL, Seel RT, Macciocchi SN, Stevens SA, Raziano K, Ericksen JJ: The impact of diabetes mellitus on stroke acute rehabilitation outcomes. *Am J Phys Med Rehabil* 86:754–761, 2007

Robinson RG, Schultz SK, Castillo C, Kopel T, Kosier JT, et al.: Nortriptyline versus fluoxetine in the treatment of depression and in short-term recovery after stroke: a placebo-controlled, double-blind study. *Am J Psychiatry* 157:351–359, 2000

Sharma S, Oliver-Fernandez A, Liu W, Buchholz P, Walt J: The impact of diabetic retinopathy on health-related quality of life. *Curr Opin Ophthalmol* 16:155–159, 2005

Sohmiya M, Kanazawa I, Inomata N, Yonehara S, Sumigawa M, et al.: A new device to introduce self-injection of insulin by his non-dominant hand in a patient with hemiplegia. *Diabetes Technol Ther* 6:505–509, 2004

Straetmans JM, van Schrojenstein Lantman-DeValk HM, Schellevis FG, Dinant GJ: Health problems of people with intellectual disabilities: the impact for general practice. *British Journal of General Practice* 57:64–66, 2007

Thombs BD, Bass EB, Ford DE, Stewart KJ, Tsilidis KK, et al.: Prevalence of depression in survivors of acute myocardial infarction. *Journal of General Internal Medicine* 21:30–38, 2006

Uslan MM: Analysis: beyond the "clicks" of dose setting in insulin pens. *Diabetes Technol Ther* 7:627–628, 2005

Uslan MM, Burton DM, Chertow BS, Collins R: Accessibility of insulin pumps for blind and visually impaired people. *Diabetes Technol Ther* 6:621–634, 2004

Uslan MM, Eghtesadi K, Burton D: Accessibility of blood glucose monitoring systems for blind and visually impaired people. *Diabetes Technol Ther* 5:439–448, 2003

Valensi P, Girod I, Baron F, Moreau-Defarges T, Guillon P: Quality of life and clinical correlates in patients with diabetic foot ulcers. *Diabetes Metab* 31:263–271, 2005

van Harten B, de Leeuw FE, Weinstein HC, Scheltens P, Biessels J G: Brain imaging in patients with diabetes. *Diabetes Care* 29:2539–2548, 2006

Van Horn E, Fleury J, Moore S: Family interventions during the trajectory of recovery from cardiac event: An integrative literature review. *Heart & Lung: The Journal of Acute and Critical Care* 31:186–198, 2002

Vileikyte L, Leventhal H, Gonzalez JS, Peyrot M, Rubin RR, et al.: Diabetic peripheral neuropathy and depressive symptoms: the association revisited. *Diabetes Care* 28:2378–2383, 2005

Vileikyte L, Rubin RR, Leventhal H: Psychological aspects of diabetic neuropathic foot complications: an overview. *Diabetes Metab Res Rev* 20 (Suppl. 1):S13–S18, 2004

Vinik AI, Park TS, Stansberry KB, Pitteneger GL: Diabetic neuropathies. *Diabetologia* 43:957–973, 2000

Von Korff M, Katon W, Lin EHB, Simon G, Ciechanowski P, Ludman E, Oliver M, Ruttter C, Young B: Work disability among individuals with diabetes. *Diabetes Care* 28:1326–1332, 2005

Walsh SM, Sage RA: Depression and chronic diabetic foot disability. A case report of suicide. *Clin Podiatr Med Surg* 19:493–508, 2002

Wegener ST, Mackenzie EJ, Ephraim P, Ehde D, Williams R: Self-management improves outcomes in persons with limb loss. *Arch Phys Med Rehabil* 90:373–378, 2009

Wegener ST, Kortte KB, Hill-Briggs F, Johnson-Greene D, Palmer S, Salorio C: Psychological assessment and intervention in rehabilitation. In *Physical Medicine and Rehabilitation*. 3rd ed. Braddom RL, Ed. Philadelphia, Elsevier, 2007, p. 63–92

Whitmer RA: Type 2 diabetes and risk of cognitive impairment and dementia. *Current Neurology and Neuroscience Reports* 7:373–380, 2007

Wiart L, Petit H, Joseph PA, Mazaux JM, Barat M: Fluoxetine in early poststroke depression: a double-blind placebo-controlled study. *Stroke* 31:1829–1832, 2000

Williams AS: A focus group study of accessibility and related psychosocial issues in diabetes education for people with visual impairment. *Diabetes Educ* 28:999–1008, 2002

Williams AS: Accessible diabetes education materials in low-vision format. *Diabetes Educ* 25:695–698, 700, 702, 1999

Williams AS: Recommendations for desirable features of adaptive diabetes self-care equipment for visually impaired persons. Task Force on Adaptive Diabetes for Visually Impaired Persons. *Diabetes Care* 17:451–452, 1994

World Health Organization: *Towards a Common Language for Functioning, Disability and Health: The International Classification of Functioning, Disability and Health (ICF)*. Geneva, World Health Organization, 2002

World Health Organization: *International Classification of Function, Disability and Health (ICF)*. Geneva, World Health Organization, 2001

Wray LA, Ofstedal MB, Langa KM, Blaum CS: The effect of diabetes on disability in middle-aged and older adults. *J Gerontol A Biol Sci Med Sci* 60:1206–1211, 2005